Color Atlas of Operative Techniques in

Head and Neck Surgery

Face, Skull and Neck

Jatin P. Shah MD, MS(Surg), FACS

Attending Surgeon
Head and Neck Service
Memorial Hospital
New York
Member
Memorial Sloan-Kettering Cancer Center
New York

Wolfe Medical Publications Ltd.

To
My parents, Sarla and Premanand Shah,
for giving me the opportunities they never had
My wife, Bharti,
for bearing with me in my quest for what I want to be
and
My daughter, Mili,
a constant source of joy for making it all worthwhile.

Cover illustration by
David Purnell, MA, AMI
New York.

Copyright © Jatin P. Shah, 1987
Published by Wolfe Medical Publications Ltd, 1987
Printed by BPCC Hazell Books Ltd, Aylesbury, England
UK ISBN 0 7234 0844 0

Reprinted 1991

For a full list of other atlases published by Wolfe Publishing Ltd,
please write to the publishers at: Brook House, 2–16 Torrington Place, London WC1E 7LT, England

Contents

Foreword

Surgery of the head and neck has become an increasingly complex and varied "regional" surgical sub-speciality incorporating knowledge, skills and expertise of divergent surgical disciplines including general surgery, otolaryngology, plastic surgery, neurosurgery, oral and maxillofacial surgery and prosthodontics in order to successfully cope with the varied and complex neoplasms of the head and neck. In their inexorable growth, these tumors respect neither structure nor physiological functions. Increasingly broad training and experience are mandatory for the surgeon who will undertake the satisfactory investigation and treatment of these varied neoplastic processes.

In the first volume of his proposed series entitled, *Head and Neck Surgery — Color Atlas of Operative Procedures*, Dr Shah has compiled a selected group of operative procedures on the skin of the face, skull and paranasal sinuses and neck. His text describes the preparation and planning for surgery, the details of the technical procedure and follow up care and the photographs actually taken by the author, amply illustrate the basic principles and highlights of the operative procedures. However, in a larger sense, Dr Shah has emphasized the epitome of the surgeon's art and craft, that is, the attention to detail and technical excellence. He amply describes and illustrates in a well organized fashion the important steps in assessing the extent of disease, treatment planning and the technical steps required in the various minor and major surgical procedures in order to achieve a successful outcome. The multiple components of management including careful patient and disease assessment, attention to details in planning extirpation and reconstruction and rehabilitation are appropriately described, illustrated and emphasized. In his preface, Dr Shah acknowledges the advantages and disadvantages of the single authored text but gives us a beautifully illustrated and documented description of his philosophy and techniques. The need for training and experience in allied disciplines is well illustrated. One of the most important attributes of a "compleat" surgeon must be his technical proficiency and excellence, both of which are amply documented in this volume. The compilation and publication of this material has been a monumental effort and the author is to be congratulated for the magnitude and excellence of the result and the publisher for bringing all this together in a superb book for our edification and education. This first volume is an excellent introduction of more to come and beautifully illustrates the continuing and ever paramount importance of the craft of surgery.

Elliot W. Strong, MD, FACS
Attending Surgeon
Chief Head and Neck Service
Memorial Sloan-Kettering Cancer Center
New York

Acknowledgements

Many individuals have played a significant role in the development of my career as a head and neck surgeon. I gratefully acknowledge my indebtedness to my colleagues and peers for their encouragement, support and contributions towards my knowledge and experience in the field of head and neck oncologic surgery.

I must, however, take an exception and mention the names of a few individuals who have played a significant role in my career development and the feasibility of bringing about this book to a reality. The late Dr Manubhai D. Patel was amongst the first who impressed upon me the importance of superb technical surgery. It was he to whom I remain indebted for learning the finer aspects of surgical techniques. Dr A.B. Kothari, my former teacher and guide, deserves special mention, particularly for his interest in my career at an early stage. Dr Hollon W. Farr deserves my heartfelt gratitude for planting the seed of head and neck surgery in my mind years ago that ultimately lead to my interest in this surgical specialty. His support and encouragement were very instrumental during the early years of my training and clinical practice. Dr H. Randall Tollefsen was responsible for training me as a head and neck surgeon and particularly getting me interested in the field of operative photography. His encouragement and instructions in the early years became very useful in bringing about this operative atlas to a reality. To him I am gratefully indebted. Dr Frank P. Gerold, my former teacher and present colleague, has always amazed me with his courage and judgement in dealing with complex head and neck oncologic problems. I have learned many things from him and I am thankful to him for the knowledge shared.

Elliot W. Strong, the Chief of the Head and Neck Service at Memorial Sloan-Kettering Cancer Center practically for the entire period of my career in the specialty of head and neck surgery is one individual to whom I remain most indebted. He took an active interest in fostering my career development in the field of head and neck oncologic surgery. He has been most helpful in every professional endeavor that I have undertaken and has remained a source of encouragement and idealism. I want to express my most sincere gratitude to him, a learned colleague, and a dear friend.

Mrs Octavia Mack deserves special mention for her diligence in typing the manuscript in time, in spite of her other responsibilities in the office.

Preface

This book is addressed primarily to the aspiring head and neck surgeon who has already obtained broad basic training either in the field of general surgery, otolaryngology or plastic surgery. Head and neck surgery over the years has evolved into a very complex specialty demanding expertise in various surgical disciplines and exposure to numerous allied specialities. Thus, a modern day head and neck surgeon should have additional training of one to two years, specifically devoted to the field of head and neck oncologic surgery, after his basic surgical qualification. During this training period he should have had exposure to maxillofacial prosthodontics, neurosurgery, microvascular surgery, radiation oncology, medical oncology, biostatistics and basic research methodology. While clinical training in all these fields is necessary, surgical expertise is essential to carry out the complex surgical procedures for head and neck tumors safely and successfully. During the past decade quantum leaps have taken place in the technical aspects of head and neck oncologic surgery. The introduction of microsurgical reconstructive techniques, myocutaneous flaps, new approaches to skull base and craniofacial surgery, laser technology, etc. all have contributed significantly to the development of new operations and improvement of the technical details and safety of established procedures.

The operative procedures demonstrated in this book are all as practiced by the author. Thus, clearly they express the opinions, methodology and technique of one individual. While there may be some advantage to a multi-authored book of this nature, a clear concept and uniform methodology of surgical approach to various problems does not develop in a multi-authored book. To that extent there is clear advantage to following an approach developed by one individual with many years of an extremely busy head and neck practice. Nearly all procedures shown in the book are those performed by the author on his patients. In many instances the author has specified his choice of handling a particular problem with other approaches mentioned for the sake of completeness. The technical details of each operative procedure shown here present state of the art in the field of head and neck oncologic surgery.

This color atlas is quite a different approach to demonstration of technical aspects of head and neck operations. Operative atlases with line drawings do indeed demonstrate anatomic and technical details graphically. However, in such books appreciation of the complexity of anatomy and the three dimensional aspects of seeing "real life" anatomy are lacking. This color atlas clearly demonstrates anatomy in the living, as encountered during each of the operative procedures. The sequential photography of each of the operative procedures was performed by the author, himself, to maintain the "surgeon's view" of the operative field. Where necessary, line drawings are used to complement the exposure of a complex surgical field.

It is obviously impossible for an operative atlas on techniques of head and neck surgery to be either complete or permanently up to date, any more than can a dictionary. New words are being coined while new meanings are assigned to old words, likewise new operative procedures are being revised and refined. The current volume is actually an epitome of the greater portion of my surgical experience during the past two decades on the Head and Neck Service at Memorial Sloan-Kettering Cancer Center. I do however, welcome readers' comments for only by such process may knowledge be advanced.

1: Operating Room Setup and Anesthesia for Head and Neck Surgery

Physical characteristics of the operating room

Head and neck surgery consists of operative procedures ranging from the relatively simple to the highly complex. Therefore operating room characteristics for these operations should be able to meet all contingencies. The operating room should be large enough to provide free movement of personnel and equipment during the operative procedure. Laminar airflow is desirable to minimize contamination of wounds through floating bacteria and droplet infection. Ideally, the operating room should be interposed between the 'green core' and the 'grey core'.

The green core is that area in the operating room suite to which operating room personnel only, in appropriate operating room attire with mask and cap, have access. There is no flow of patient traffic through this area to the operating room. Sterile operating room equipment such as instruments and other accessories are brought into the operating room through the green core. The grey core should be located diagonally opposite the entrance to the operating room via the green core. Entrance of patients and personnel handling the patients to the operating room should be through the grey core. Thus, a patient is brought into the operating room through the grey core and discharged from the operating room to either the recovery room or patient's own room via the grey core entrance.

Satisfactory lighting through ceiling-mounted lights is important to minimize clutter on the floor. It is also desirable to have suction ducts and electrical connections—oxygen and nitrous oxide delivery systems and access outlets—available through suspension cylinders from ceiling to avoid clutter and allow for free movement of personnel.

Equipment

The operating rooms designed for conducting head and neck surgical procedures should contain all possible equipment needed both for complex procedures and to meet all contingencies. Thus, at least two sets of suction-duct systems or portable suction equipment should be available at all times. An electrocautery unit is necessary for smooth and successful execution of complex head and neck operations; an operating microscope as well as laser equipment are also an integral part of the technological backup necessary. Also, equipment for suspension of the larynx, support of head for operative procedures in prone positions and other ancillary equipment and attachments for the operating room table are important. Surgical instruments infrequently used in routine head and neck procedures should be made available within the operating room in sterile packages for ready access as and when necessary. High-speed drills and saws are routinely used for surgery of the mandible and facial skeleton and these should be available on demand when necessary, as should appropriate dermatomes for harvesting skin grafts. Complete listing of all necessary instruments is beyond the scope of this book.

Operating Room Floor Plan

The position of various equipment in the operating rooms should be relatively constant for the day-to-day smooth conduct of operative procedures. Thus, the positions of the operating table and equipment should be standardized so that they remain the same throughout various procedures. In a square operating room it is best to have the operating room table in a diagonal plane to provide free flow of movement of personnel on either side of it. Also, it is desirable for the head end of the operating table to remain in one place unless otherwise indicated by special circumstances. Transfer of equipment and personnel on both sides of the operating table should accommodate both right-handed and left-handed surgeons. Location of cabinets, laser equipment, operating microscopes, trolleys and suction machines, etc. should be individualized depending upon the operating room setup in a given environment, the available equipment and the personal preferences of those using this equipment daily. The general overview of a head and neck operating room during the conduct of a surgical procedure is shown in (1).

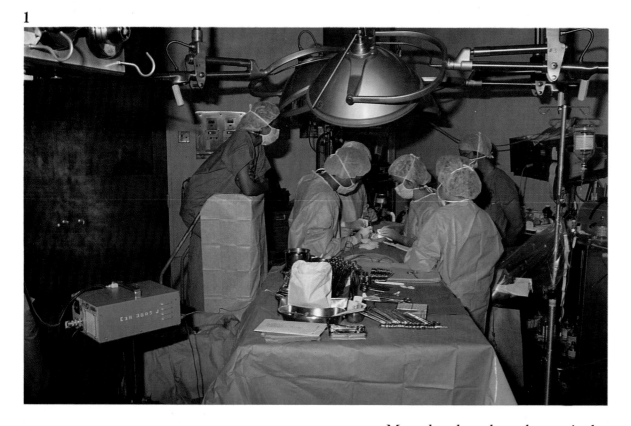

2

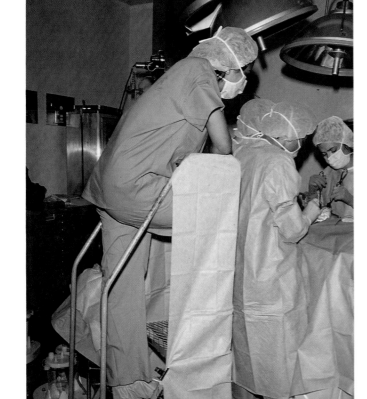

Most head and neck surgical procedures can be conducted with a single surgical team consisting of the operating surgeon and his first and second assistant surgeons. A scrub nurse and a circulating nurse are also necessary, as are an anesthesiologist preferably with one assistant if surgical procedures are to be conducted under general anesthesia. An orderly must be available on call at all times. Several complex operations require more than one surgical team due to different types of expertise, as well as occasional simultaneous working of two teams. Examples of such complex operations include surgery of the skull base, extrathoracic pharyngolaryngoesophagectomy with gastric transposition, and the resection of advanced head and neck tumors with immediate reconstruction using free microvascular skin, intestinal or bone grafts. When multiple surgical teams are involved, the plan of the surgical procedure and its sequence should be discussed with the operating room nurses and the responsible operating surgeons to ensure smooth conduct of the procedure.

If there are observers or students watching the surgery, their positions must be specifically designated to avoid unnecessary crowding in the operating room. The use of an observer's stand, as shown in (2), is ideal as it places the observer at a level higher than the floor of the operating room. These observer stands isolate the observer from the operating team but still maintain the sterility of the personnel involved in the operative procedures and provide a satisfactory view of the surgical field. Alternatively, a ceiling-mounted camera with a television monitor placed in a remote room with two-way communication can also work satisfactorily.

Setup for Surgical Procedures

It is vital that the position both of individuals involved in each surgical procedure, and the equipment used in such surgical procedures, are also relatively constant and standardized. This will avoid unnecessary delay in starting the operation, and also eliminate confusion about location of equipment during the operating procedure.

Setup for General Open Head and Neck Operations

Since most operations on the upper aerodigestive tract and paranasal sinuses are considered clean-contaminated, antibiotic coverage is necessary for the patient before placement of the incision. The patient is brought into the operating room with a satisfactory intravenous line and the first dose of antibiotics is given just prior to induction of general anesthesia. Following this, and appropriate placement of the anesthetic tube and its connections, the surgical team positions itself as outlined in (3). For a right-sided operative procedure, the operating surgeon stands on the right side of the patient with his first assistant situated at the head end of the table, and his second assistant directly across from him on the left side of the patient. The endotracheal tube and its connecting ducts are isolated by sterile transparent drapes between the first and second assistants and connected to the anesthetic equipment. The patient's contralateral arm is kept abducted at 90° and isolated out of the sterile field to give the anesthesiologist access to intravenous line and blood pressure monitoring, etc. The anesthesiologist should be located in the vicinity of the outstretched left arm, but away from the endotracheal tube and its connections to maintain a sterile field; thus, appropriate securing of the endotracheal tube is necessary while the patient is being draped.

The scrub nurse stands on the right or left side of the patient with the Gerhardt instrument table brought over the operating table up to the level of the umbilicus. The electrocautery machine is positioned behind and between the operating surgeon and the scrub nurse. Suction tubing and basin should be placed between the operating surgeon and the first assistant to provide access for both. Two waste disposal buckets are necessary: a large one is placed directly across from the scrub nurse, so that she can see its contents; a small one is put between the operating surgeon and his first assistant, so

3

S	Surgeon	1	Anesthesia machine
A1	First Assistant	2	Electrocautery
A2	Second Assistant	3	Suction basin
AN	Anesthesiologist	4	Waste bucket
N	Nurse		

that they can drop soiled linen, gauze and instruments directly into the bucket. Although this setup is relatively standard for most head and neck procedures, the positions of personnel and equipment are reversed for left-sided procedures.

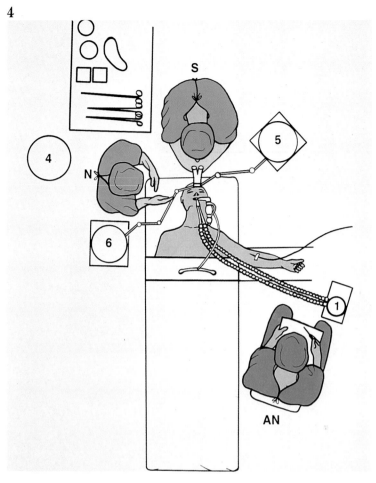

S Surgeon   **4** Waste bucket
AN Anesthesiologist   **5** Operating microscope
N Nurse   **6** Laser
1 Anesthesia machine

Setup for Endoscopic Surgery

A sterile field is not mandatory for endoscopic laryngeal microsurgery. This includes the use of the laser in surgical procedures of the endolarynx. The setup and positioning of personnel necessary for both types of surgery is shown in (4)—the operating surgeon is at the head of the table with the scrub nurse on the right-hand side of the patient; instruments are kept on the table on the right-hand side. The endotracheal tube and its connections to the anesthetic machine are positioned along the patient's chin and left arm with the anesthesiologist situated on the patient's left-hand side for good access to the arm, anesthetic equipment and machine. The operating microscope is placed to the left of the patient for access by the operating surgeon; the laser assembly and laryngeal suspension equipment are on the right-hand side of the patient, so the scrub nurse can adjust the controls, as necessary. Since most modern operating rooms have a television camera attachment on the microscope, the remaining surgical team and observers can watch the surgery on a television screen away from the operating microscope.

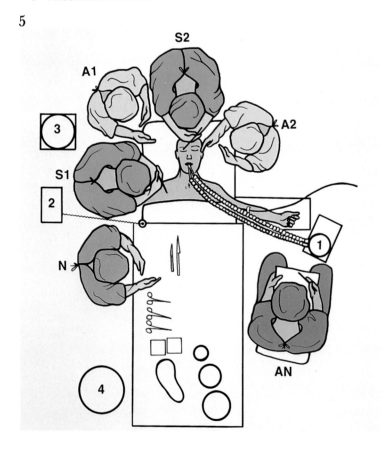

Setup for Two-Team Craniofacial Surgical Procedures

Simultaneous surgery for tumors involving the skull base by both neurosurgeon and head and neck surgeon requires proper planning of the operating sequence to avoid confusion and crowding at the operating table (5). The patient is prepared and draped for simultaneous activity by both the neurosurgical and the head and neck surgical teams, although many stages of this operation are performed sequentially by one team at a time. When both teams are working simultaneously, the head and neck surgeon is placed at the right-hand side of the patient for a right-sided lesion, his first assistant situated

S1 Head and neck surgeon   **N** Nurse
S2 Neurosurgeon   **1** Anesthesia machine
A1 First assistant   **2** Electrocautery
A2 Second assistant   **3** Suction basin
AN Anesthesiologist   **4** Waste bucket

between him and the neurosurgeon, who is at the head end of the operating table, and the neurosurgical assistant is directly across from the head and neck surgeon on the left-hand side of the patient's head. The scrub nurse is placed directly adjacent to the head and neck surgeon on the right-hand side of the patient. The position of the anesthesiologist, as well as anesthetic, electrocautery and suction equipment are shown in (5). There are two sets of electrocautery equipment: bipolar for the neurosurgeon, and unipolar for the head and neck surgeon. Two sets of suction tubing are also necessary for this complex operative procedure.

Setup for Simultaneous Operations for Resection and Reconstruction with Two Surgical Teams

These complex operations require two independent surgical teams with the operating surgeon, his assistant and a scrub nurse for each aspect of the procedure (6).

For a pharyngolaryngoesophagectomy with gastric transposition, planned for a left-sided lesion, the head and neck surgeon is positioned on the left side of the patient's head with his assistant at the head end of the table. The endotracheal tube and its connections are brought along the outstretched right arm, so that the anesthesiologist, who is situated on the right-hand side of the patient's head and above the outstretched right arm, has good access. The abdominal surgeon is placed on the patient's right-hand side below the outstretched arm with his assistant directly opposite. The scrub nurse for the head and neck team is situated obliquely at the left-hand side of the patient, with her instrument table while the scrub nurse for the abdominal surgical team has her instrument table covering the feet of the patient over the operating table. This positioning of the personnel involved in this operation provides maximum access and exposure to the respective surgical teams without unnecessary crowding of hands in the surgical field or crossover of instruments from one field to another.

When a head and neck resectional surgical procedure is in progress simultaneously with harvesting of a free microvascular skin, visceral or bone graft, the surgical teams again have to be totally independent. The head and neck team continues to work on the head and neck area, while the microvascular surgical team operates on the abdomen, groin, thigh, arm or foot as indicated. To enable simultaneous conduct of these procedures, all areas of the patient must be prepared and draped.

It is important that all personnel involved in these surgical procedures know their respective positions and can work in harmony from their respective locations. Positional diagrams must be included in the operating room manual to be used by nurses, anesthesiologists and surgical assistants.

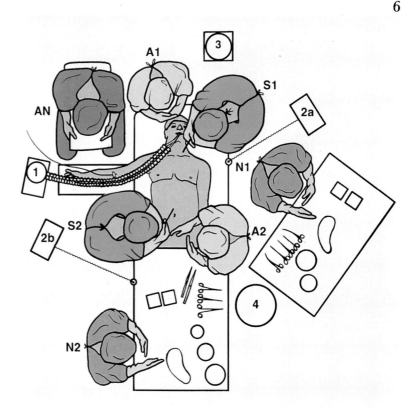

6

S1	Head and neck surgeon	1	Anesthesia machine
S2	Thoracic surgeon	2a,2b	Electrocautery
AN	Anesthesiologist	3	Suction basin
N1	Head and neck nurse	4	Waste bucket
N2	Thoracic nurse		

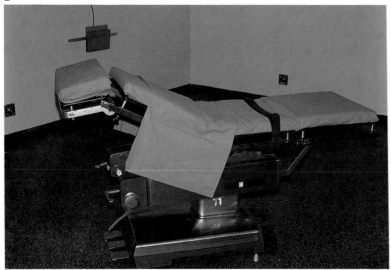

Position and Draping of the Patient

In head and neck surgical procedures, the patient must be placed on the operating table in such a way that extension of the head in a partially propped-up position is possible (1). An electrically controlled operating table is desirable, but one with manual controls is equally satisfactory, provided that it offers similar ease in positioning. The head end of the operating table should be hinged in two sections. A drawsheet is placed on the table over the mattress prior to placing the patient on the operating table. The standard position required for most head and neck surgical procedures means that the table be hinged at the patient's waist at approximately 30° with the headboard dropped at least 35° to provide extension to the neck; so patient would be in a semisitting position with the neck extended for most procedures on the neck, face or oral cavity. Extension of the head is usually not necessary in procedures involving surgery of the paranasal sinuses.

Under appropriate premedication, the patient is placed supine on the operating table and positioned on the table as previously described (2). The patient is asked whether his position is comfortable, without any pressure points causing discomfort. For surgery on the right side, the right arm is placed close to the body and tucked under the drawsheet to prevent it dropping off the operating table under anesthesia (3). Proper care should be taken to see that both the wrist and arm are not under any heavy pressure or tightly bound under the drawsheet.

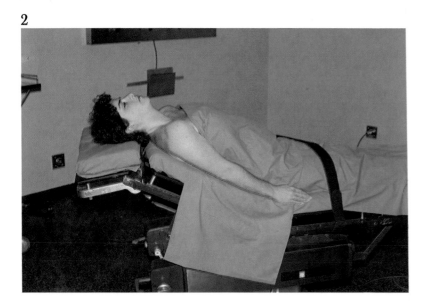

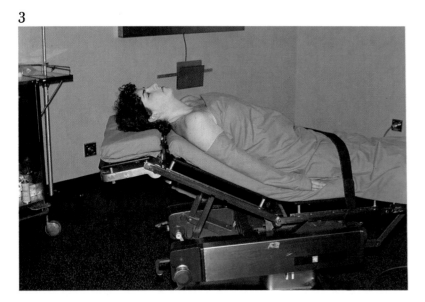

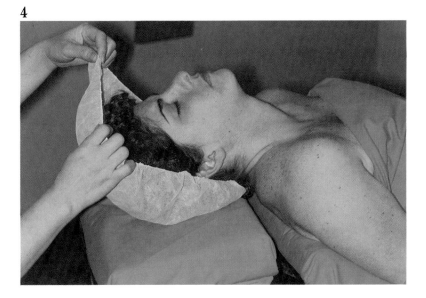

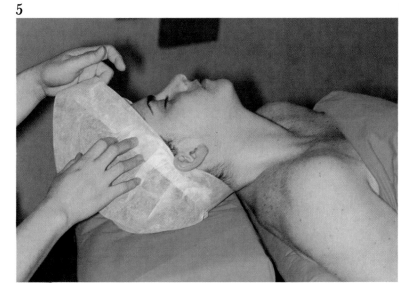

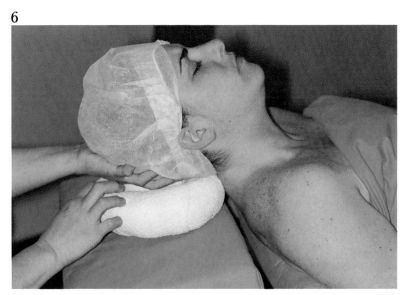

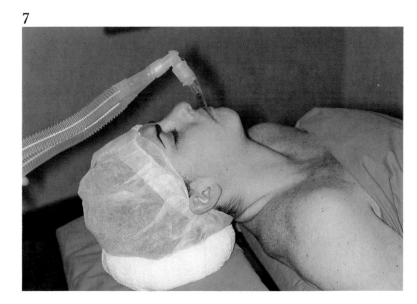

A surgical cap covers the patient's hair (4); shaving of the hair along the trapezius muscle in the posterior part of the neck is often necessary on surgical procedures of the neck, as is shaving of the sideburns for surgery of the parotid gland.

A paper tape then secures the cap to the skin right around the hairline (5), so that it does not fall off during surgery. The pinna of the ear on the side of surgery is exposed in the surgical field, but the contralateral pinna is covered by the cap.

A cotton ring cushion made with fluff and Kerlix bandages is used to support the head and prevent it from rolling from side to side (6). Now the patient is ready for induction of general anesthesia and establishment of an appropriate endotracheal airway for connection to the anesthetic equipment.

The choice of orotracheal or nasotracheal intubation, and appropriate tubes, should be decided by both surgeon and anesthesiologist prior to induction of general anesthesia (7) to facilitate smooth running of the operative procedure. The endotracheal tube is secured with appropriate adhesive tape to the side of the face opposite the surgical field and outside the sterile field. The operating surgeon must be present in the operating room during this time to facilitate both induction of general anesthesia and positioning and connecting the anesthetic equipment.

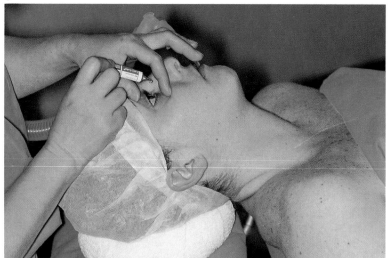

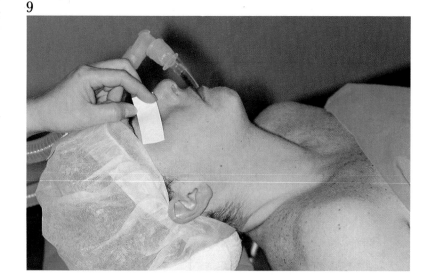

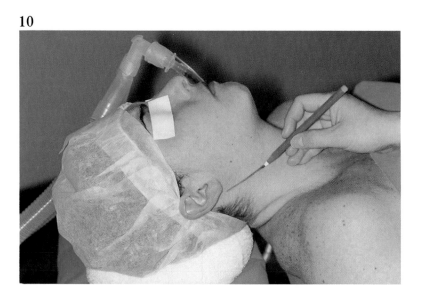

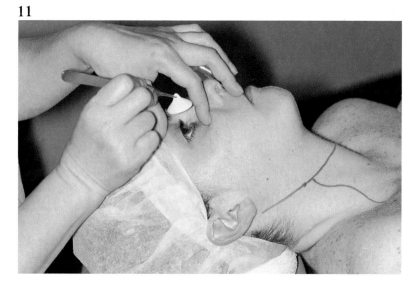

The eyes are protected by instilling methylcellulose (lacrilube) eyedrops or ointment in the conjunctival sac to prevent dryness of the cornea (8). The upper eyelid is carefully closed and maintained closed with elastic microfoam adhesive tape (9).

The proposed surgical incision, and all potential extensions, are now marked out to provide a guide for preparation of the skin in the sterile field (10). The circulating nurse prepares the skin with bacteriostatic agents to include all potential incisions in the sterile field.

If, however, the eye and eyelids are to be included in the sterile field, then it is desirable to use a ceramic corneal shield which protects the cornea by resting on the sclera, and allows preparation of the eyelids and the conjunctival sac with bacteriostatic solution used for the skin (11). This should be done very carefully otherwise corneal abrasion will result during placement or removal. The upper eyelid is retracted enough to expose the sclera all around the cornea, and at this point the corneal shield is held with a fine-toothed forceps and slid under the upper eyelid without touching the cornea. Once it is in that position it is dropped and both the upper and lower eyelids are allowed to return to normal position, thus preventing any direct injury to the cornea.

12

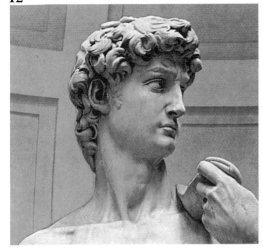

13

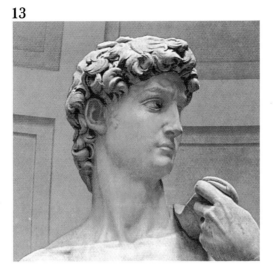

14

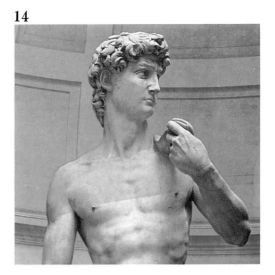

15

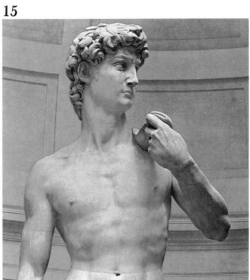

16

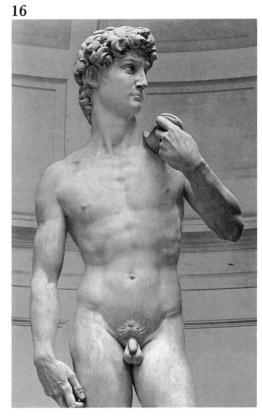

Various bacteriostatic solutions can be used for cleansing and preparation of the skin, including alcohol, Cetavlon, Betadine, etc.; the choice is best left to the operating surgeon and the practices of each institution. Generally, the areas to be prepared should include not only the desired field for the operative procedure planned, but also its possible extensions **(12)**. For example, the surgical preparation by bacteriostatic agents necessary for a parotidectomy includes preparation of the skin from the hairline of the forehead, including the skin in front and behind the pinna of the ear, the ipsilateral side of the face and the entire neck on the side of surgery up to the clavicle.

For surgery of facial and skin lesions and surgery on paranasal sinuses, the entire face on both sides should be prepared from hairline to clavicle **(13)**.

For surgical procedures on the oral cavity and neck dissections, including tracheostomy, preparation should extend from a line joining the tragus to the ala of the nose down to the nipples **(14)**.

If use of a myocutaneous flap is anticipated, preparation should go well below the costal margin to the umbilicus. Where two surgical teams are working simulta-

neously, the entire surgical field of both sides, including the intervening skin, is prepared with bacteriostatic solution. Thus, for a craniofacial procedure, the scalp is shaved and the entire head from the vertex up to the nipple line is prepared **(15)**.

For a pharyngolaryngoesophagectomy with gastric transposition, the skin is prepared from a line joining the tragus to the nose down to the groin, and includes the intervening skin **(16)**. However, if a microvascular surgical team is harvesting a graft from the abdomen or iliac crest, then it is unnecessary to prepare the intervening skin since the two surgical fields will remain separate through all parts of the operation.

17

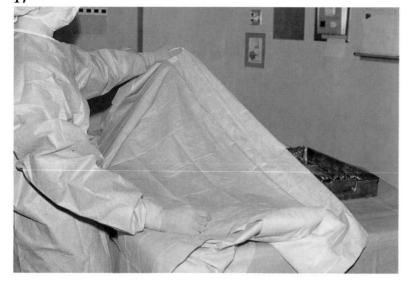

18

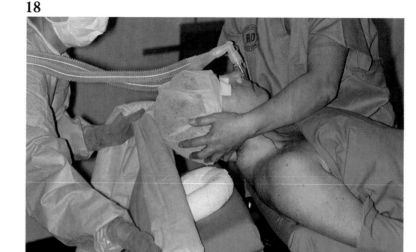

19

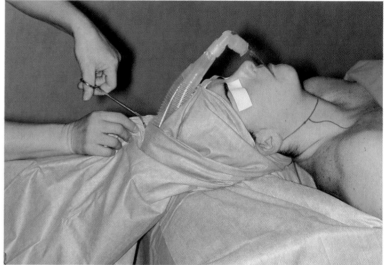

20

Once the skin is scrubbed and prepared with bacterio-static solution, draping of the patient for the surgical field begins. Isolation of the head with a proper head drape requires the use of two sheets folded and laid one over the other with a margin of approximately 10 cm left between the folded edges of the two drapes (17). This allows the lower drape to rest on the table, while the upper drape is wrapped round the patient's head over the cap so that the head can be rotated on either side without breaking a sterile field. These drapes are laid open and properly positioned by the scrub nurse on the instrument table before draping begins.

Once these drapes are properly aligned, the scrub nurse lifts both drapes simultaneously and places them under the patient's head over the cotton ring cushion. The circulating nurse helps to lift the head without contaminating the prepared skin (18). The anesthetic tubing must be held up in the air while this is taking place. The head is lifted up and flexed enough to provide access to the back of the neck well up to the shoulders on both sides.

Both drapes are placed flat on the headboard. The patient's head is then placed back on the drapes, and the upper drape is wrapped round the patient's head covering the cap and the entire hairline (19). Attention should again be paid to prevent buckling of the pinna on either side. The ipsilateral pinna is exposed in the sterile field, but the contralateral pinna is included within the head drape, which is secured snugly over the cap. The ends of the drape are held in position with a towel clip.

The anesthetic tubings are now placed over the folded head drape and two sides of the drape sheet are folded over the tubing securing it with another towel clip in a position to avoid kinking (20). This maneuver completes the head drape.

21

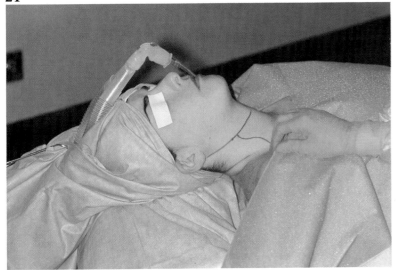

22

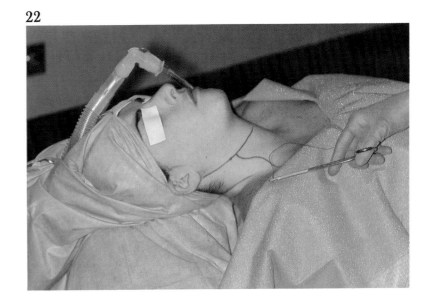

23

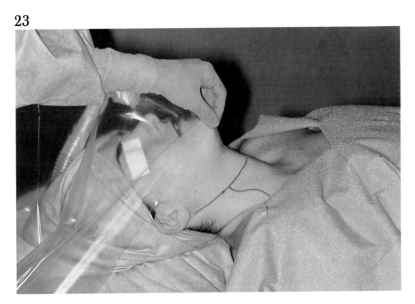

24

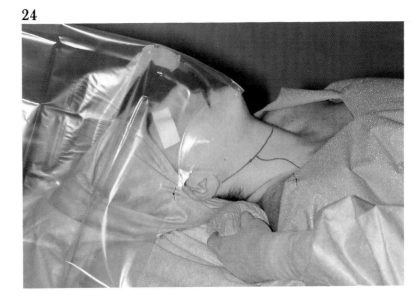

Next, a split sheet is placed by the operating surgeon on the anterior surface of the patient's body covering it entirely **(21);** it is secured in proper position with a silk suture taken through the skin over each shoulder near the acromioclavicular joint **(22).** This provides exposure of the area within the sterile field as necessary.

The exposed anesthetic tubing and the upper part of the head are now isolated by a sterile transparent plastic drape; this provides both visualization of the anesthetic tubing connections and eyes during the operation, and access to all these areas by the anesthesiologist. The self-adhering edges of the plastic drape are applied to the skin where desired.

In **(23),** where the draping is done for a neck dissection, the transparent drape is applied from the midpoint of the chin to the upper part of the pinna onto the head drape. Similarly, the plastic drape is applied on the opposite side, and is secured with a silk suture to the head drape on both sides just above the pinna. The far end of the plastic drape is applied to the anesthetic equipment so that the entire anesthetic tubing remains under continuous vision during the operation.

A crush towel (absorbent paper towel opened and rolled into a round ball) is inserted into the space behind the nape of the neck on either side, to prevent blood dripping under the patient's shoulders **(24).**

The completed preparation of the skin and draping of the patient for a neck dissection is shown in **25.** Note that although a large area of the skin is prepared by bacteriostatic solution, the sterile field exposes only a limited area to accommodate the incision. The purpose of preparing a larger field is to maintain a sterile margin of skin under the drapes in case the incision needs to be extended on either side. The surgical team now takes their appropriate positions before beginning the operation.

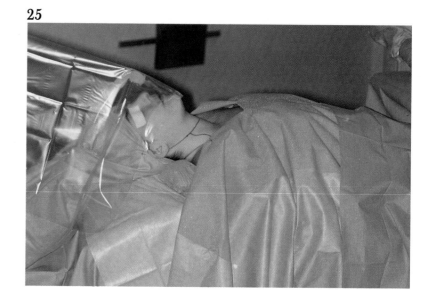

25

Anesthesia for Head and Neck Surgery

Head and neck surgical procedures are all major procedures to the anesthesiologist. As the airway can often be invaded by the surgical procedure an endotracheal tube is necessary in general anesthesia. Once anesthesia is induced, and the patient is prepared and draped for surgery, the anesthesiologist must work in a restricted area with only limited access to the endotracheal tube, so the anesthetic equipment should allow free movement of the head and an unobscured operative field. If a patient shows signs of respiratory obstruction preoperatively, or has partial trismus, the endotracheal tube should be introduced under topical anesthesia while the patient is still awake and in command of his own airway. If this is not feasible, then an airway should be secured by performing a preliminary tracheostomy under local anesthesia; this is also advisable in those patients who have bulky, friable tumors in the oropharynx, hypopharynx or larynx, and those with complete trismus.

Upon arrival in the operating room the patient should have a satisfactory intravenous line with preferably a number 18 gauge needle or angiocath introduced into a peripheral vein in the contralateral arm. A satisfactory intravenous channel must be used for administration of anesthetic agents, intravenous fluids and blood or blood products. Details of the anesthetic techniques and agents used are not described here.

It is important, however, to have adequate knowledge of the anesthetic endotracheal tubes available and desirable for certain operative procedures **(1).** Most frequently used oral endotracheal tubes are transparent cuffed with an inflatable balloon; they come in a shape which conforms to the curve of the upper air passage, and have a low pressure balloon that seals the airway and provides an airtight anesthetic delivery system (i). However, where a semirigid tube is not desirable, an anode tube is used; this is a soft, very flexible rubber tube with a wire coil incorporated within its wall. It is also available with a cuff containing an inflatable balloon (ii).

For those procedures using a laser, either metallic flexible endotracheal tubes or rubber tubes covered with an aluminum foil are used to prevent perforation of the tube with the laser and its consequent hazards. The rubber tube should have aluminum foil wrapped over it from the proximal end of the balloon all the way up to the proximal end of the tube; this reflects the laser beam and prevents rupture of the tube causing an explosion (iii).

For nasotracheal anesthesia, special tubes that conform to the curve of the nasal air passage into the larynx are available **(2).** These tubes require special connections to prevent kinking between the tip of the nose and

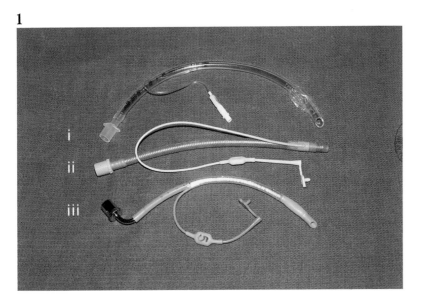

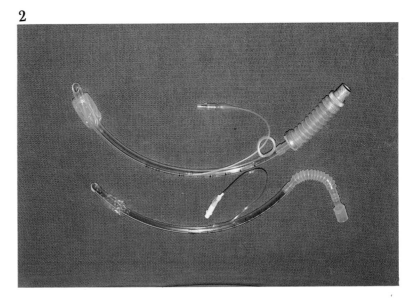

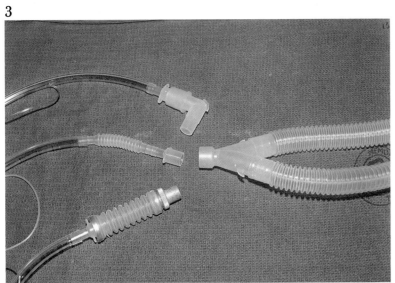

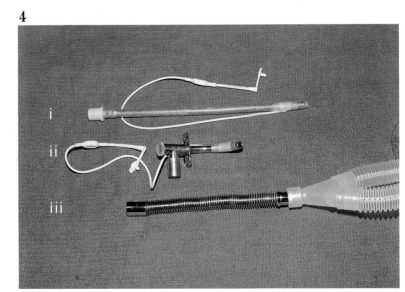

the anesthetic tubing (3): rubber resins or accordion-type plastic, or right-angled elbow-joint type connectors are used, each of which has a special application depending on the individual situation. The anesthesiologist should have all types of tube available.

For a preliminary tracheostomy, an endotracheal tube through the tracheostomy site is necessary for delivery of anesthesia (4). If the tracheostomy site is to be exposed within the sterile field, anode tubes are used, as they can be sterilized and are flexible enough to conform to the curves necessary during draping of the patient (i). On the other hand, if the tracheostomy site is

not to be included within the sterile field, then a regular Sklar metallic tracheostomy tube with a balloon, or a Shiley Silastic tube with inflatable balloon, can be used (ii). A flexible metallic resin connector is necessary to connect the tracheostomy tube to the anesthetic equipment (iii). If an anode tube is used for delivery of anesthetic agents during the operative procedure, it is removed at the end of the operation, and either a Sklar or a Shiley tracheostomy tube is introduced; it is secured in position with silk suture applied to the skin, or an umbilical tape around the neck.

2: Basic Surgical Techniques

Biopsy

It is advisable to establish an accurate histological diagnosis prior to treatment planning of any neoplastic process in the head and neck area. No special precautions are necessary for superficial lesions of the skin, which are easily accessible to an open punch biopsy, or lesions in the oral cavity (1), for which biopsy under topical or local anesthesia can be performed.

A variety of biopsy forceps are available, and use of these depend upon the location of the lesion and the amount of tissue (2 to 4) available to obtain a representative sample. In 2, Healey (i) and Moser (ii) biopsy forceps are shown. Curved laryngeal biopsy forceps is shown in (3) and angled biopsy forceps for the nasopharynx is shown in (4) attached to a Storz fiberoptic nasopharyngeal telescope. Alternatively, a simple scalpel may be used to obtain a wedge of tissue from the tumor for pathological diagnosis. Accurate diagnosis cannot be established if the tissue removed is scanty, has crush effect, or is not from a 'representative' part of the lesion. For squamous carcinomas, it is generally recommended that a biopsy is obtained from the periphery of the lesion (5), so that the pathologist can demonstrate a zone of invasion in the normal tissues. However, this is not mandatory, as adequate sampling of tissue from the center of the tumor is equally satisfactory to establish a clear histological diagnosis. A punch biopsy using a circular drill type of punch is recommended by some for skin lesions, but if this does not extend through the entire thickness of the lesion, an accurate histological interpretation of the lesion (for example, melanoma) will not be obtained. For lesions of the skin in particular, it is desirable to use a sharp scalpel and obtain a long sliver of the lesion through its full thickness.

If a skin lesion is only a few millimeters in diameter, and the possibility of skin cancer is suspected, then an excisional biopsy rather than an incisional biopsy is preferred, followed by a subsequent excision for treatment. On the other hand, larger lesions are best dealt with in the appropriate way under controlled circumstances in the operating room. An accurate histological diagnosis must be however established prior to induction of general anesthesia for surgical excision.

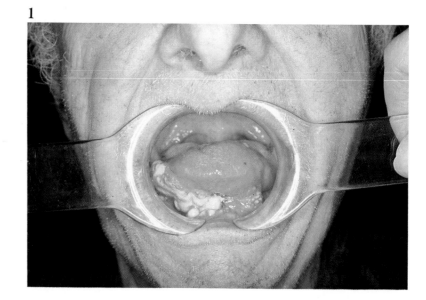

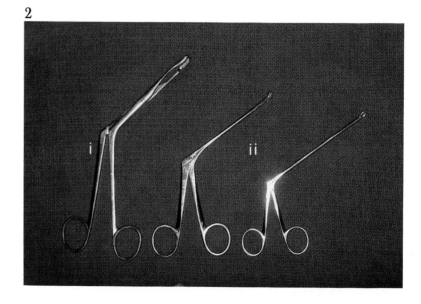

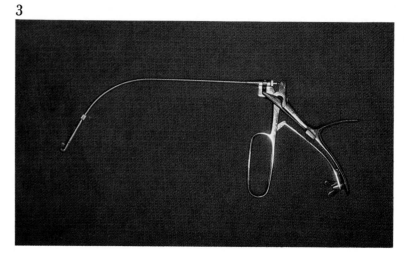

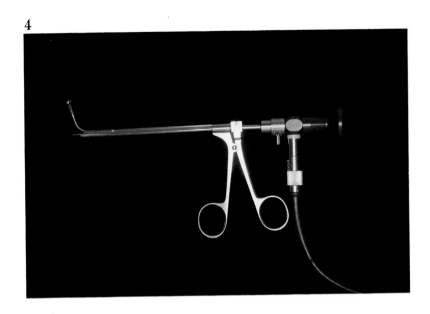

4

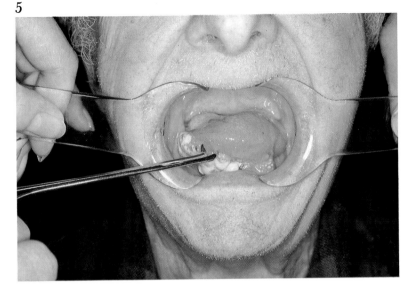

5

Needle Aspiration Biopsy

Subcutaneous or submucosal masses, which are not accessible on the surface for biopsy with a punch, should be considered for needle aspiration biopsy. Although in the past a large-bore needle was used to obtain tissue, currently fine needle aspiration biopsy is preferred. Successful biopsy depends on two people: (1) the individual who performs the needle aspiration biopsy, who should be familiar with the technique; and (2) the cytopathologist, whose experience is vitally important to interpret accurately the tissue provided. Thus, cervical lymph nodes which are clinically felt to be metastatic in nature are eminently suitable for fine needle aspiration; and neoplastic processes or masses involving the thyroid gland, salivary glands, and soft tissue tumors in the neck or masses presenting in the submucosal region of the upper aerodigestive tract should all be aspirated for tissue diagnosis.

The biopsy technique is simple, and requires a 10 cc syringe with a number 22 gauge needle (**1**). The skin is sterilized with a bacteriostatic solution such as alcohol or Betadine. The mass is fixed with the fingers of one hand and biopsy is performed with the other. Prior to insertion of the needle in the mass, approximately 1 cc of air is left in the syringe; the needle is then inserted in the mass through the skin (**2**). Suction is now created by pulling the plunger back, and under suction multiple passes of the needle are made in the center of this mass allowing a core of tissue to be withdrawn in the syringe. Prior to removal of the syringe the suction is released and the plunger allowed to rest in normal position. The syringe and needle are now withdrawn, and the aspirated material from the syringe and the needle is ex-

1

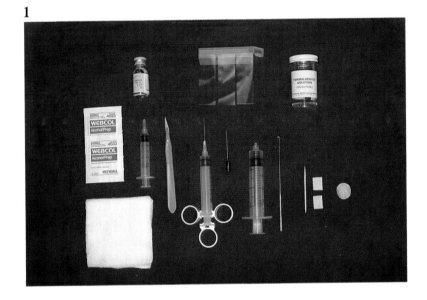

2

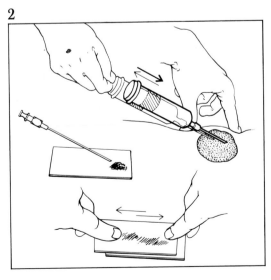

pressed on a glass slide. Dry smears are made from this material and they are either sent to the pathology laboratory for H and E (hemotoxylin and eosin) staining, or fixed in 95% alcohol for cytological interpretation. If a large amount of tissue is aspirated, the remaining tissue is sent in formalin to the pathology laboratory for appropriate processing for tissue blocks.

Caution

It is vital not to inject air into the tissues while inserting the needle into the mass. Extreme caution and care must be exercised in making multiple passes within the mass to ensure that there is no seeding of the tumor cells when the needle is withdrawn from the mass into the soft tissues or outside through the skin, since this may lead to tumor implantation. Suction on the plunger should be released prior to removal of the syringe, to allow the core of tissue lodged within the barrel of the needle to come out with the syringe. To minimize trauma, avoid using a large-bore needle. Manual pressure at the site of needle aspiration should be maintained for a few minutes to prevent hematoma. Needle aspiration should be avoided at the most tense part of a mass or at the 'head' of an apparently inflammatory looking mass, to avoid formation of a sinus tract with drainage of tumorous material.

Dissection Techniques

A sharp scalpel is used for skin incisions at all times. However, the technique of subsequent deep dissection is largely dependent on personal preferences. The author prefers to use electrocautery with coagulating current to elevate skin flaps, as this greatly minimizes blood loss and provides dry clean tissue planes.

Subsequent dissection in the deeper tissues can be performed using sharp scalpel, scissors, electrocautery or laser. The author prefers to use electrocautery—pencil-type with fingertip controls—throughout all operative procedures in the head and neck area since it greatly minimizes blood loss, makes the operative field relatively dry and clean, and ensures a speedy operation. Pencil type electrocautery is shown in (3) with flat tip (i) and needle tip (ii). Excessive charring of the tissues to prevent inflammatory reaction leading to large seromas in the wound can be avoided by judicious use of electrocautery. However, the latter does not function well if the tissues are wet or flooded with blood, water or edematous fluid.

Caution

Electrocautery should not be used directly on major vessels, nor in the vicinity of important nerves. The heat generated at the needle tip is extreme (>1000 °C) and

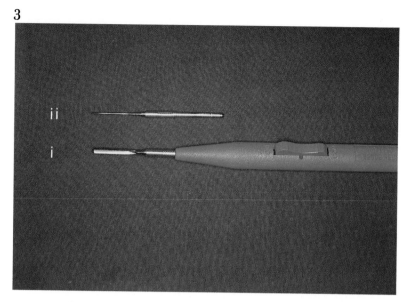

3

can produce temporary nerve damage leading to transient paralysis of the nerve where electrocautery was used. Entry into a major vessel is also likely if electrocautery is used incautiously near or on major vessels. The cautery tip should always be along the plane of dissection, remaining at an angle of 15–30° to the tissues rather than at right angles—this will prevent injuries such as buttonholes in the skin during elevation of skin flaps.

Anatomically the tissues in head and neck are in a relatively superficial plane, therefore surgical procedures can be easily performed with help from the first and second assistants. Exposure is usually not a problem if adequate incisions at the desired site are employed. Traction on the tissues applied towards the operating surgeon, and countertraction provided by his first assistant, is sufficient to allow the tissue planes to separate with electrocautery or a sharp scalpel. Blunt dissection is not desirable, and is often dangerous since it may violate clean tissue planes, cause rupture of metastatic lymph nodes or soft tissue extensions of the tumor and produce spillage in the operative field potentially causing disease to recur. Applying sharp penetrating clamps into tumor-bearing tissue is to be avoided at all times. Hemostats should be used instead, applied to grossly normal-looking tissues around the tumor to provide traction on the surgical specimen being mobilized.

Closure of Wounds

The author's personal preference for closing mucosal wounds is to use interrupted sutures of absorbable material. However, a variety of materials, both absorbable and non-absorbable, are available, and the results of interrupted versus continuous sutures vary in the hands of different surgeons. Wound closure should not be under tension, and the sutures should be placed only a few millimeters apart to avoid large gaps in the suture line and fistula formation. The skin and platysma are sutured as separate layers. Meticulous attention should be paid when using fine suture material in approximation of skin edges, and overlap during suture should be avoided. For esthetic reasons, a subcuticular suture is desirable when feasible.

Drainage of Wounds

The Penrose drain is used for small superficial wounds where only a minimal amount of serosanguinous drainage is anticipated. It is also suitable for drainage of wounds following both thyroid surgery and superficial parotidectomy. In most other instances suction drainage is desirable (4). The suction drains should be placed to provide maximum drainage from the surgical field, carefully avoiding placing them over nerves or major vessels. The perforated inner ends of the suction drains should be appropriately positioned in the wound with absorbable suture material, and the drains should be brought out through separate stab incisions, fixing their external ends with silk sutures.

4

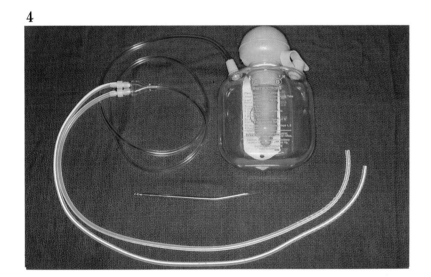

Dressings

Whenever a Penrose drain is used, a fair amount of serosanguinous discharge is to be anticipated through the wound which will require medium-size absorbent dressings. Pressure dressings are usually not necessary unless there is undue oozing from the entire wound during the course of the operation or at the time of closure, and they are only used if hemostasis is adequate prior to wound closure. When applying dressings care must be taken to avoid undue pressure on the eye, pinna of the ear, or on the airway. No pressure dressings should be left longer than 48 hours following application. Dressings are usually not necessary when suction drains are used.

The patency of suction drains should be checked very carefully during the final stages of wound closure, and clots in the drainage system should be cleared. The wound should be irrigated with saline with the suction drains functioning during closure of the wound. The skin flaps should be completely flat on final closure of the skin incision. If the suction drains are clogged with clot, they will not function and this will result in the development of hematoma leading to further bleeding, and the need to re-explore the wound for hemostasis. So it is essential that the suction drains remain patent and functioning prior to, during, and immediately after closure of the wound. They should be maintained on high negative pressure suction for the first 24 hours following surgery to allow the skin flaps to remain down and adhere to the deep tissues.

Preoperative and Postoperative Care

Preoperative Care

Open head and neck operative procedures are considered clean-contaminated surgical procedures, and therefore all patients require prophylactic antibiotic coverage, administered immediately prior to administration of general anesthetic and maintained for a period of at least 48 hours postoperatively. Establishing an adequate airway may become necessary in those patients who have obstructing lesions. In such instances, preliminary tracheostomy under local anesthesia is performed to establish a safe airway prior to induction of general anesthesia. All patients undergoing major head and neck surgical procedures should receive instructions regarding their postoperative status, care of the tracheostomy and feeding tubes, the need for deep breathing exercises and early ambulation.

Postoperative Care

Postoperative care of patients following major head and neck surgical procedures is relatively simple when no major body cavities are invaded. Generally patients are ambulatory within 24 hours after surgery. Early ambulation is not only important but essential to facilitate pulmonary toilet and self-care. Suction drains must be patent and functioning immediately postoperatively. Care of the oral cavity and intraoral suture line is important, and patients must be taught self-care with the use of gravity-controlled, frequent oral irrigation. Hydrostatic power sprays using hydrogen peroxide and saline in the oral cavity should be performed at least twice in 24 hours. Nasogastric feeding may be started as early as 1 day postoperatively. Once the patient has stabilized, the Foley catheter (if present) and intravenous lines are disconnected. The patient is then taught to feed himself, take care of his tracheostomy tube and encouraged to become mobile.

3: Facial Skin Lesions

Introduction

Small lesions of the skin of the face are excised in the direction of the cleavage planes which are at right angles to the pull of the facial muscles. A brief review of the skin lines of the face is important prior to embarking on excision of a facial skin lesion. Generally, an elliptical incision is best suited for small lesions. Configuration of the facial skin lines and potential directions for elliptical incisions are shown in (1). Meticulous attention should be paid to approximation of subcutaneous tissues using absorbable interrupted sutures, and the skin should be closed with fine sutures which can be removed as early as 4 days postoperatively. Alternatively, one may elect to use a subcuticular suture, particularly in the area of the eyelids.

The most common malignant lesions of the skin of the face are basal cell carcinomas, squamous cell carcinomas, and melanomas. Occasionally, one may see rare lesions such as a keratoacanthoma, Merkel cell tumor and sweat gland carcinoma. If the extent of excision is such that a primary closure through an elliptical defect is not possible, then one must consider the applicability of split-thickness or full-thickness skin grafts, or local flaps.

Application of split or full-thickness skin graft is best suited to that part of the face with minimum facial motion, such as the lateral aspect of the bridge of the nose or the temple. Similarly, a skin graft can be used in the parotid region because the facial movement in this area is minimal and cosmetic disfigurement is minimal. The most suitable donor sites for obtaining full-thickness skin grafts are from the retroauricular or supraclavicular areas.

Flaps from the immediate neighborhood of the defect are most desirable from both the functional and esthetic point of view. Primary closure of the donor site defect can usually be accomplished with ease by proper planning of local skin flaps. For example, a triangular defect can usually be covered with a rotation flap. A variety of other flaps are available for closure of facial skin defects, the most applicable of which are the swinging rotation flap, advancement rotation flap and the rhomboid flap, etc.

Excision of Small Lesions by Elliptical Incisions

The facial muscles of expression and the lines of tension on the skin of the face are shown here in (2). By asking the patient to grimace, the line of direction of the long axis for elliptical incision is established. These lines are horizontal on the forehead and around the bridge of the nose and the outer canthus of the eye. Near the cheek the tension lines run obliquely or perpendicularly, near the lips they run radially from the mouth opening, and on the chin they run horizontally on the midline and obliquely perpendicular at the sides. On the sides of the neck the wrinkles and tension lines run obliquely downward and forward. Horizontal elliptical excision of a small growth of the lower eyelid or the upper eyelid is perfectly suitable, but larger excisions in this way from the lower eyelid tend to result in ectropion.

1

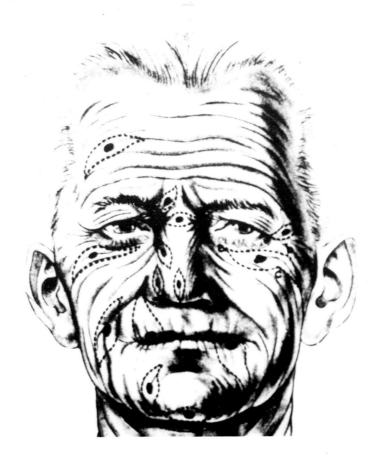

2

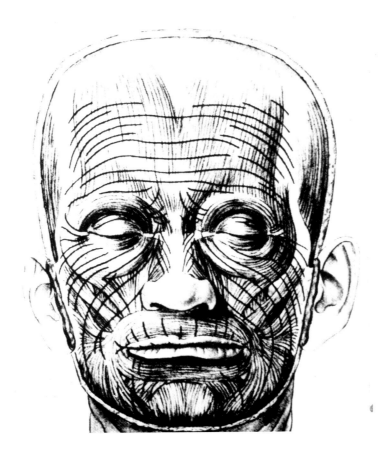

Excision and Full-Thickness Skin Graft on the Nose

The operative technique described below is for a patient who presented with Hutchinson's melanotic freckle on the side of the nose (1). The procedure is performed under general anesthesia. It is vital to estimate carefully the size of the surgical excision prior to embarking on the operative procedure. Good lighting and occasional optical magnification is necessary when examining subtle skin lesions such as this to assess accurately the extent of the tumor and the desired excision. Difficulties in estimating the extent of the excision are often encountered in patients who present with lentigo maligna, or morphea type of basal cell carcinomas.

The desired extent of excision is marked out with a skin marking pen and its dimensions are measured (2). If possible, a paper template of the anticipated surgical defect should be obtained to outline the area of skin graft required. The surgical defect should not be considered as final, however, until after frozen sections are obtained from the margins of surgical excision to ensure the adequacy of the resection.

The ideal donor site for the size of defect in this patient is from the skin of the supraclavicular region. A transverse elliptical incision is made of the desirable dimensions (larger than the anticipated defect) in the loose skin in the supraclavicular fossa posterior to the sternomastoid muscle (3). The skin is incised with a scalpel through its full thickness but not through the subcutaneous fat or platysma. Using a sharp scalpel and fine hook retractors the full-thickness skin graft is harvested remaining just deep to the dermis (the so-called 'white layer' of the skin). No fat should be retained on the skin graft, and attention should be paid to remain in the same plane of subdermal dissection so that the thickness of the graft is uniform. If any fat deposits are harvested inadvertently on the skin graft, they should be excised with sharp scissors. The skin graft is preserved in a wet sponge soaked with saline solution for subsequent use. The resulting defect at the donor site is closed primarily in two layers after adequate hemostasis is obtained. If the skin graft is larger than 3 cm at its widest point then there is some tension on the suture line, and undermining the skin edges may be necessary to facilitate closure. However, this part of the skin of the neck will heal adequately in spite of some tension on the suture line. If such is the case, then the sutures on the skin should be left for approximately 2 weeks.

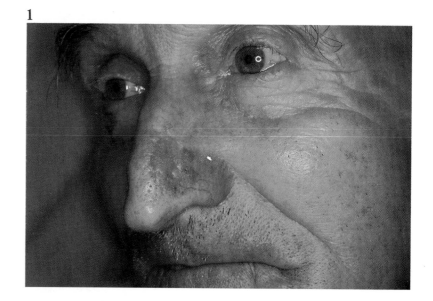

1

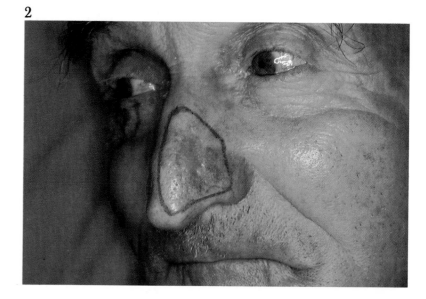

2

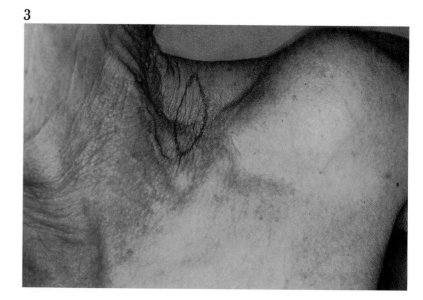

3

4 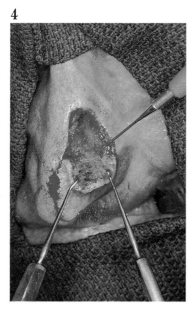 **5** 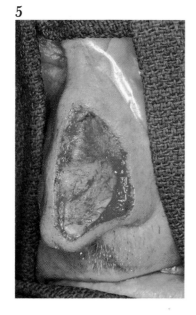 **6** 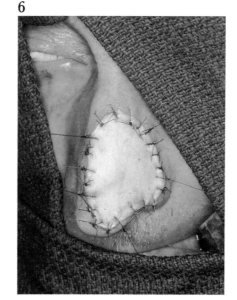 **7**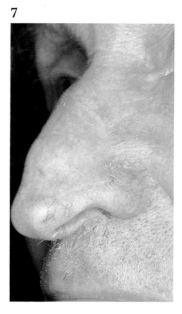

Attention is now focused to the site of tumor excision. The area of the surgial excision is prepared and draped in the usual fashion (**4**). A skin incision is made using a number 15 scalpel through the previously marked outline, circumferentially through the full thickness of the skin but remaining superficial to the nasal cartilage underneath. Brisk bleeding from the skin incision is to be anticipated due to the rich blood supply of nasal skin. Fine, sharp hooks and a suction with Frazier suction tip to keep the area of advancing surgical excision dry are used. Once an edge of the skin is elevated, the remainder of the dissection proceeds using needletip electrocautery to give a precise plane of excision without causing excessive charring or burning of tissues. Applying adequate traction on the surgical specimen with the skin hook as shown in (**4**) is important. This will provide a uniform plane of excision remaining deep to the dermis and the soft tissues but over the cartilage. Bleeding is to be anticipated from branches of the nasolabial artery and the subdermal plexus of vessels. In general the hemorrhage can be controlled with electrocautery, but occasionally ligation of the branches of the nasolabial artery may be necessary.

After the surgical specimen is excised and complete hemostasis achieved, several frozen sections are obtained from the margins of the surgical defect to ensure the adequacy of excision (**5**). A frozen section is also obtained from the depth of the surgical field as its deep margin. Once adequacy of surgical excision is confirmed by the pathologist, then the previously harvested full-thickness skin graft is brought to the surgical field, and appropriately tailored to fit the surgical defect. A single-layered closure using non-absorbable suture material is performed paying meticulous attention to approximating accurately the skin edge to the full-thickness skin graft (**6**). Accurate approximation of epidermis to epidermis is of utmost importance for a desirable esthetic result. Several interrupted skin sutures are applied, and

every third suture is left with a long end which will be subsequently used to tie a bolster dressing.

After the entire skin graft is sutured in place, several stab incisions are made in the center of the graft to drain any serosanguinous material that may accumulate beneath the graft. Following this a bolster dressing is applied—xeroform gauze is wrapped over plain gauze and a bolster of appropriate size is placed over the skin graft; the long edges left on select sutures are now tied over the bolster to keep it taut over the skin graft. The sutures should not be tied too tight otherwise the edges of the skin on the surgical defect will 'tent' and cause necrosis or disruption of sutures. Antibiotic ointment is applied at the edges of the suture line.

Postoperatively some crusting and minor clots are to be anticipated along the suture line, and these must be cleared to prevent sepsis. Massive hematoma under the skin graft is unlikely because of the bolster dressing, but occasionally small amounts of blood clot can accumulate under the skin graft. The bolster dressing should be inspected daily and the suture line kept clean with hydrogen peroxide to clear crusts and clots. The bolster dressing is removed on the 7th postoperative day and the skin graft left open. Over the next 2–3 days the remaining skin sutures can be removed.

The skin graft may initially look purplish-blue because of small amounts of underlying hematoma, but as it heals its color will change. Initially the skin graft is quite pale compared to the pinkish skin of the nose due to its minimal capillary vascularity. However, as vascularization continues the skin graft takes on an essentially normal color similar to that of the nasal skin. The postoperative appearance of the skin graft in this patient at 6 months is shown in (**7**). Since sensations on this skin are absent, the patient must avoid trauma to prevent ulceration and infection. The esthetic result for this kind of skin graft is excellent with no specific donor site deformity.

Excision of Large Skin Carcinoma on the Temple With Full-Thickness Skin Graft Coverage

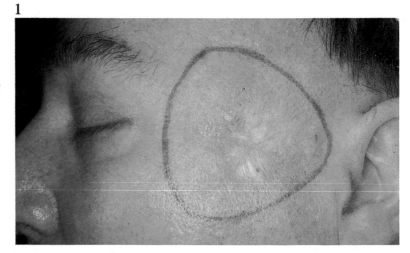

A large area of relatively non-mobile skin on the side of the face such as the temple is best suited for excision with repair using a full-thickness skin graft. The patient shown in (1) presented with a superficial but recurrent multifocal epidermoid carcinoma involving a large area of the skin extending from that overlying the lateral aspect of the orbit to the front of the ear. Excision of this lesion was performed in the usual way remaining in a subcutaneous tissue plane but meticulous attention was paid to avoid injury to superficial branches of the facial nerve, which are identified and carefully preserved. If, however, the tumor infiltrates through the soft tissues then deliberate sacrifice of these terminal branches of the facial nerve may be necessary.

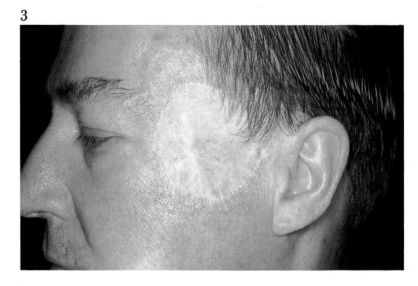

A full-thickness skin graft is harvested from the right supraclavicular fossa. The skin graft is sutured in place with multiple interrupted non-absorbable sutures, and multiple stab wounds are made in the skin graft for drainage, a procedure often called 'pie crusting' (2). A bolster dressing is applied over the skin graft, but in this instance it was retained in position by separate silk sutures taken through the normal skin on the periphery of the surgical defect. Because of the large size of the skin graft, if long ends are left on the sutures between the skin graft and the surgical defect, then the skin edges are likely to 'tent' leading to a possible hematoma.

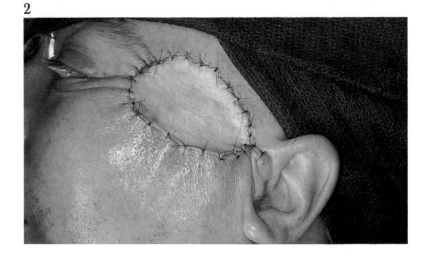

Postoperative appearance of the patient at approximately 6 months following surgery is shown in (3). Although the color of the skin graft still does not match the normal adjacent skin, the esthetic result is quite acceptable. Surgical defects of larger dimensions on the skin of the side of the face can be covered using full-thickness skin grafts. These can also be used in patients who develop multiple skin cancers and in whom the potential development of new skin cancers is high. In those patients where mobilization of local flaps is ill-advised, full-thickness skin grafts can be considered.

Local Skin Flaps

When repair of a surgical defect demands more adequate full-thickness reconstruction, local flaps are best suited for this purpose. The blood supply of facial skin and soft tissues is extremely rich, as the terminal branches of the external carotid artery provide a major source of blood to the facial skin. In addition to this, there is an extensive subdermal anastomotic network which facilitates the use of several random flaps with relative ease. Some flaps carry an identifiable axial blood supply while others are more random. Examples of axial skin flaps are: nasolabial, glabellar, Mustardé cheek, and temporal forehead; examples of random flaps are: cervical, rhomboid, and bilobed.

Reconstruction With a Glabellar Z Plasty

A skin lesion located in the center of the forehead is best suited for elliptical excision with primary closure, giving a midline vertical scar. However, when the lesion is off the midline and when an elliptical excision leaves a surgical defect likely to produce forehead asymmetry by primary closure, then a Z plasty may be considered. The lesion, as shown in (1), measures 2×1.5 cm and is a recurrent basal cell carcinoma. Surgical excision of this lesion is performed in the usual way, going through full thickness of the skin of the forehead but remaining superficial to the underlying frontalis muscle. Adequacy of surgical resection is confirmed by frozen section of margins.

A Z plasty is outlined so that the surgical defect will distribute tension on both sides of the midline equally leaving a symmetrical forehead with well-balanced eyebrows. Skin incision is made through the outlined area as shown in (2), and the triangular flaps of skin developed at the upper and the lower part of the mobilized area are transposed so that the upper triangle is shifted to the right-hand side while the lower triangle is shifted to the left-hand side to fill the surgical defect. Tension on the suture line of the surgical defect is now distributed in such a way as to balance the forces of traction on both sides of the midline.

Meticulous attention to detail is necessary in closure of the subcutaneous tissues (3). Fine chromic catgut sutures are taken through the subcutaneous tissue and the knots are buried. Subcutaneous sutures should be placed so that they enter the undersurface of dermis on both sides at the same level, to facilitate approximation of the skin edges with fine nylon sutures without tension. No dressings are necessary, but Bacitracin ointment is applied to the suture line.

The same patient's postoperative appearance is shown approximately 1 year later (4). Although the scar is visible, the eyebrows are well balanced and the midline of the forehead is not distorted. Similar Z plasties distribute the lines of tension well on the edges of the scar thus preventing formation of a hypertrophic scar.

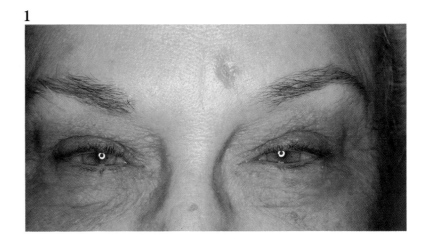

1

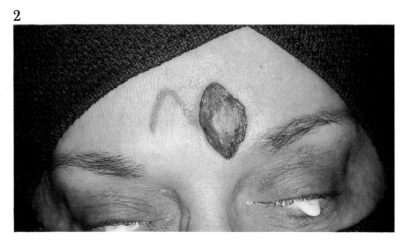

2

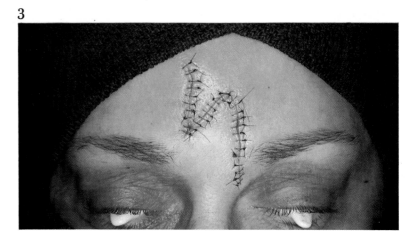

3

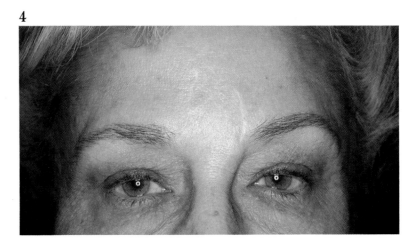

4

Glabellar Flap

This flap is best suited for reconstruction of surgical defects at either the bridge or the upper half of the nose. It is an axial flap which derives its blood supply mainly from the supratrochlear artery and also from the dorsal nasal branches. The flap can be quickly elevated and lined with split thickness on its undersurface to provide coverage of through-and-through defects of the nasal dorsum. Extreme care must be taken with incisions for this flap. The upper portion of the incision is carried down to the periosteum, proximal mobilization of the root of the flap near the nasofrontal angle is only through the skin, and the deeper dissection on the undersurface of the flap is done bluntly to avoid injury to the supratrochlear vessels. Meticulous attention should be paid to this part of the dissection to avoid any inadvertent injury to the supratrochlear artery, and it is best done under direct vision, very slowly and carefully. The flap must be outlined longer than actually necessary. Since the flap is to be turned 180°, some length is lost in its rotation, but in spite of this it must be rotated without any tension so as not to compromise its blood supply.

The patient shown in (1) has multifocal squamous cell carcinomas involving the skin of the bridge of the nose and the glabellar region. The skin is freely mobile over the underlying periosteum.

The area of proposed excision is marked with an outline of the proposed glabellar flap which will derive its blood supply from the left supratrochlear vessels (2). The skin flap is taken all the way up to the hairline to give adequate length; if further length is necessary it is desirable not to use the hair-bearing area of the scalp as growth of hair on the front of the nose is most unsightly, and other methods of reconstructing the surgical defect should be considered.

Since both eyes are in the operative field, the corneae are protected using ceramic corneal shields (3). The patient is under general anesthesia with an endotracheal tube passed through the oral cavity. Skin, subcutaneous tissue and the underlying fascia are incised at right angles to the plane of the skin through the circumference of the planned excision. Elevation of the lesion-bearing skin is performed using sharp skin hooks and fine needlepoint electrocautery. A Frazier suction tip is used to keep the field dry during mobilization of the surgical specimen, which can be done rapidly with electrocautery. Hemostasis is thereafter obtained with either electrocoagulation or ligation of bleeding points as necessary. Frozen section control of the margins of the surgical defect is obtained at this point to ensure that surgical resection is adequate. The surgical defect in this patient (3) is such that no generous pedicle for the

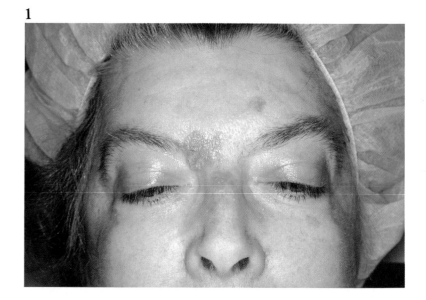

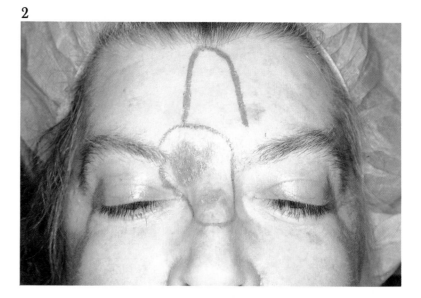

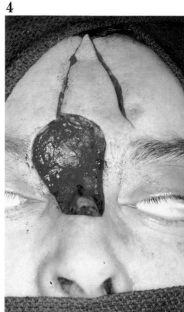

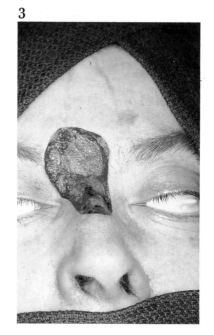

glabellar flap is available, except for the left supratrochlear vessels.

Skin incisions are made (4) at the previously outlined area for the flap. The apex of the flap is sharply angled to facilitate closure of the donor site. Raising of the flap begins at its most distal part elevating the tip and working proximally. Incision of the right side of the skin flap is completed first up to the surgical defect to prevent injury to the left-sided supratrochlear vessels and carried up to the periosteum. The remaining flap is retracted on the left side and carefully elevated while palpating and preserving the supratrochlear vessels on its undersurface. Elevation of the flap is necessary up to the margin of the orbit and the supratrochlear foramen on the left side, where the incision on the left side of the flap is completed and the flap fully elevated.

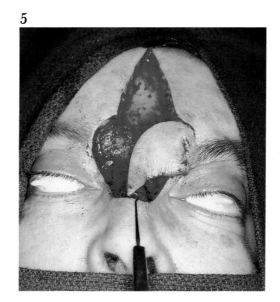

The flap is now rotated 180° to see whether it will fill the surgical defect satisfactorily (5). If not then further mobilization of the flap becomes necessary to avoid tension on its suture line and compromise of its blood supply. The tip of the flap is trimmed away and closure of the surgical defect using this rotated glabellar flap begins with subcutaneous 3-0 chromic catgut interrupted buried sutures. After appropriate mobilization of the lateral areas of the surgical defect, the skin flap is tailored to fit the surgical defect. The forehead is mobilized on both sides to allow primary closure of the donor site defect with a straight midline vertical closure.

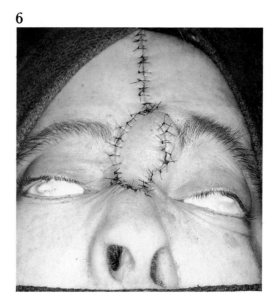

Closure of the skin is performed with 5-0 nylon interrupted sutures without any tension (6); at 180° rotation the skin flap will leave a 'dog ear'. Here, extreme caution must be exercised not to compromise the blood supply of the flap. If there is any risk to the supratrochlear artery, then the dog ear is best left alone at this point for revision at a later date.

Postoperative appearance of the patient approximately 1 year following surgery is shown in (7). The skin flap has set well in place with well balanced eyebrows on both sides and satisfactory coverage of the skin and soft tissue defect at the bridge of the nose. Closure of the donor site leaves an esthetically acceptable midline vertical scar.

A modification of this procedure is an island glabellar flap where the flap is tunneled under an intact bridge of skin at the glabella, keeping its blood supply intact on the vascular pedicle containing the supratrochlear artery and vein. However, elevation of an island flap in this fashion is risky and has very limited application.

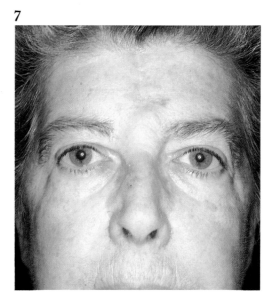

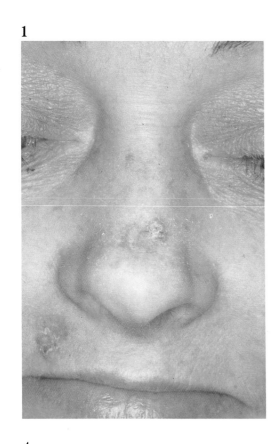

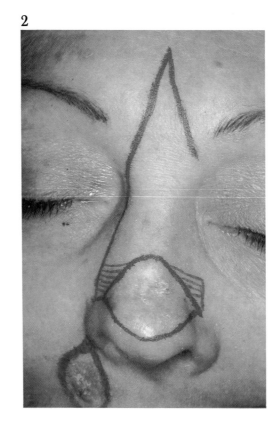

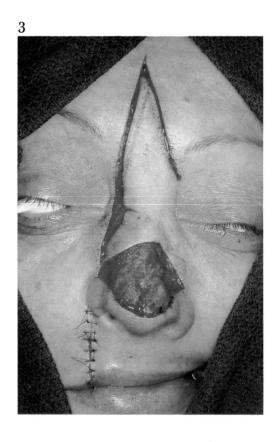

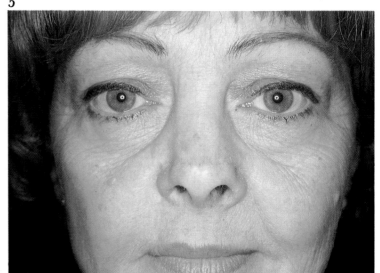

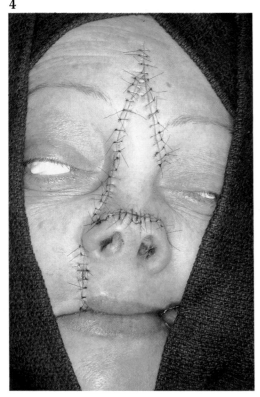

Excision and Repair With a Sliding, Rotation, Degloving Nasal Flap

Full-thickness surgical defects of the skin on the front of the lower half of the nose present considerable problems for esthetic repair. The ideal substitute for the excised skin in this area is the nasal skin itself. The patient shown in **(1)** has two separate basal cell carcinomas on the skin of her face: the one on the skin of the upper lip was excised and repaired primarily with an elliptical excision; that on the nose was a deeply infiltrating lesion measuring 2.5 × 2 cm. Although the underlying cartilages were not involved, the lesion had infiltrated through the skin and the underlying soft tissues.

The plan of surgical excision and reconstruction is marked out in **(2)**. The degloving flap is outlined in such a fashion that the incision to mobilize the flap is on the right side along the nasolabial fold going up to the glabellar region. The apex of the flap is on the midline with its left limb remaining symmetrical to the right limb.

Excision of the lesion is performed in the usual way. In this particular patient a generous amount of underlying soft tissues were excised down to the cartilage and nasal bone **(3)**. An adequate surgical excision was confirmed by frozen section control of margins. The degloving flap is mobilized by extending the incision on the right side along the nasolabial fold up to the apex of the outlined mark. The left limb of the flap is also elevated by an incision beginning at the apex and stopping at the medial margin of the left eyebrow. The flap is elevated to lift it off the nose and nasal bones entirely, and is mobilized well to the left side of the nose carefully preserving the left nasolabial artery.

The flap is then ready for rotation and sliding caudad to fill the surgical defect. The corners of the flap at both sides, as previously outlined in the skin markings, are sacrificed and closure of the flap to the surgical defect at the tip of the nose is performed using interrupted 3-0 chromic catgut subcutaneous buried sutures **(4)**. The remaining closure of the incision is performed in the usual way so that the defect at the superior end of the flap in the center of the forehead is closed like a 'V'–'Y' plasty. Closure of the defect at the tip of the nose in the midline is difficult since it significantly lifts the tip of the nose cephalad, and elevation of the tip of the nose in this way gives a 'piggy' nose deformity. However, with passage of time the tip of the nose drops to its normal configuration and the eventual esthetic result is very acceptable.

Postoperative appearance of the patient approximately 18 months later is shown in **(5)**. Note that the surgical incision is barely perceptible, the tip of the nose has dropped down and symmetry of the nares on both sides is restored, and the reconstructed nose has regained its essentially normal configuration. The degloving flap is of limited application in very large defects at the tip of the nose, as are the mobility of this flap and its capability to slide and rotate. Although the blood supply to the flap is generous its flexibility to fill the surgical defect is not very good, and therefore extreme caution should be exercised in deciding to use this flap for repair of nasal skin defects. Configuration of the nose in itself is also an important consideration for the application of this flap—for example, a patient with a nose pointing downward with a large hump would not be a suitable candidate.

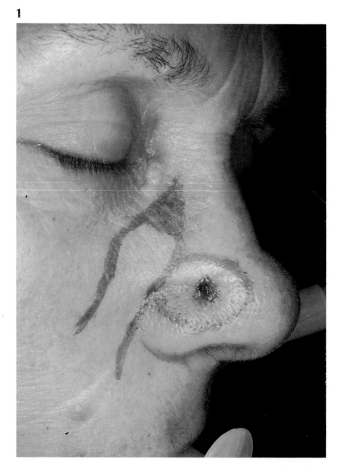

1

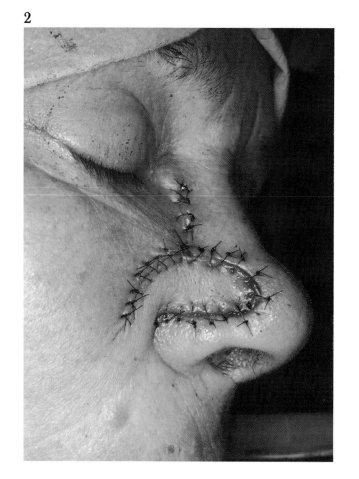

2

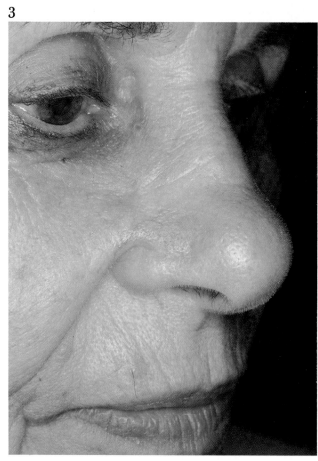

3

Nasolabial Flap

The nasolabial flap is an axial flap deriving its blood supply from the nasolabial artery, one of the terminal branches of the facial artery. The width:length ratio can be as much as 1:5 in select circumstances. The nasolabial flap is a highly reliable and very versatile flap; it is generally employed in reconstruction of surgical defects resulting from excision of skin cancers on the side of the nose, or the ala of the nose, as well as for full-thickness reconstruction of excised nasal ala, philtrum and columella.

Inferiorly Based Nasolabial Flap

Since the vascular supply of the nasolabial flap is through the nasolabial artery, it would appear logical to have the flap based inferiorly. The elevated distal part of the flap is rotated downward and anteriorly to fill the surgical defect. However, the length of the flap used in this way is limited since the skin at the root of the nose near the medial canthus is rather tight and little flexibility is available for closure of the donor site defect.

The site of surgical excision and the outline of the proposed nasolabial flap are marked out prior to excision (1). Appropriate measurements should be taken with a gauze to see that the flap is of adequate length and will rotate without any kink. Even though the flap is required to fill a circular defect, its apex is made triangular to allow primary closure of the donor site defect. Surgical excision of the lesion is performed using electrocautery but saving the underlying cartilage, as on this patient.

If, however, a through-and-through excision is necessary, then the nasolabial flap *elevated in this way* is not satisfactory. Once the adequacy of surgical excision is confirmed by histological evaluation of the surgical defect margins, then the nasolabial flap is elevated. Incision is made along the previously marked outline of the proposed nasolabial flap. *It is important to note that the lateral aspect of the surgical defect becomes the medial edge of the proposed skin flap.*

Elevation of the flap is begun superiorly near the apex of the triangular tip. Increasing thickness of the flap is retained as dissection proceeds proximally, so that adequate soft tissue coverage will be available to repair the surgical defect satisfactorily. During this maneuver, however, it is important to note that the flap should remain superficial to the underlying facial musculature. Brisk bleeding from branches of the nasolabial artery is usually encountered, and these vessels require clamping and ligation. Delicate handling of the flap is essential during elevation so that injury to the nasolabial artery is prevented, although sharp dissection is recommended. A sufficient length of the flap should be elevated to avoid any kinking or tension on the suture line.

Following elevation of the flap and achievement of complete hemostasis, the flap is rotated anteroinferiorly to fill the surgical defect on the nose. Several interrupted inverting 4-0 chromic catgut sutures are used to secure the flap to the surgical defect (2), and the flap is trimmed appropriately to shape it to the surgical defect. Prior to skin closure, the donor site defect is closed by mobilization of the skin of both the cheek and nose which is approximated with subcutaneous chromic catgut sutures and 5-0 nylon for skin. Skin closure between the skin flap and the nose is performed either using 5-0 or 6-0 interrupted nylon sutures. If the flap is small, then horizontal mattress sutures on both sides are not advisable since they may compromise the axial blood supply of the flap causing necrosis of the tip; half buried sutures, as described by Gillies, are recommended. These sutures begin on the skin of the nose, come through the dermis at the surgical defect, are taken horizontally through the dermis of the skin flap and then brought back out through to the dermis and the nasal skin. The knot, therefore, is on the nose side, while the intradermal suture in the skin flap remains parallel to the axial blood supply of the flap. This is an excellent suture technique and is ideally recommended for small flaps with axial blood supply such as this patient's skin flap.

Edema of the flap and slight duskiness is not unusual on the first postoperative day. Although the flap may look dusky or bluish, its vascularity is guaranteed; the discoloration is usually due to venous congestion, but the arterial blood supply of the flap is usually intact. Satisfactory healing of the skin is achieved in approximately 5–7 days when the skin sutures can be removed. Excessive fat retained on the flap will result in a 'fat flap'; this may require defattening under local anesthesia, but is not recommended for at least 6 months to a year. If sufficient care is taken to match the thickness of the flap to the thickness of the surgical defect with appropriate excision of excess fat from the flap at the time of the closure, one can avoid a 'fat flap' complication. Postoperative appearance of the patient several months later shows an excellent cosmetic result with essentially very little facial deformity at either the donor site or along the nasolabial skin crease (3).

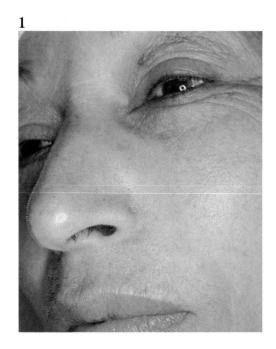

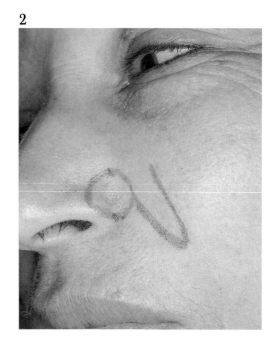

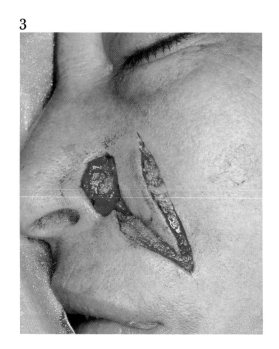

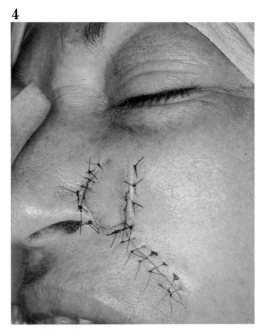

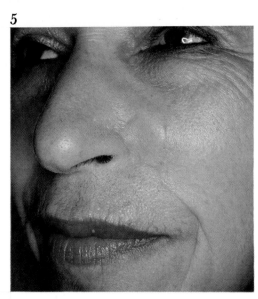

Superiorly Based Nasolabial Flap

Although the axial blood supply of the nasolabial flap is derived from the nasolabial artery, anastamotic communications between the angular branch of the anterior facial artery and vessels coming from the infraorbital foramen provide adequate blood supply to a superiorly based nasolabial flap.

A patient with recurrent basal cell carcinoma involving the lateral aspect of the ala and the nasolabial skin fold is shown preoperatively in (1). This lesion was treated previously by electrodesiccation and curettage.

The plan of surgical excision and repair using a superiorly based nasolabial flap is shown in (2). An adequate circumferential excision is carried out in the usual way with control of margins by frozen section studies, and the nasolabial flap is elevated keeping the medial incision along the nasolabial skin crease (3). The generous amount of fat in the subcutaneous tissue is kept attached to the nasolabial flap for appropriate trimming prior to closure of the surgical defect.

The flap is elevated up to its base and is rotated anteromedially to fill the surgical defect. The flap is trimmed appropriately and closed in two layers with 4-0 chromic catgut interrupted subcutaneous sutures and 6-0 nylon half-buried skin sutures (4). The donor site is primarily closed with advancement of the skin edges.

The patient is shown approximately 1 year postoperatively in (5); the excellent esthetic result is achieved by the superiorly based nasolabial flap for repair of lateral alar defect. The nasolabial fold skin crease is maintained in its normal position without any esthetic deformity at the donor site.

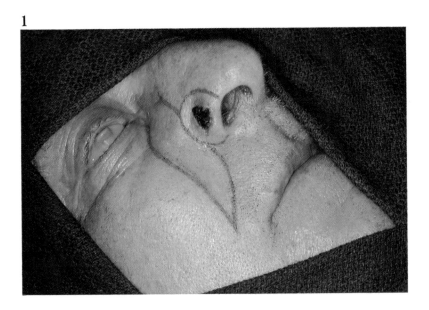

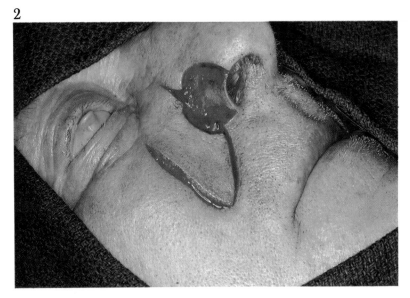

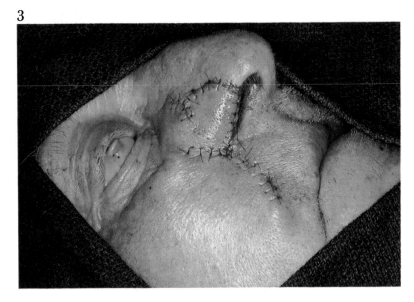

Superiorly Based Nasolabial Flap for Defect of the Ala Including Its Free Edge

Skin carcinomas of the ala involving the alar cartilage but not the underlying mucosa can be excised with the cartilage, carefully preserving the underlying mucosa. The nasolabial flap here provides an excellent choice for repair of alar defect.

A patient with basal cell carcinoma of the skin of the ala adherent to the alar cartilage is shown in (1). The underlying mucosa was intact. Surgical treatment required a circumferential excision including the free edge of the ala at the mucocutaneous junction. The nasolabial skin flap is outlined along the nasolabial skin crease, and the flap is superiorly based.

A surgical defect with excision of the ala to the alar groove, and including the alar cartilage but sparing the mucosa of the nasal vestibule, is shown in (2). The mucocutaneous junction of the ala is excised along with the surgical specimen. After ensuring adequacy of the surgical excision by frozen section study of surgical defect margins, the nasolabial flap is elevated, and rotated anteriorly and medially to fill the surgical defect. The flap is trimmed as necessary to obtain satisfactory contour. A suture line between the lateral edge of the skin flap and the mucosa reconstituted the free alar margin in this patient.

The skin flap had to be rotated anteriorly and an angulation in its long axis required an excision of a small wedge in its middle third (3). The donor site defect is closed primarily by appropriate mobilization.

The postoperative appearance of the patient approximately 6 months later (4) shows very satisfactory reconstruction of the alar defect including the free margin.

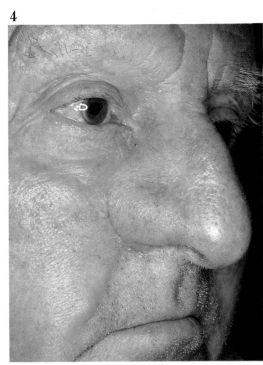

Nasolabial Flap Reconstruction for Through-and-Through Defect of the Alar Region

1

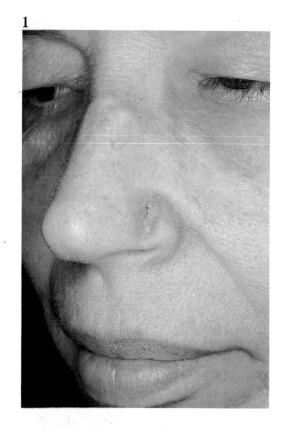

2

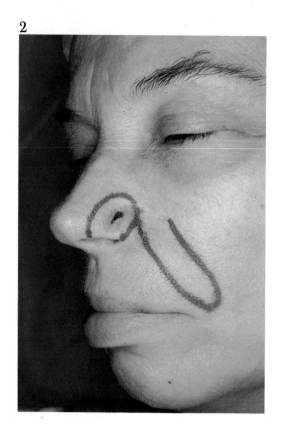

3

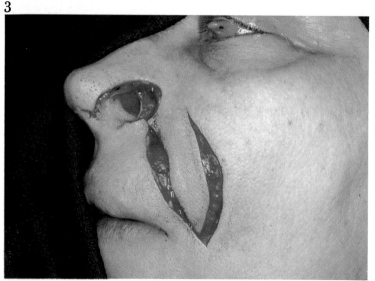

4

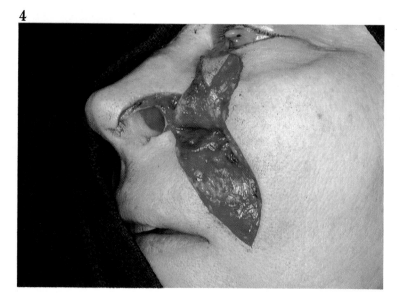

Recurrent basal cell carcinoma involving the skin of the ala and through the alar cartilage and nasal mucosa into the nasal vestibule is shown in **(1)**. The patient had previously received electrodesiccation and curettage on two occasions.

A surgical excision plan requiring a through-and-through resection of the ala of the nose including the underlying mucosa, and a proposed nasolabial flap for reconstruction of the surgical defect providing external and inner lining, is shown in **(2)**.

The excision is completed showing a through-and-through defect **(3)**. The nasolabial flap is elevated based superiorly on the anastomotic branches between the nasolabial artery and the vessels from the infraorbital foramen. The flap is elevated lateral to the nasolabial crease with a generous amount of fat on the undersurface.

The distal quarter of the flap is completely defatted leaving only the skin and dermis behind **(4)**. The tip of the flap is now turned over itself to provide for an inner lining and the free edge of the ala, and maintained in this inverted fashion using interrupted chromic catgut sutures. The entire distal part of the flap is now brought into the surgical defect and sutured in three layers.

The skin of the tip replacing the mucosa is sutured to the mucosa of the nasal vestibule with interrupted chromic catgut sutures **(5)**, and subcutaneous sutures set the flap in the surgical defect. The skin closure is performed with interrupted fine nylon sutures.

The postoperative appearance of the patient following minor revision for defattening of the flap is shown in **(6)**, at 1½ years after surgery. The nasolabial flap used in this way is ideal for repair of a through-and-through defect of the alar region of the nose **(7)**. The flap is folded over itself to replace the free edge of the ala and is esthetically quite acceptable. Cartilage support is usually not necessary unless the alar defect extends from the tip of the nose to the region of the nasolabial crease.

5

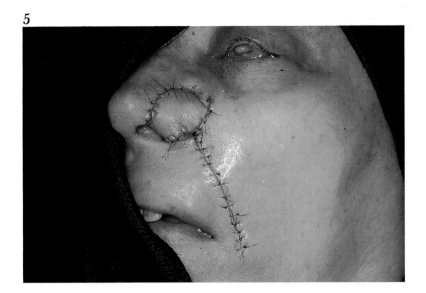

6

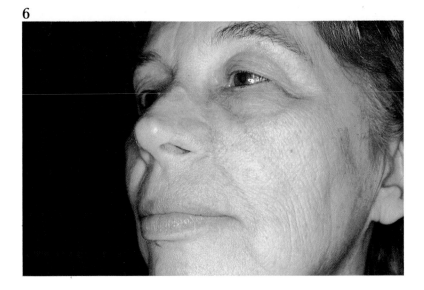

7

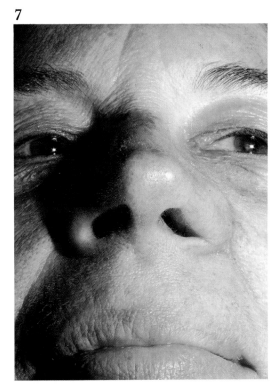

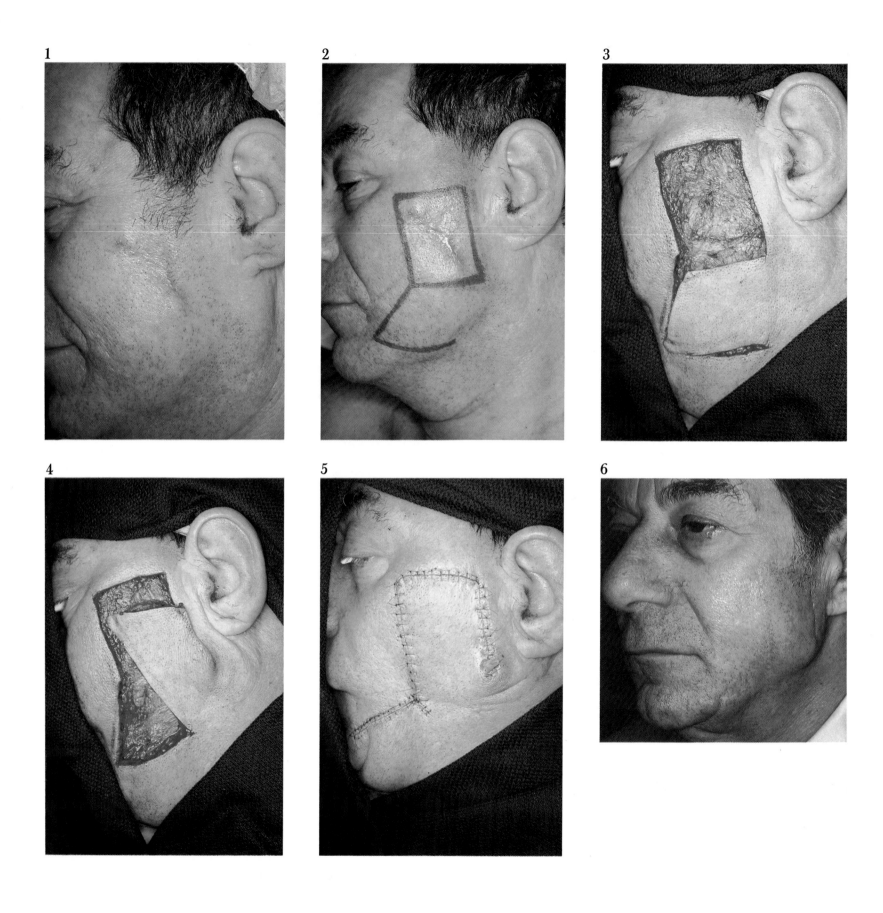

Rhomboid Flap

This versatile geometric flap was described by Limberg, a mathematician. It can be used in many areas of the body and provides a satisfactory closure of moderate-sized surgical defects; it is particularly useful in closing lax skin without tension.

A patient with recurrent basal cell carcinoma following previous surgical excision is shown in (1). The rhomboid flap outline should be made such that the donor site closure line will match facial skin lines (2). A surgical defect of any shape can be converted to a rhomboid, thus allowing design and elevation of this flap. Surgical excision of the recurrent cancer is carried out to include the subcutaneous tissue but superficial to the muscular layer. In this particular patient, terminal branches of the facial nerve remain at risk because of their proximity to the deep margin of the surgical specimen. These branches must be preserved by meticulous dissection, unless tumor invasion is demonstrated, in which case they should be sacrificed.

A surgical specimen has been removed and the flap is elevated (3). It should now be mobilized enough to allow for easy rotation to fill the surgical defect; if there is any tension on the suture line the outline of the flap is extended further.

The flap is now rotated, cephalad, to fill the surgical defect (4), which is closed in two layers using 3-0 chromic catgut interrupted inverting sutures for subcutaneous tissue and 5-0 nylon for skin (5). The triangular defect at the donor site is closed primarily by mobilization of the skin edges and its approximation. A small Penrose drain is left in the subcutaneous plane and brought out at the edge of the skin incision. Light dressings are applied.

The postoperative appearance of the patient approximately 9 months following surgery (6) shows excellent coverage of the surgical defect with minimal donor site deformity. As a result of elevation and transfer of this flap, all the facial musculature is maintained intact, so the patient has normal facial expression with no distortion.

The rhomboid is a random flap and therefore has limited application for coverage of larger-size defects. It is a highly reliable flap, and when properly planned as to placing the incisions for flap elevation the eventual esthetic result is excellent.

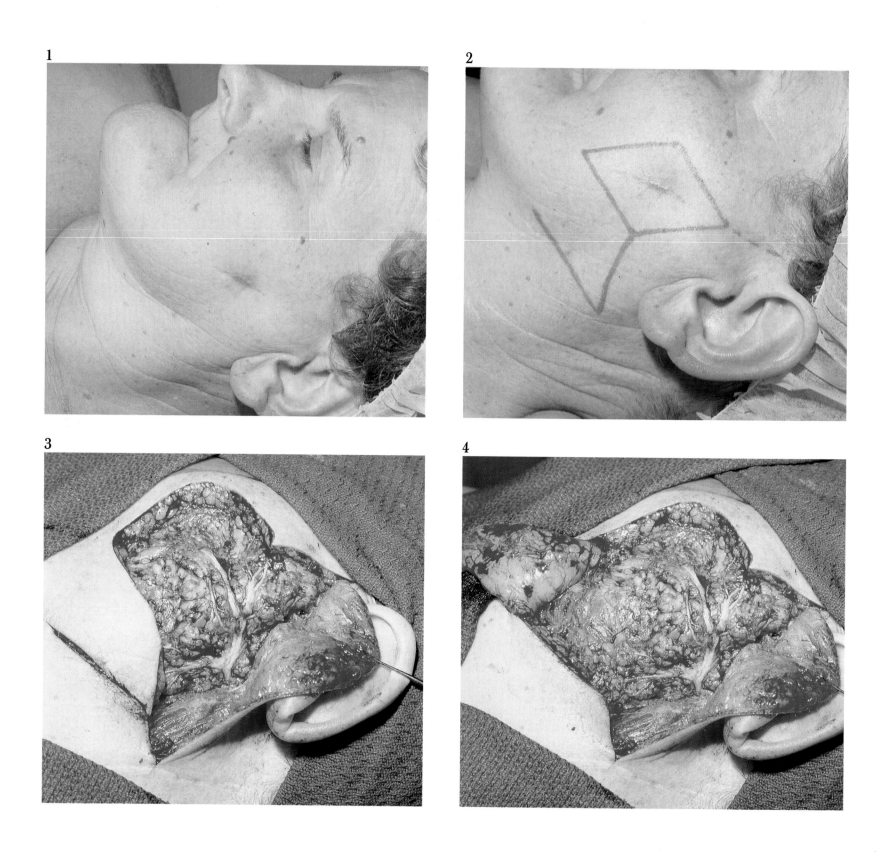

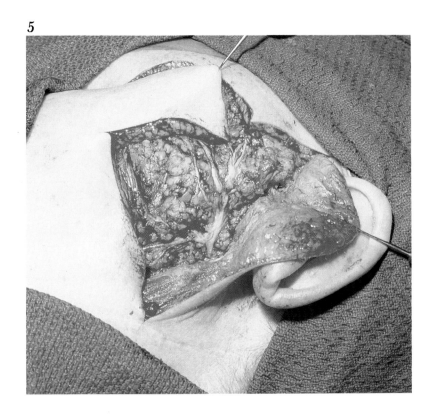

5

Anteriorly Based rhomboid flap

A patient with a superficial malignant melanoma involving the skin of the cheek is shown in **(1)**; she had undergone excisional biopsy of the tumor for diagnosis. The plan of surgical excision and elevation of rhomboid flap for transfer cephalad to close the surgical defect is shown in **(2)**. Because of the proximity of the tumor to the terminal branches of the facial nerve, a superficial parotidectomy was performed requiring extension of the incision up to the pinna in the preauricular region.

Surgical defect with excision of the skin of the cheek at the site of the primary melanoma, in conjunction with superficial parotidectomy with dissection and preservation of the facial nerve in its entirety, is shown in **(3)**. The rhomboid skin flap has been elevated, and retracted to show the entire surgical field following excision of the tumor and superficial parotidectomy **(4)**. The flap is now rotated cephalad to fill the surgical defect with appropriate closure of the remaining skin and the donor site defect **(5)**. A small Penrose drain is left in.

The postoperative appearance of the patient approximately 5 days later **(6)**, and 1 year after surgery **(7)** shows an excellent esthetic result.

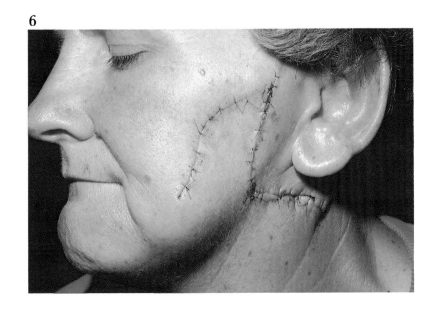

6

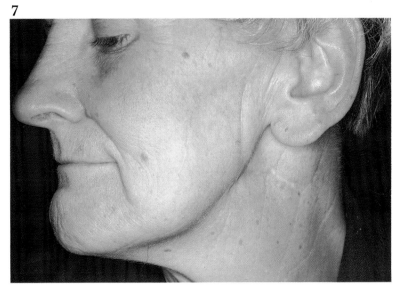

7

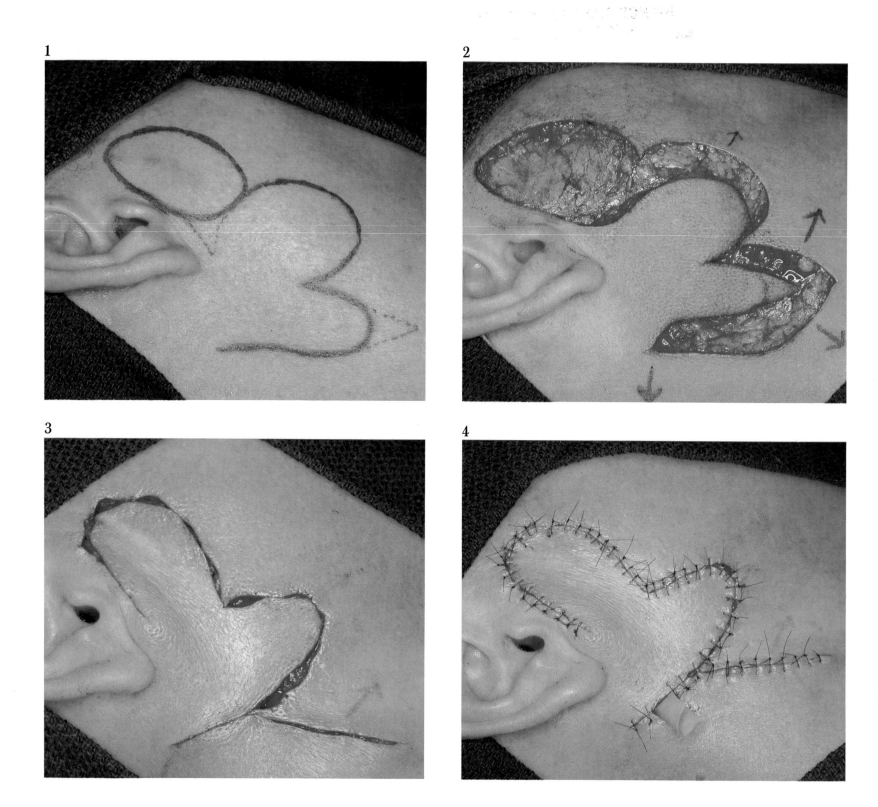

Bilobed Flap

The bilobed flap is a random flap, but is excellent for coverage of medium-size surgical defects throughout the body. The principle of 'borrowing from Peter to give it to Paul' is exemplified in the design and elevation of this flap.

A patient who has undergone excisional biopsy of a superficial malignant melanoma of the skin of the preauricular region is shown in (1). The patient is 28 years old and has relatively tight skin which does not allow use of a cervical flap without secondary repair. Outline of the surgical excision and proposed elevation of the bilobed flap is shown in (1). One principle of using a bilobed flap is that the first lobe of the flap, which is to fill the surgical defect, is approximately 80% of the latter's size; and the second lobe is approximately 80% of the defect at the site of the first lobe. Thus, the first lobe fills the surgical defect, while the second lobe fills the defect at the site of the first lobe, and the defect created at the site of the second lobe is closed primarily by mobilization of the skin edges. The principle is that of diminishing the size of both the flaps from the surgical defect for closure.

Surgical excision of the preauricular skin is completed and the bilobed flap is elevated (2). By careful planning of the surgical incisions, the scar is hidden in both the preauricular skin crease and the upper cervical neck crease. Two wedges of skin are excised to prevent dog ears, the first wedge at the point of rotation of the first lobe of the flap and the surgical defect as shown in (1), and the second wedge at the apex of the second lobe to convert a circular into a linear defect.

The bilobed flap is now rotated cephalad to fill both the surgical defect of the excision and that created by the first lobe. Inverting interrupted subcutaneous chromic catgut sutures set the flap properly (3). The subcutaneous sutures take tension away from the skin sutures, and bring the skin edges as close as possible.

The final closure shows skin sutures in place with a small Penrose drain brought out through the posterior aspect of the donor site incision (4). Light dressings are necessary for serous drainage, expected for 48–72 hours.

The postoperative appearance of the patient approximately 1 month later shows satisfactory healing of the wound (5). Accurate anticipation of the size of the surgical defect and appropriate planning of the bilobed flap usually give a very gratifying esthetic result.

5

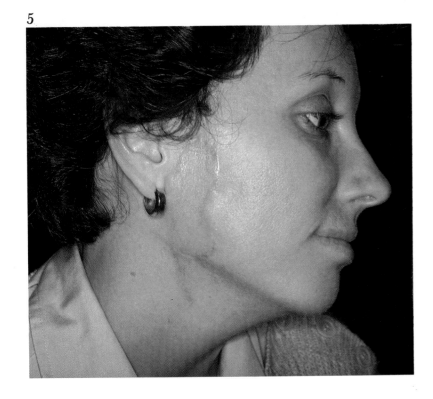

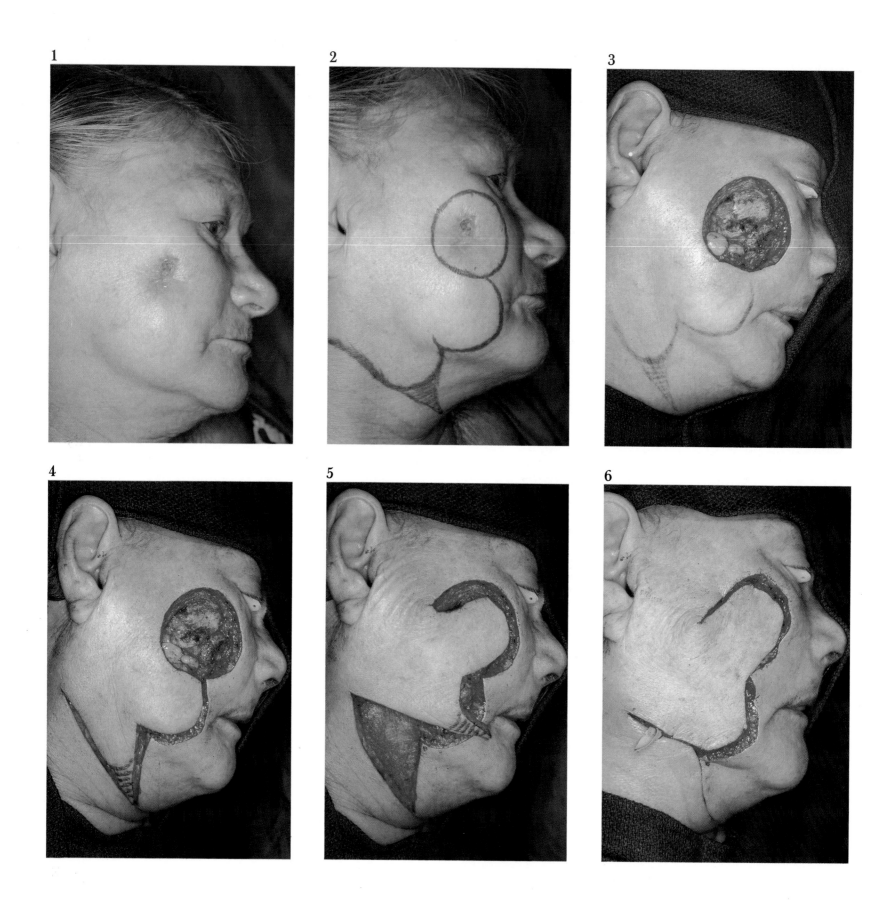

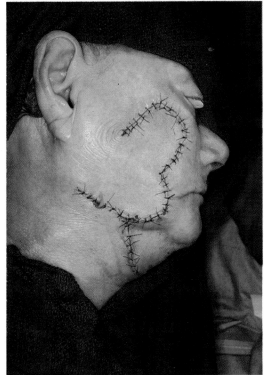

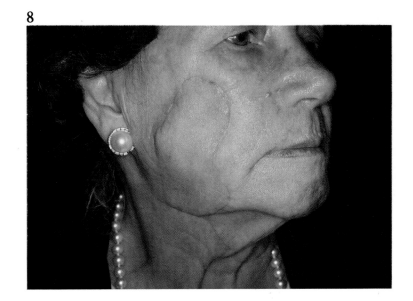

flap (4). The second lobe of the flap has a triangular apex to facilitate closure of the donor site deformity, and this will be excised when the flap is rotated. The flap is elevated posteriorly far enough to allow easy rotation cephalad.

The flap is now rotated cephalad so the first lobe of the bilobed flap fills the surgical defect at the site of excision, while the second lobe fills the defect created by the first lobe (5). The surgical defect in the upper part of the neck created by the second lobe will be closed primarily by mobilization of the skin of the neck. Interrupted chromic catgut sutures are taken for subcutaneous tissue to distribute tension appropriately and set the flap in the surgical defect accurately (6). The triangular apex of the second lobe is excised and subcutaneous sutures are taken at this point. Mobilization of the neck skin in the lower part allows closure of the donor site defect in the upper part of the neck. A small Penrose drain is inserted and brought out through the posterior aspect of the incision line in the neck.

Final skin closure using interrupted nylon sutures for approximation of skin edges is shown in (7). To achieve the best esthetic result, the skin must be accurately approximated.

The postoperative appearance of the patient approximately 1 month following surgery (8) shows satisfactory closure of the surgical defect with minimal donor site deformity due to alignment of the transverse scar in the upper part of the neck along the facial skin lines. Bilobed flaps used in this fashion provide a very readily available tool for the closure of sizeable defects laterally in the cheek. The flap works best in patients who have excess or lax skin providing easy rotation of both flap and donor site deformity leaving a transverse scar along the upper skin crease in the neck.

Bilobed flap for anterior cheek defect

The bilobed flap can also be used very effectively on defects of the cheek anteriorly. Surgical defects of the skin and soft tissues of the cheek overlying the zygoma and the buccinator muscle are very well suited for reconstruction using a bilobed flap.

The patient shown here (1) has a recurrent basal cell carcinoma involving the skin and subcutaneous tissues, though not the underlying buccinator muscle. The area of skin at risk around the tumor measures approximately 5 cm in diameter.

The plan of surgical excision and reconstruction using a bilobed flap is outlined here (2). A circular disk of skin measuring 5.5 cm is outlined around the ulcerated lesion for surgical excision. The bilobed flap is also outlined using skin of the lower part of the cheek and the upper part of the neck for rotation cephalad to cover the surgical defect with closure of the donor site defect along the upper skin crease in the neck.

The surgical excision is completed showing the defect exposing the zygoma in the upper part of the surgical field and the buccinator muscle, as well as other facial muscles in the lower part of the defect (3). Adequacy of surgical resection was confirmed by frozen section of margins from both periphery and depth of the surgical defect. The buccal branch of the facial nerve had to be sacrificed due to its proximity to the undersurface of the surgical specimen.

The bilobed flap is elevated, superficial to the facial musculature but keeping all the subcutaneous fat on the

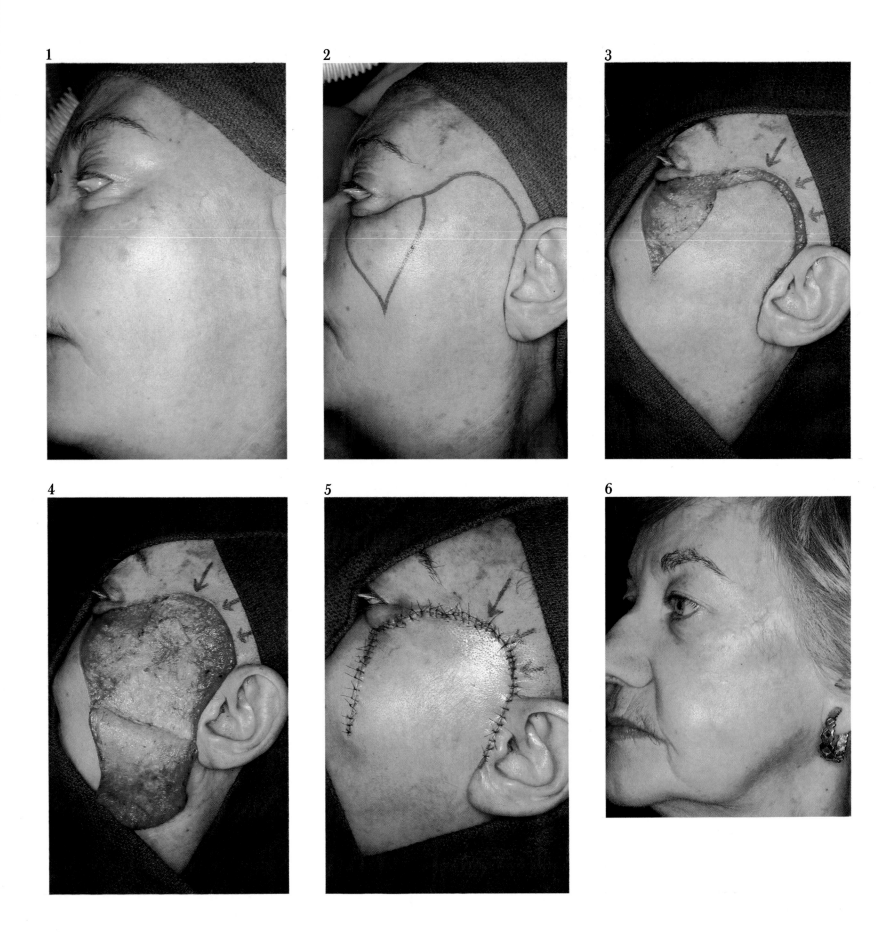

Mustardé Advancement Rotation Cheek Flap

Skin defects resulting from surgical excision of lesions involving the skin in the infraorbital region of the cheek and medial part of the cheek are best suited for repair using a Mustardé flap. The major blood supply of this skin flap is from the posterior branches of the facial artery with the wide pedicle of the flap remaining inferiorly.

A patient with a Hutchinson's melanotic freckle and *in situ* melanoma presenting on the skin of the cheek in the infraorbital region is shown in **(1)**. The plan for surgical excision with outline of the anticipated surgical defect and the incision outline for elevation of the Mustardé flap is shown in **(2)**. The superior margin of the surgical defect and the Mustardé flap are kept as close to the tarsal margin as possible, depending on the location of the lesion and the surgical defect. Surgical excision is carried out depending on the histology of the primary tumor and its necessary resection thickness.

Excision of the tumor is completed, preserving the orbicularis oculi and its nerve supply but carefully excising a generous margin of underlying fat **(3)**. Skin incision is taken for elevation of the Mustardé flap. In the preauricular region the incision is usually taken cephalad towards the temple so that the line of tension along the suture line draws the lower lid cephalad rather than caudad to prevent drooping of the lateral canthus of the eye. The incision is then carried into the preauricular skin crease, and if additional mobilization is necessary it can be extended into the retroauricular region like a bilobed flap. The skin flap is elevated superficially to the parotid gland but carefully preserving the underlying subcutaneous tissues on the flap to avoid any compromise of its blood supply. Sufficient mobilization of the flap up to the angle of the mandible is often necessary to avoid tension on the suture line.

Mobilization of the skin of the forehead and temporal region is often needed to facilitate closure. Arrows on the skin shown in **(4)** point to the line of maximum tension in carrying out closure of the donor site defect. Here the skin flap is elevated and retracted downward to show the extent of mobilization prior to its advancement and rotation for closure of the surgical defect. The flap is now advanced medially and rotated inferiorly to allow closure.

Inverting chromic catgut interrupted subcutaneous sutures are made to bear tension on the suture line **(5)**, and the sutures must be placed between the skin flap and the skin of the temporal region and forehead to balance the suture line. Maximum tension line again is as shown by the arrows in the preauricular and temporal region **(5)**. A small Penrose drain is brought behind the lobule of the ear posteriorly.

The postoperative appearance of the patient approximately 9 months later **(6)** shows the excellent esthetic result achieved by this technique.

Another patient with *in situ* melanoma of the skin of the infraorbital region is shown in **(7,)** and the plan of surgical excision and elevation of the Mustardé flap is outlined in **(8.)** Note that the intended skin flap takes the incision line cephalad in the temporal region, as mentioned above, so that the suture line in the region of the lateral canthus pulls upward rather than downwards. The lateral aspect of the skin incision for the flap is taken in the preauricular skin crease.

7

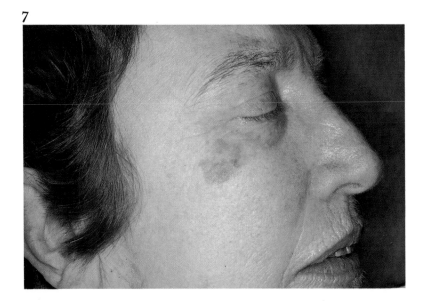

8

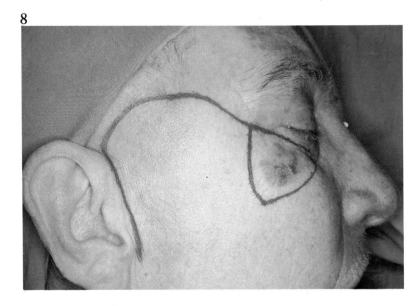

9

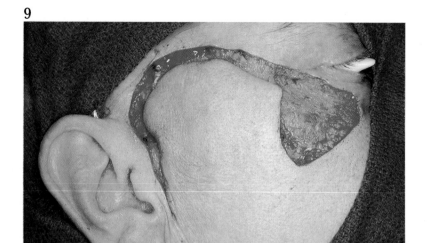

10

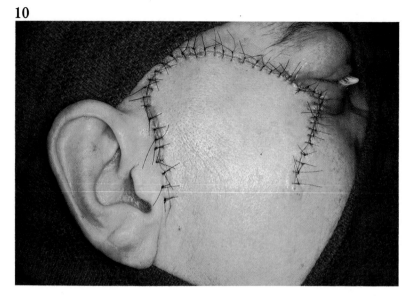

11

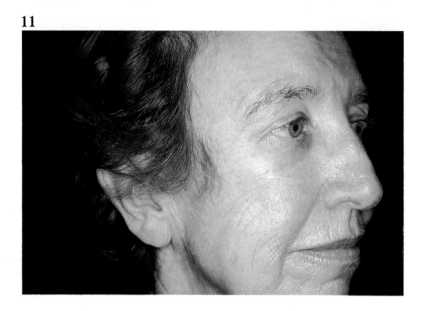

The surgical specimen is excised and the skin flap elevated as described above (9). With anterior advancement and a caudad rotation, the skin flap is brought to fill the surgical defect and allow for satisfactory closure (10). The postoperative appearance of the patient approximately 1 year later (11) shows an excellent esthetic and functional result.

The Mustardé flap is very useful for closure of defects of the cheek in the infraorbital region, or the medial aspect of the cheek in the region of the nasolabial crease. However, the dimensions of this flap are limited so very large resections of the cheek are not suitable for repair with the Mustardé flap. Generally, surgical defects of one-third the width between the medial canthus and the tragus of the ear are suitable for closure. Larger defects of the cheek can be closed using a bilobed flap technique, with the Mustardé flap as the first lobe, and the second lobe developed from skin of the postauricular area and transferred in front of the ear. Occasionally, minor skin loss may result in the temporal region where maximum tension is present on the suture line. However, if blanching and tension on the suture line is appreciated at the time of wound closure, the lateral incision may be taken further down in the skin of the neck or in the postauricular region to minimize tension and prevent skin necrosis.

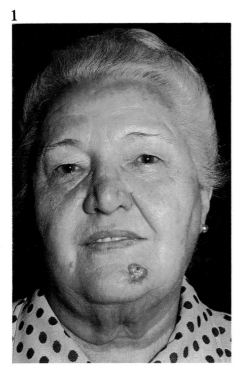

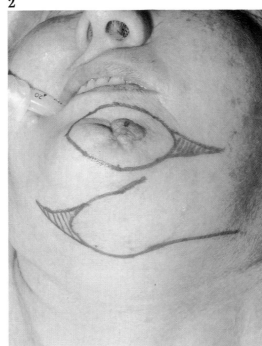

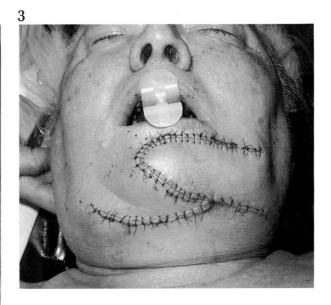

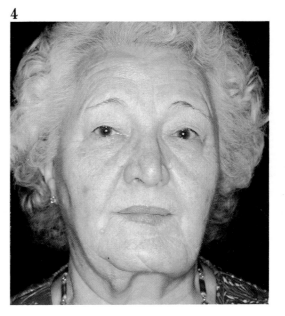

Cervical Flap

Skin defects resulting from excision of lesions of the skin of the chin or the lower part of the face present a problem best handled by reconstruction using a cervical flap. The transverse-oriented cervical flap is a random flap, so the length to which it can be elevated with ease without compromise of blood supply is limited. Generally, a width:length ratio of 1:3 is the maximum that a random flap can tolerate.

A patient with a recurrent nodular basal cell carcinoma involving the soft tissues and the underlying musculature of the chin is shown in (1). The plan of surgical excision and elevation of flap for transfer to cover the surgical defect is shown in (2). Two triangular wedges of skin had to be excised to fill the surgical defect and provide satisfactory closure at the donor site defect. Surgical excision in this patient was carried down to the bone because of the depth of the tumor infiltration, so the cervical flap required inclusion of the underlying subcutaneous tissue and platysma to provide substance. Meticulous attention should be paid to the dissection, identification and preservation of the mandibular branch of the facial nerve during elevation of the proximal part of the cervical flap.

Closure of the surgical defect is performed in two layers using 3-0 chromic catgut interrupted inverting sutures for subcutaneous layer and 5-0 nylon for skin (3). The donor site defect is closed similarly by mobilization of the skin of the lower part of the neck.

The postoperative appearance of the patient approximately 1½ years following surgery is shown in (4). A satisfactory esthetic result is accomplished in a one-stage procedure for a sizable defect of the skin of the chin. Minor revision and defattening of the flap can be undertaken to enhance the esthetic appearance of the patient if necessary.

1

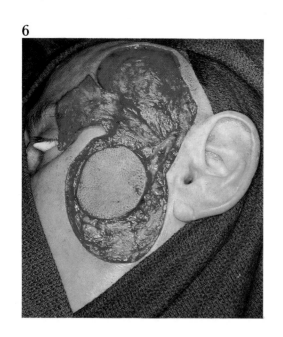

2

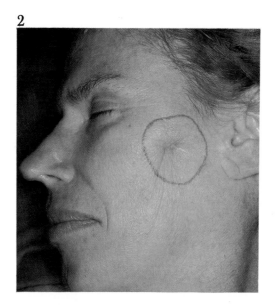

3

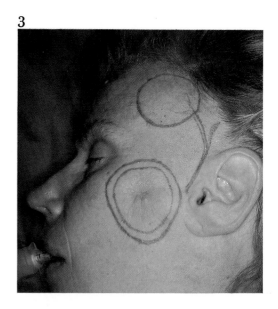

4

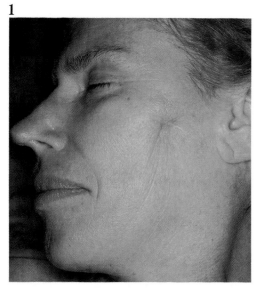

5

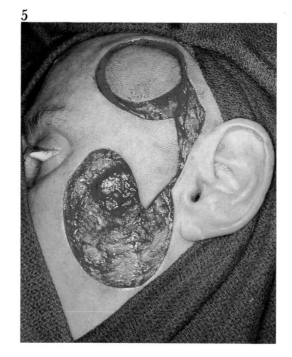

6

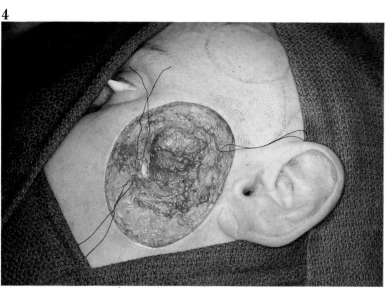

7

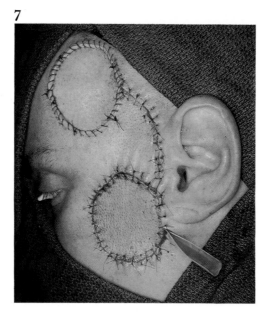

8

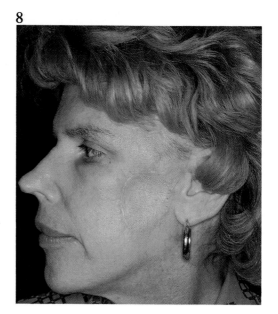

Island Pedicle Flap

Island pedicle flaps with their own vascular pedicles are isolated in various locations in the head and neck area. One of the most versatile and easily available island pedicle flap is that based on the superficial temporal artery and vein, usually on the anterior branch which provides blood supply to the forehead. This flap is elevated from the lateral aspect of the forehead.

Its advantages include fairly regular and identifiable artery and vein, a long vascular pedicle, and thick forehead skin to provide for replacement of excised skin and soft tissues. Also, the color match is excellent for coverage of facial surgical defects.

Its disadvantages are that the size of the flap is limited, and occasionally may be hair-bearing. It is important to ensure smooth rotation of the pedicle since a kink in the vascular pedicle of the flap can result in disaster with complete loss of flap.

A patient with a recurrent basal cell carcinoma who had previous curettage and desiccation, as well as surgical excision of this lesion performed elsewhere is shown in (1). The lesion is indurated and adherent to the underlying zygoma.

An outline of the extent of palpable induration around the area of recurrent tumor is shown in (2). The intended surgical excision would include a through-and-through resection of all soft tissues including a portion of the zygoma to obtain satisfactory margins around the primary tumor.

The plan of surgical excision and repair showing the incision at the site of the primary tumor is shown in (3). Location of the vascular pedicle for the proposed flap with bifurcation of the superficial temporal artery shows the blood supply to the island flap, the outline of which is measured to match the surgical defect.

The surgical defect in (4) shows both buccal and temporal branches of the facial nerve which are isolated and preserved. The branches of the zygomatic division of the facial nerve immediately beneath the tumor, including a portion of the underlying zygoma, were sacrificed deliberately. The surgical defect shows a through-and-through three-dimensional excision of the recurrent basal cell carcinoma; all margins of resection, including peripheral and deep, were checked at this point to ensure adequacy of excision.

The island pedicle flap is now isolated with a circular disk of skin from the forehead on the vascular pedicle from the anterior branch of the superficial temporal artery and vein (5). The flap is now rotated caudad along with the vascular pedicle to fill the surgical defect (6). Meticulous attention to detail must be paid during elevation of the skin flap and its vascular pedicle to avoid any injury to it. Branches from the vascular pedicle that are not important to the nourishment of the flap are sacrificed without compromising the lumen of the arterial and venous pedicle. During rotation of the flap and its setting in the surgical defect, any kink in the pedicle must be avoided, but if there is any kinking further mobilization of the vessels is undertaken to correct it.

The flap is sutured to the edges of the surgical defect in two layers with a small Penrose drain brought out through the suture line (7). The donor site defect is closed with split thickness skin graft applied over the temporalis fascia, held in position with a bolster dressing.

The postoperative appearance of the patient approximately 9 months after surgery is shown in (8). Although excellent coverage of the surgical defect is obtained, the esthetic result is not as pleasing as one would like to see, largely due to loss of underlying zygoma and masseter muscle causing lack of soft tissue support; this in turn causes lack of fullness and sunken appearance to the cheek.

Island pedicle flaps are excellent for coverage of certain surgical defects resulting from loss of skin and soft tissues in the region of the nose or the side of the cheek. However, extreme caution and skill must be exercised in anticipation of the size of both the surgical defect and the elevated skin flap. Meticulous attention should be paid to the extremely careful and skilful dissection of the vascular pedicle with gentle hands, as injury to the vascular pedicle would mean loss of the flap. Those branches of the vessels that are not necessary for the vascularity of the flap are sacrificed, but short stumps of these vessels must be left attached to the main vascular pedicle so that the lumen of the feeding artery and draining vein is not compromised. Similarly, extreme care must be exercised during transport of the flap and its rotation to avoid any kinking or torsion. Transport of island flaps generally manifest venous congestion in the first 48 hours, but as long as capillary filling is present the flap will survive.

Where there is extreme venous congestion and engorgement causing compromise of the blood supply of the flap, a technique of flap phlebotomy may be vital to the survival of the flap. In island flaps where venous drainage is unsatisfactory, as shown by bluish discoloration and edema in the immediate postoperative period, but where arterial blood supply is intact, as shown by blanching, flap phlebotomy may be indicated. If venous blood is drained from the congested flap immediately postoperatively to maintain perfusion of the flap, then these otherwise doomed flaps can be salvaged. A technique of flap phlebotomy using multiple needle punctures on the skin of the flap with a number 22 needle is recommended. This will provide immediate drainage of congested, dark venous blood and improve perfusion of the flap. Strict sterile conditions must be maintained for absorbing the oozing of venous blood in sterile dressings until new venous channels are established.

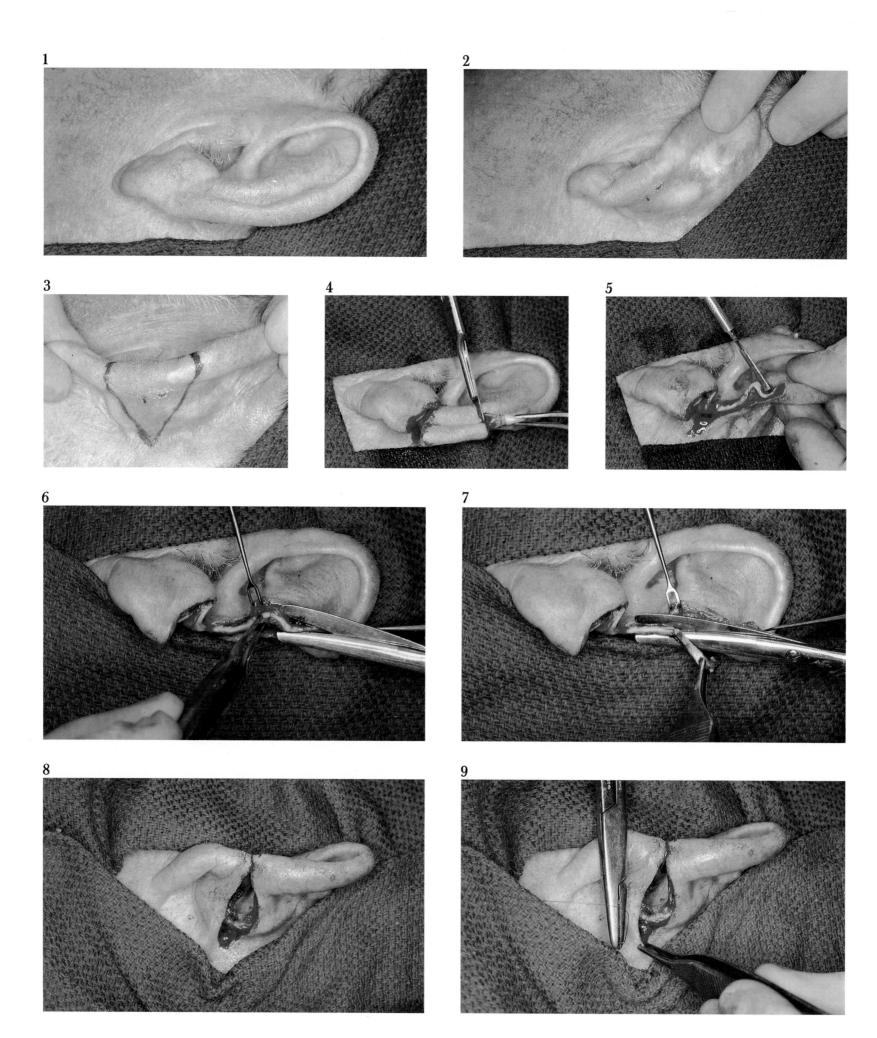

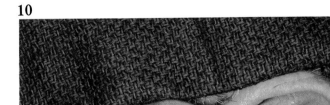

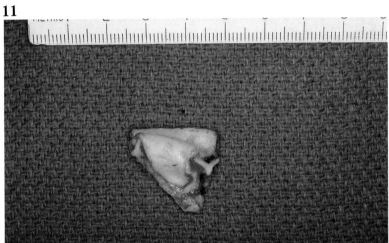

Wedge Excision of the External Ear

Malignant tumors of the skin of the external ear often invade the underlying cartilage or perforate through to present on both sides of the external ear. These lesions require a through-and-through excision of a portion of the pinna to remove the tumor satisfactorily. Surgical defects resulting from excision of one-third of the vertical height of the pinna are suitable for primary closure by approximating the edges of the surgical defect. The height of the pinna is reduced, but the esthetic result is acceptable.

The preoperative appearance of the anterior surface of the pinna (1) of a patient with a recurrent basal cell carcinoma involving the underlying cartilage mainly presenting on the posterior aspect. The lesion involves the helix and the underlying cartilage (2).

A plan of surgical excision is outlined by an incision drawn to resect a wedge of the ear with the apex of the wedge in the retroauricular skin crease (3). A similar incision is marked out on the anterior aspect of the pinna so that the apex of the surgical defect meets at approximately the same point both anteriorly and posteriorly. Excision is made with a sharp knife taken through and through the predrawn skin incision (4). A wedge of the pinna is excised, including the skin of the anterior aspect, the cartilage beneath as well as the skin of the posterior aspect until the two skin incisions meet at the apex of the wedge.

Following removal of the surgical specimen, brisk hemorrhage is encountered from the dermal vessels, but this is easily controlled by electrocoagulation of the bleeding points from the cut edges of the pinna (5). Once hemostasis is obtained, an extra margin of the cartilage is removed to facilitate skin closure.

The skin edges usually retract over the cartilage immediately following excision of the tumor (6). The extruded portion of the cartilage is excised using a sharp scissors, so that during closure the cartilage ends do not push against each other causing excessive tension on the skin suture line (7). A strip of cartilage is thus excised from both the upper and the lower margins of the surgical defect.

Closure of the surgical defect is begun by first taking one nylon skin suture at the margin of the helix from the upper part of the surgical defect to the lower part of the surgical defect to provide accurate approximation of the edges of the helix of the pinna (8). This suture is not tied but held in position and retracted laterally to facilitate skin closure. Both posterior and anterior skin is closed separately in two layers. No attempt is made to suture the cartilage ends, so the closure consists exclusively of skin sutures anteriorly and posteriorly (9).

Bacitracin ointment is applied to the skin edges on the suture line and a light dressing is applied (10). These skin sutures are left in for approximately 2 weeks for satisfactory healing and secure scar before removal of the stitches.

The surgical specimen in (11) shows a through-and-through wedge of the pinna with the skin of its anterior aspect, the underlying cartilage and the skin of the posterior aspect encompassing the entire tumor.

Wedge excision of the pinna is a very acceptable and satisfactory operative procedure for lesions requiring through-and-through excision of any parts of the external ear. Primary closure is possible for defects not exceeding one-third of the vertical height of the pinna. Larger defects are not suitable for primary closure.

4: The Lips

Introduction

Surgical treatment of tumors of the upper and lower lip is highly sophisticated. The lips are complex, anatomical structures lined with labial mucosa inside the vermilion border and the skin externally. The lips are responsible for speech function, and facial expressions and functions of the oral cavity—smiles, grimaces, puckers, etc. are largely produced by the lips. Functionally, competency of the lips and oral commissure is vital to prevent drooling. Blood supply to the lips is derived from superior and inferior labial arteries. Control of the intricate musculature of the upper and lower lip is provided totally by the buccal and mandibular branches of the facial nerve.

The most frequently encountered tumors arising on the lips are: squamous cell carcinomas, basal cell carcinomas, and rarely carcinomas arising from minor salivary glands as well as melanomas and sarcomas. Preneoplastic leukoplakia of the mucosa over the vermilion border of the lip often also demands surgical intervention. Tiny, superficial lesions involving the vermilion border of the lip are easily amenable to elliptical excision generally performed under local anesthesia with very gratifying esthetic and functional results. Natural skin creases on the vermilion border are in a radial direction along the circumference of the mouth; so elliptical excision is therefore planned accordingly, and the resulting scar virtually merges with the natural skin lines leaving a very pleasing esthetic result.

Lip shave

The most important indications for a lip shave operation are areas of leukoplakia with keratosis and superficially invasive or *in situ* carcinomas. The entire vermilion border of the upper or lower lip may have to be removed with this clinical entity if both upper and lower lips are involved. For this operation to be successful, the diseased areas of the lip must be confined to the mucous membrane and not be infiltrating in nature. Adjacent mucosa of the labial surface of the lip may be removed. The operation can be combined with V excision of the lip where superficial involvement has a specific area of deep infiltration.

Lip shave operation with V excision for carcinoma of the lower lip

The patient shown here (1) has a nodular, infiltrating squamous cell carcinoma of the vermilion border of the lower lip on the right side measuring approximately 1.5 cm on its surface. He also has diffuse areas of leuko-

plakia involving the vermilion border of the lower lip as shown (1). Except for the palpable nodule at the site of the infiltrating cancer, the remaining lesion is only superficial.

1

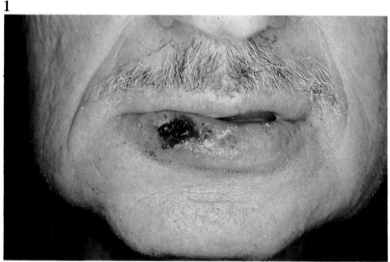

2

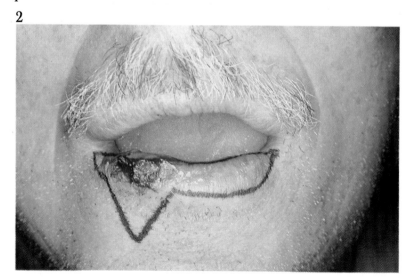

3

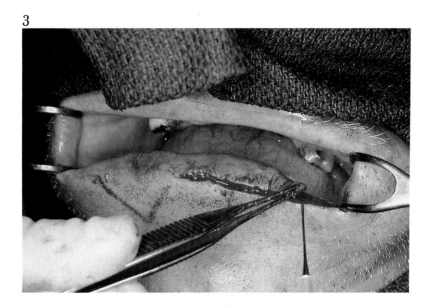

4

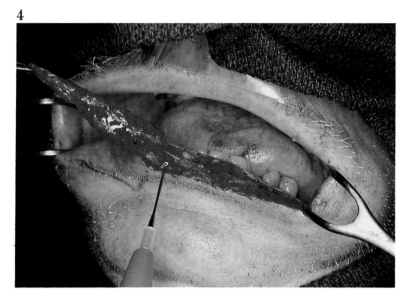

5

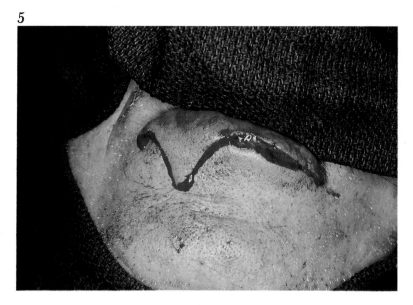

The outline of the proposed surgical excision calls for a V excision at the site of the palpable nodule, in conjunction with lip shave procedure for excision of the complete vermilion border of the lower lip (2). The operation can be performed under local or general anesthesia. If local anesthesia is used, the entire lower lip is infiltrated with 1% Xylocaine with epinephrine, 1 in 100 000, and the extent of surgical excision must be marked out with a skin marking pen prior to infiltration of anesthesia. The author prefers general anesthesia because it allows more satisfactory control of the operative procedure, and avoids any distortion in the configuration of the mucocutaneous junction of the lip.

The operation begins with the lip shave part of the procedure first (3). A skin incision is made at the mucocutaneous junction of the lower lip beginning on the left side and up to the left border of the proposed V excision. A similar incision is made on the mucosal aspect of the lower lip following the outline as marked before. Brisk bleeding from this area should be expected and therefore use of a suction with a hand-controlled Frazier suction tip is preferable for a dry field. A toothed Adson forceps is then used to grasp the tip of the surgical specimen on the left side, and remainder of the dissection proceeds with the use of fine needletip electrocautery and coagulating current. Dissection now proceeds in a relatively superficial plane taking as little of the underlying musculature as possible, but ensuring that no buttonholes take place through the mucosa of the surgical specimen.

As the specimen is mobilized towards the right side, dissection continues keeping uniform thickness of the excised specimen until the left limb of the V excision is reached (4). Complete hemostasis is obtained at this stage of the operation by electrocoagulating the bleeding points which are usually from the dermal as well as the mucosal edge of the surgical defect.

At this point, using a number 15 scalpel, a skin incision is made along the previously marked out V, then carried across to the right side near the commissure of the mouth and completing the entire length of the incision on the mucosa posteriorly (5). The remainder of the surgical excision is then completed again using electrocautery, which at the site of the V, performs a through-and-through wedge of the lower lip excising the underlying musculature and the overlying mucosa posteriorly. Usually, the labial artery can be easily identified, clamped, divided and ligated to minimize brisk hemorrhage from the vessel. Pulling on the specimen must be avoided, as it is pulled too hard during the dissection unnecessary quantities of the labial musculature is sacrificed resulting in a notched deformity at the site of the surgical resection.

6

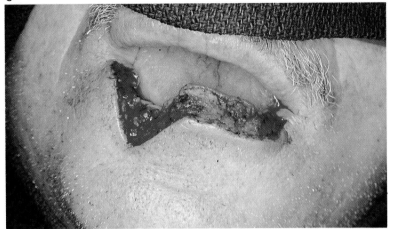

7

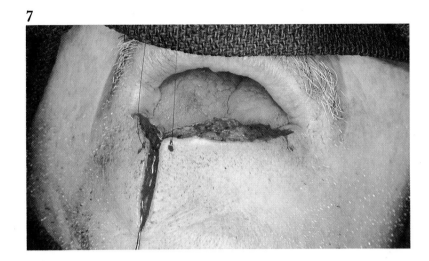

8

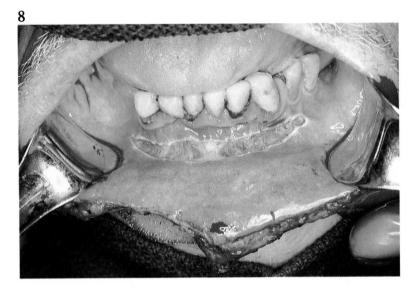

9

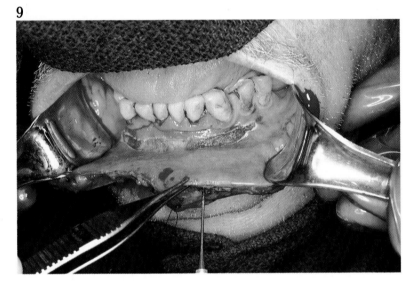

The surgical defect resulting from this excision is shown in **(6)**. The labial artery will require ligation at both ends of the defect of V excision. Adequacy of surgical excision is confirmed by frozen section control of surgical defect margins. Meticulous attention should be paid to absolute hemostasis, otherwise bleeding and hematoma will pose a problem postoperatively.

Closure of the surgical defect begins at the apex of the V excision approximating the muscular layer with interrupted chromic catgut sutures **(7)**. However, prior to this a fine nylon suture is taken through the edge of the skin defect at both ends of the V excision defect of the lower lip, placed and held tight, but with no knots. This will allow accurate approximation of the vermilion edges to avoid a notching deformity or inaccurate approximation of the vermilion border of the reconstructed lower lip. Tension is now applied to the ends of this skin suture to allow both the surgical defect to collapse, and accurate placement of the muscular sutures. Once the muscular layer is closed, the dynamic reconstruction for maintenance of competency of the oral cavity is accomplished.

Attention is now focussed on mobilization of the labial mucosa which will be used in reconstruction of the new vermilion surface **(8)**. The oral cavity is opened generously, and large Richardson retractors placed at the oral commissure on both sides to expose the gingivolabial sulcus. Electrocautery is used to place an incision in the gingivolabial sulcus as shown here. The labial mucosa is placed under tension by retracting it, while the incision in the gingivolabial sulcus is made with electrocautery, to allow easy separation of the mucosa covering the gum and the lower lip.

An Adson forceps is now used to grasp the upper edge of the labial mucosa and, using electrocautery, submucosal dissection of this bipedicled, labial mucosal flap is undertaken **(9)**. Meticulous attention is paid to the technique of dissection in the submucosal plane, otherwise buttonholes would result in the mucosa if the flap is too thin, or unnecessary musculature of the lower lip would be taken with the flap if it is kept too thick. The accurate plane of dissection is such that some minor salivary gland tissue will be on the mucosal flap while the musculature remains intact. The entire flap is mobilized through the length of the incision in the mucosa of the gingivolabial sulcus; so thus this becomes a bipedicled, labial, mucosal flap of the lower lip.

10

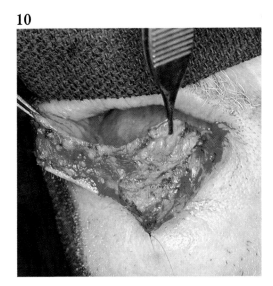

11

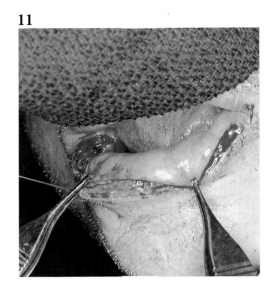

12

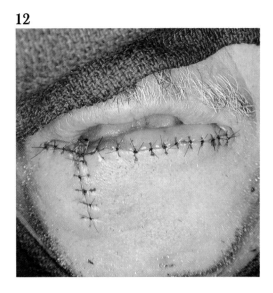

13

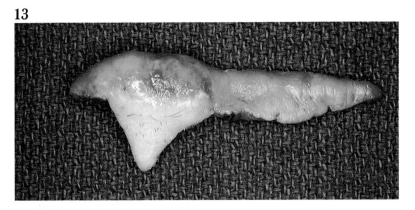

14

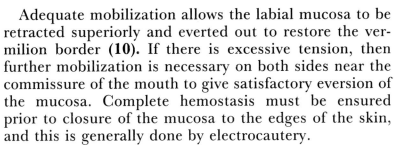

15

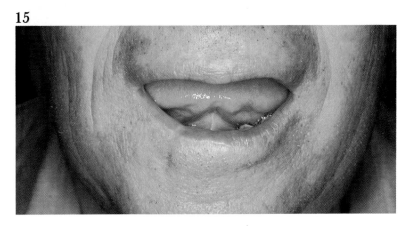

Adequate mobilization allows the labial mucosa to be retracted superiorly and everted out to restore the vermilion border **(10).** If there is excessive tension, then further mobilization is necessary on both sides near the commissure of the mouth to give satisfactory eversion of the mucosa. Complete hemostasis must be ensured prior to closure of the mucosa to the edges of the skin, and this is generally done by electrocautery.

Closure of the labial mucosal flap to the edges of the skin of the lower lip is performed in a single layer with non-absorbable suture material **(11).** Extreme care must be exercised for accurate approximation between the mucosal and the skin edges to restore a new mucocutaneous junction of the vermilion surface. Some trimming of the mucosa may be necessary at the two lateral edges of the surgical defect.

The entire vermilion border is thus restored with the mucosa of the lower lip. Finally, the skin closure at the site of the V excision is completed with interrupted, non-absorbable suture material **(12).** The mucosal defect created in the gingivolabial sulcus, intraorally, is left open to heal by secondary intention.

The surgical specimen in **(13)** shows complete stripping of the lower lip in conjunction with a V excision at the site of the infiltrating cancer—note full-thickness resection of the lip with complete excision of the vermilion border in areas of diffuse leukoplakia.

The postoperative appearance of the patient approximately 8 weeks following surgery is shown in **(14)**—note complete restoration of the normal configuration of the lips and commissure with the mouth closed. At the site of the V excision only a linear, vertical scar is noticeable.

On opening the mouth, the mucocutaneous suture line becomes apparent **(15).** The substance of the lower lip is preserved, and a satisfactory vermilion border is restored. Accurate approximation of the musculature of the lower lip prevents any notching at the site of repair of the V excision defect, and competency of the oral commissure has remained intact.

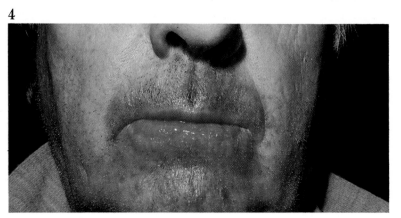

Extensive lip shave procedure for a superficial carcinoma of the lower lip

The patient shown in (1) presented with a hyperkeratotic superficially infiltrating squamous carcinoma involving nearly four-fifths of the vermilion border of the lower lip. On palpation, the lesion had no infiltrative component in the underlying musculature. An extensive lip shave procedure with resection of only a small amount of lip musculature was planned.

Surgical defect following a radical lip shave procedure encompassing the entire tumor is shown in (2). Adequacy of resection is confirmed by frozen section control from margins of the surgical defect.

Mucosa of the lower lip is advanced in the manner described above, and it is everted out for closure with the skin margin of the surgical defect (3). Interrupted non-absorbable suture material is used for approximation of the labial mucosa to the skin restoring the new vermilion surface.

The postoperative appearance of the patient approximately 1 month following surgery (4) shows the restored vermilion border with preservation of the substance of the lip, maintenance of the oral commissures and competency of the oral cavity. One disadvantage of an operation of this kind is that the lower lip shows a relatively wet and more pink color of the reconstructed, new vermilion border.

A V excision can be safely performed with satisfactory primary closure for tumors of the lower lip which require excision of up to one-third of the length of the lower lip. Although the size of the mouth is reduced, the functional and esthetic appearance is quite acceptable with this procedure. If, however, more radical resection requiring sacrifice of a larger portion of the lower lip is indicated, then V excision is not satisfactory.

Poor results can be expected with inadequate closure of the muscular layer of the lower lip, inaccurate approximation of the mucocutaneous junction of the vermilion border, and improper approximation of the edges of the mucosa and skin. If there is loss of tissue at the vermilion border due to superficial necrosis, then indentation and notching at the site of surgery results, a defect similar to that seen in patients with unsatisfactory repair of cleft lips.

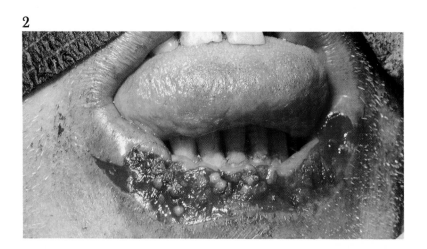

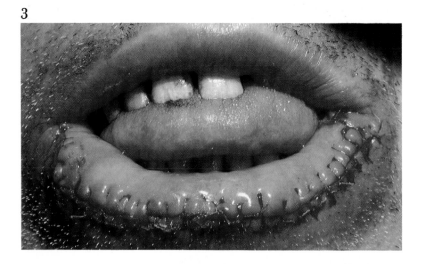

Abbe–Estlander flap repair

When more than 30% of the width of the lip is resected, reconstruction of the lip requires mobilization of a flap from the opposite lip (1). When approximately two-thirds of the lower lip has been excised, it can be reconstructed by borrowing tissue equivalent to half the surgical defect from the upper lip. The technique has been popularized by Abbe for reconstruction of the upper lip, and Estlander for the lower lip.

The patient illustrated for this operation (2) is an elderly gentleman with a deeply infiltrating squamous carcinoma of the lower lip involving the underlying musculature and the adjacent vermilion border warranting excision of nearly half the lower lip.

When the mouth is open, the lesion appears to be clear of the oral commissure on the right side, and therefore no specific measures are necessary for its restoration (3). Reconstruction of the oral commissure requires special attention and techniques described later in this chapter (pp. 75 and 76).

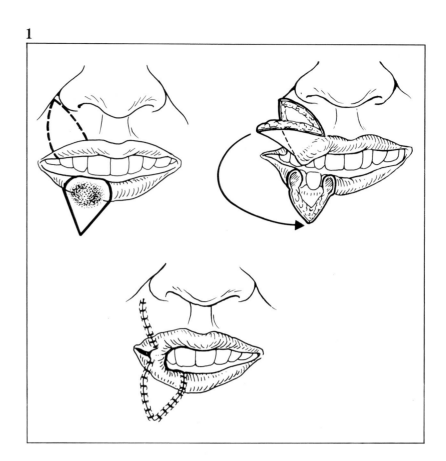

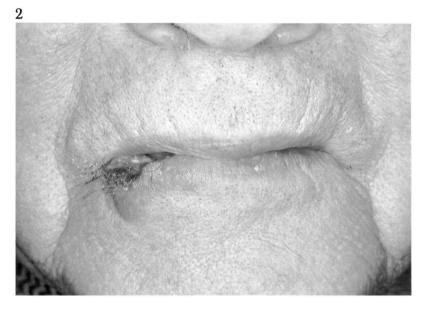

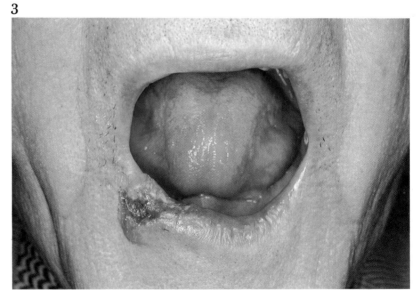

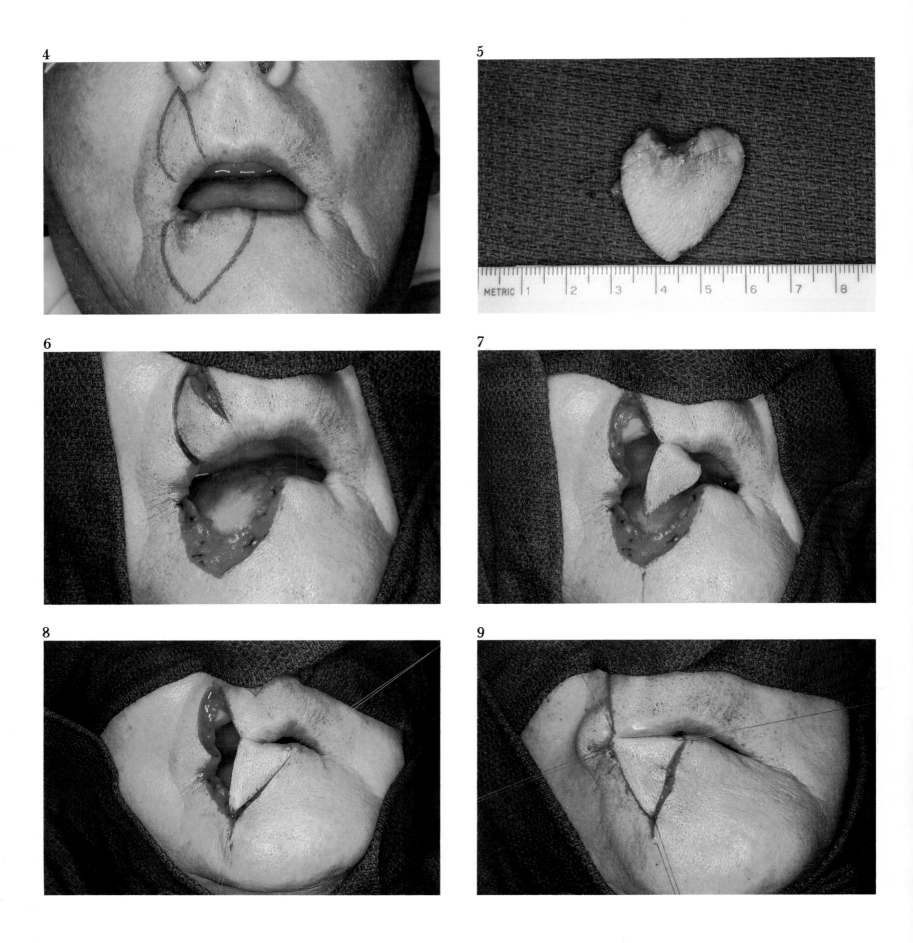

The proposed line of excision of the lower lip is marked out (4). Note that the long axis of the V excision is planned in such a fashion that a generous portion of the area of tumor involvement is excised while there is some sacrifice of the skin and the underlying musculature. A 1 cm margin at each end is desirable for deeply infiltrating tumors. A through-and-through excision is performed so that a triangular piece of mucosa, similar to the triangular piece of skin, is excised with the specimen. The principle of Abbe–Estlander flap repair is such that the width of its base is half that of the width of the base of the surgical defect. The flap is marked out on the upper lip on the same side, and can also be obtained from the opposite side of the upper lip if that is felt to be more appropriate. The long axis at the site of closure is kept along the radial skin lines around the oral cavity. Incision at the site of surgical excision is taken with a number 15 scalpel through both skin and mucosa. The remaining excision is completed using electrocautery, and a through-and-through wedge excision with the underlying musculature is made. Note that while the specimen is being mobilized it should not be grasped and pulled too hard, otherwise an undue amount of muscle of the lower lip would be excised due to stretch and pull, and this will lead to division of the muscle beyond the intended site of resection.

The surgical specimen (5) shows a through-and-through resection of the lower lip at the site of the tumor. The adequacy of surgical resection is confirmed by frozen section control from surgical defect margins.

Skin incision is now made at the previously marked outline of the Abbe–Estlander flap, on the lateral aspect carried through both the musculature of the upper lip and the mucosa extending from the vermilion border up to the apex of the flap (6). Mobilization of the medial margin of the flap, however, is done with extreme caution, care and delicacy, beginning at the apex of the flap working towards the vermilion border, in order to avoid any injury to the labial artery. As mobilization of the flap towards the vermilion border proceeds, it is desir-able to separate the musculature of the upper lip with a hemostat and divide small segments of the muscle fibers with scissors a little at a time. Once the labial artery is identified, the other attachments of the musculature of the upper lip around the labial artery are divided under direct vision still keeping the mucosa of the vermilion border intact. Thus, the contents of the pedicle of the flap would be the labial artery, its accompanying vein and the musculature between the artery and the vermilion border as well as the latter's mucosa. Labial mucosa on the medial aspect of the flap is also divided, from the apex of the flap up to the vermilion border.

The Abbe–Estlander flap, thus mobilized, derives its blood supply from the thin pedicle which remains attached to the upper lip (7). The flap is rotated 180° to fill the surgical defect in the lower lip. Setting and approximation of the flap into the defect of the lower lip begins by accurate approximation of the vermilion edges of the flap and the lower lip. Two fine nylon sutures are taken through the vermilion edges between the Abbe–Estlander flap and the surgical defect in the lower lip (8), held tight and retracted to allow accurate placement of the flap in the surgical defect. The muscular layer of the flap and the lower lip is now sutured together with interrupted 3-0 chromic catgut sutures. Extreme care must be exercised in placing the catgut suture between the right side of the edge of the flap and the musculature of the lower lip near the commissure of the mouth to avoid any injury to the pedicle of the flap and the labial artery.

Once the muscular layer is completed, closure of the donor site defect in the upper lip is undertaken first (9). The mucosal layer is closed with interrupted chromic catgut sutures followed by a muscular layer of interrupted 3-0 chromic catgut sutures. Accurate approximation of the vermilion border is not possible because of the still-attached pedicle of the flap. Skin closure is, however, completed in as accurate a manner as possible to avoid discrepancy between the commissure and the vermilion border of the upper lip.

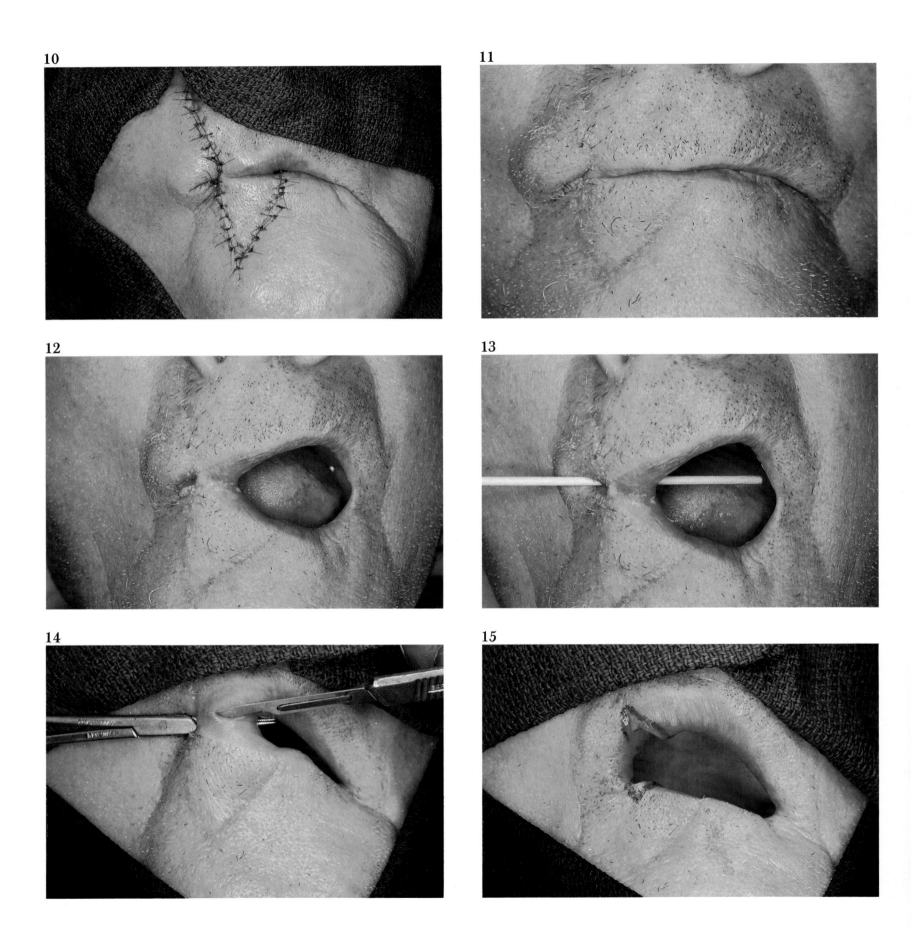

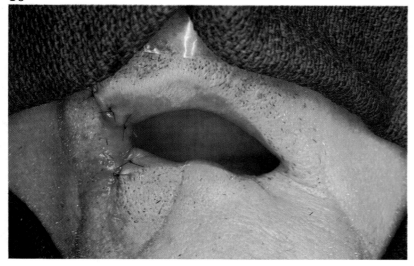

Skin sutures of 5-0 nylon are taken for closure of the skin incision of the upper lip as well as the lower lip **(10)**. Chromic catgut interrupted sutures are employed for closure of the mucosa of the flap and the labial mucosa of the lower lip. The flap thus remains attached to the upper lip through its pedicle leaving a bridged pedicle between the upper and the lower lips. The patient must be warned preoperatively about this bridge so that in the immediate postoperative period he does not inadvertently traumatize, disrupt or tear the pedicle of the flap. Because of the compromised size of the mouth, the patient has to resort to liquid foods and a blenderized diet due to inability to open the mouth completely. Skin sutures may be removed at approximately 1 week. In the immediate postoperative period, the flap may look bluish and dusky, usually due to venous congestion. However, as long as capillary filling is present, the flap will survive and remain viable in its entirety.

The postoperative appearance of the patient at approximately 3 weeks after surgery is shown in **(11)**. Note that the skin incision at the donor site in the upper lip has healed very well with almost an imperceptible scar. The flap is set well and has filled the defect very adequately restoring the continuity of the lower lip and the configuration of the mouth. On asking the patient to open the mouth, the bridged pedicle of the Abbe–Estlander flap becomes evident **(12)**—continuity of the mucosa of the vermilion border between the flap and the upper lip is demonstrated very vividly.

A wooden stick passed through the opening between the oral commissure and the bridge of the pedicle of the flap demonstrates the vascular pedicle derived from the upper lip **(13)**. In approximately 3 weeks' time, the circulation of the flap through neovascularization is satisfactory enough to allow division of the bridged pedicle. However, prior to undertaking the division, the vascularity of the flap must be checked by applying compression on the bridged pedicle with a hemostat or a rubber band. If the flap turns blue, then division of the pedicle should be delayed. Slight discoloration of the flap is to be expected on compression of the pedicle, but one must be able to confirm the presence of capillary blanching following this.

Division of the bridged pedicle is relatively simple, and can be done under either local or general anesthesia. A hemostat is passed through the lateral opening of the oral cavity and under the bridge **(14)**. A number 15 scalpel is taken, and direct transaction of the pedicle is performed releasing the upper lip from the attachment to the lower lip. The only bleeding in this maneuver is from the labial artery which is clamped and ligated.

Minor wedge excisions are performed to match and revise the raw areas at the site of the divided pedicle with appropriate primary closure of the resultant surgical defects **(15)**. Accurate approximation of the vermilion edges at both the upper and lower lip is vital for satisfactory esthetic reconstruction of the lips **(16)**. Although the size of the mouth is reduced to a certain extent, symmetry is maintained and excellent functional and esthetic reconstruction of the lip is provided by this flap.

When the oral commissure must be sacrificed along with excision of the lower lip tumor, then a non-bridged Estlander flap can be employed. This will, however, result in rounding of the commissure which will require a secondary repair to re-establish the configuration of the commissure and enlarge the opening of the oral orifice. This is performed in the manner described by Gillies. The Abbe–Estlander flap can be used in reverse when a lesion of the upper lip is excised, whereupon the flap is raised from the lower lip.

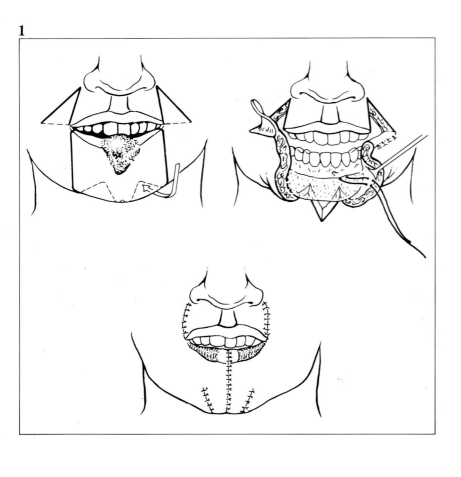

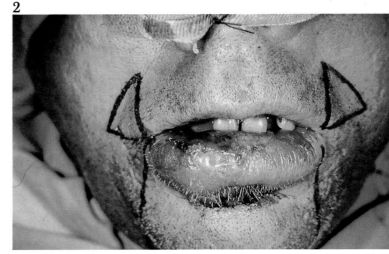

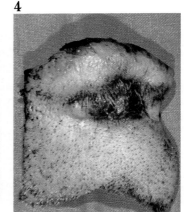

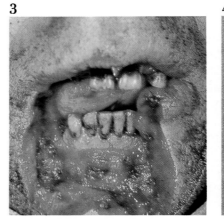

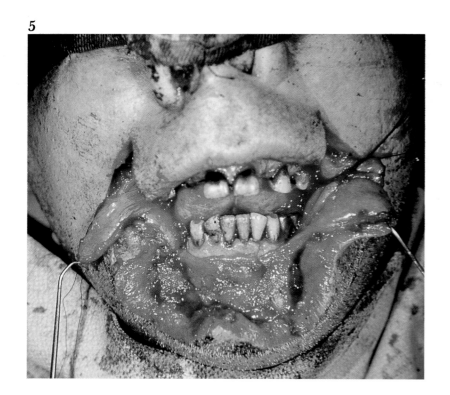

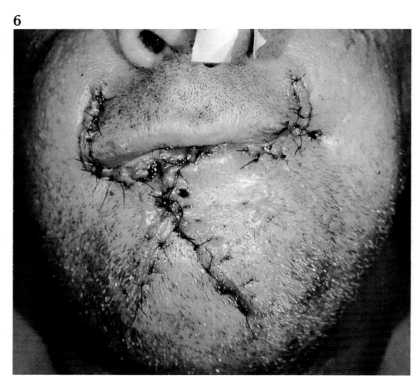

Note: pictures **2** to **8** courtesy of Elliot Strong, MD.

Bernard reconstruction of the lower lip

This operation is designed for tumors that are too extensive for either a simple V excision or reconstruction using an Abbe–Estlander flap **(1)**. The lower lip may be excised in its entirety along with soft tissues and skin of the chin, with the resulting defect closed by lateral cheek flaps to form a new lower lip. In order to set back the commissures and to prevent fish-mouth deformity, triangles of skin are excised from both sides of the upper lip, preserving the mucous membrane, to help form a new vermilion border. The distinct advantage of this operation is its ability to reconstruct nearly the whole lower lip in a single-stage procedure. An obvious disadvantage is reduction in the size of the orifice of the oral cavity and a 'permanent smile' deformity of the lips particularly in the edentulous patient.

The patient in this operative procedure has a large primary squamous cell carcinoma involving the entire thickness of the lower lip with extension to involve the skin and soft tissues of the upper part of the chin **(2)**. The area of excision is outlined along with the intended wedges of the skin to be excised from the upper lip near the nasolabial skin crease to facilitate advancement of the Bernard flaps for reconstruction of the lower lip.

The surgical defect shows a through-and-through resection of nearly seven-eighths of the lower lip **(3)**. Note that the surgical excision on the labial surface goes right up to the gingivolabial sulcus. A generous portion of the skin of the chin and the underlying soft tissues are also resected *en bloc* with the surgical specimen.

The surgical specimen in **(4)** shows the extent of resection around the primary tumor. When a significant portion of the skin of the chin is excised, it is important to plan the lower incision on the chin in such a way that the advancement flaps will allow satisfactory closure.

Generally, a triangular-shaped excision is preferred to facilitate closure. However, a variety of other surgical incisions are available including double triangles, etc. to aid reapproximation of the lateral cheek flaps and repair the chin.

Triangular wedges of the skin are now excised from the nasolabial crease on both sides **(5)**. The base of the triangle extends from the commissure of the mouth up to the nasolabial crease depending upon the width of the cheek flap to be mobilized medially. After excision of the triangular wedges of the skin in this way, the mucosa from the inner aspect of these triangular wedges is incised, and the triangular flaps of mucosa of the upper lip retrieved from these locations are shifted medially. Now an incision is made in the lower gingivolabial sulcus on both sides, and both cheek flaps are mobilized medially. In the center of the initial surgical defect, the apex of the triangular part of the skin of the chin is mobilized in the inferior part to provide a satisfactory closure, and closure of the musculature of the lip on both sides is performed with interrupted chromic catgut sutures. The triangular wedges of the mucosa from the upper lip are everted and rolled inferiorly to provide the new vermilion surface. Mucosal closure is completed inferiorly in the gingivolabial sulcus. The full-thickness wedges created in the upper lip at the commissure are closed in three layers on each side.

The immediate postoperative appearance of the patient shows completed closure with the reconstructed lower lip **(6)**. The postoperative appearance approximately 1 month after surgery shows the reconstructed lower lip with restoration of both the size of the oral orifice and the vermilion border **(7)**. A close-up of the oral orifice shows satisfactory restoration of the commissure with acceptable lining of the vermilion border of the lower lip **(8)**. Edentulous patients reconstructed in this fashion show a 'permanent smile' deformity of the lips.

7

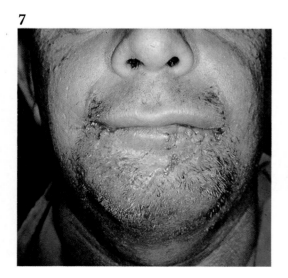

8

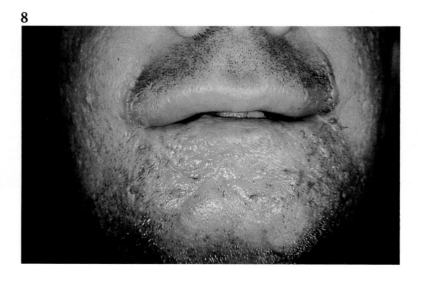

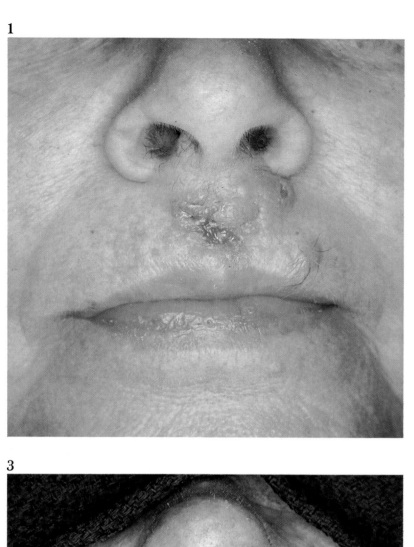

1

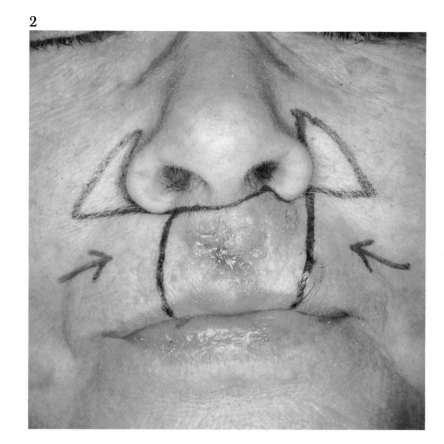

2

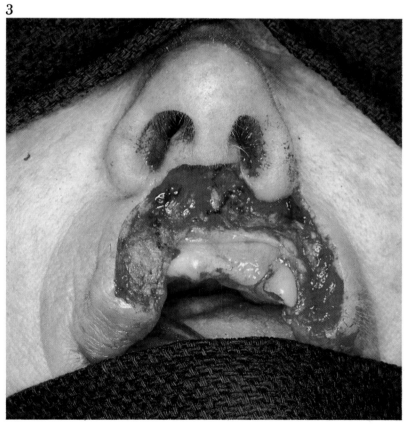

3

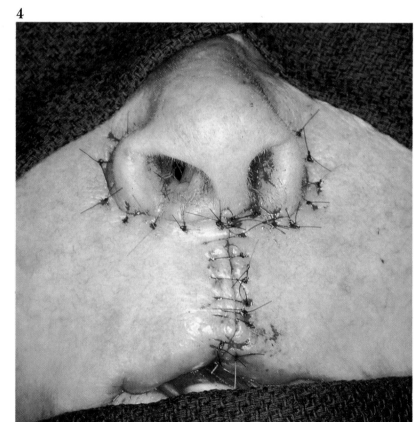

4

Burrows triangle repair of the upper lip

Full-thickness resection of the upper lip, up to one-third of its width, is easily amenable to repair by direct primary closure similar to the V excision of the lower lip. However, when a larger portion of the upper lip needs to be resected, the Burrows technique is very satisfactory for its reconstruction. The principle of surgical reconstruction is similar to the Bernard triangle repair. Triangular wedges of skin from the nasolabial crease are excised permitting lateral upper lip–cheek flaps to be mobilized medially for repair.

A patient with a primary infiltrating squamous cell carcinoma of the skin and vermilion border of the upper lip in the region of the philtrum is shown in (1). The tumor infiltrates the underlying musculature but does not perforate through the mucosa of the labial surface.

A plan of surgical excision outlined here (2) shows a through-and-through resection of the upper lip, with proposed triangular wedges of skin to be excised from the nasolabial crease adjacent to the nasal ala. The arrows indicate the extent of mobilization and medial shift of the residual upper lip on both sides showing the direction of pull.

The surgical defect following excision of the tumor (3) shows through-and-through resection of the upper lip,

leaving a large defect for repair. Note that the mucosal incision goes right up to the gingivolabial sulcus.

After excision of the triangular wedges of the skin, the lateral cheek flap and residual upper lip are mobilized medially, and a three-layered closure is performed using interrupted chromic catgut sutures for mucosa and muscles and 5-0 nylon for skin (4). If the triangular wedges are accurately placed along the side of the ala the scar of the triangular defects closure goes right along the groove of the ala and minimizes esthetic deformity. However, the size of the oral orifice is reduced and some tension on the upper lip is to be expected.

The postoperative appearance 3 months later (5) shows excellent healing and reconstruction of the upper lip, which is now distinctly smaller in length than before causing backward pull and recession in the edentulous patient. Note that the midline scar at the philtrum is well healed, so there is minimal esthetic deformity and an imperceptible scar along the nasal ala.

The same patient's appearance 8 months later following fabrication of an appropriate denture to push the upper lip out and restore the configuration of the lips is shown in (6). This is a very gratifying operation for resection of sizable tumors of the upper lip.

5

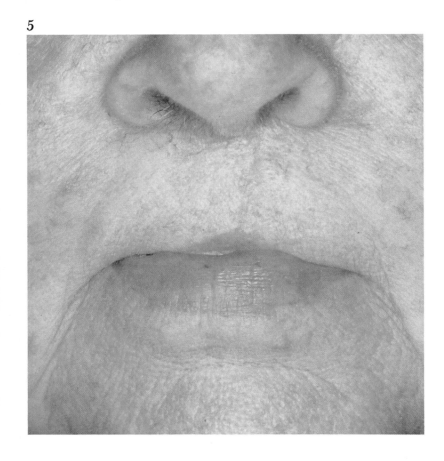

6

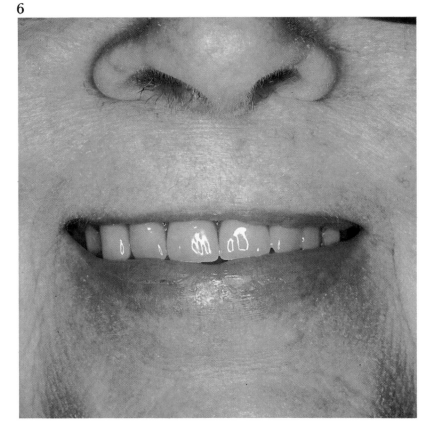

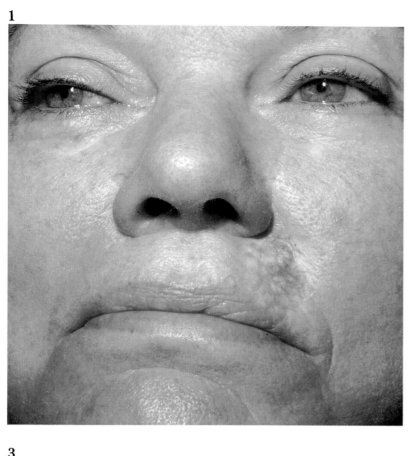

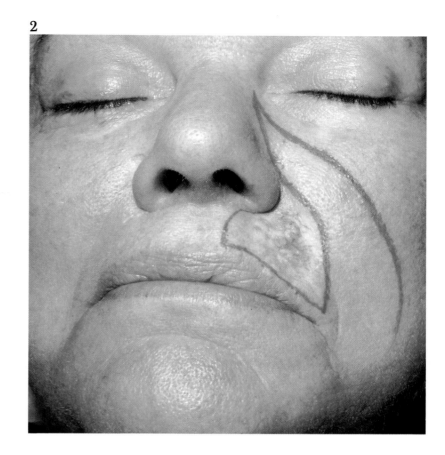

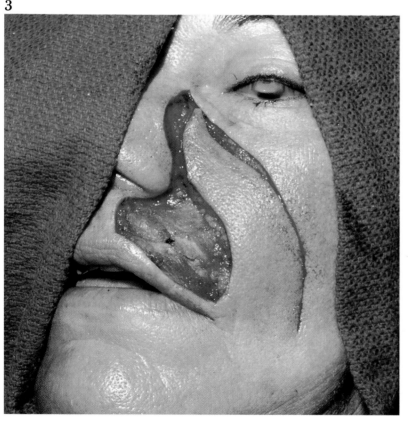

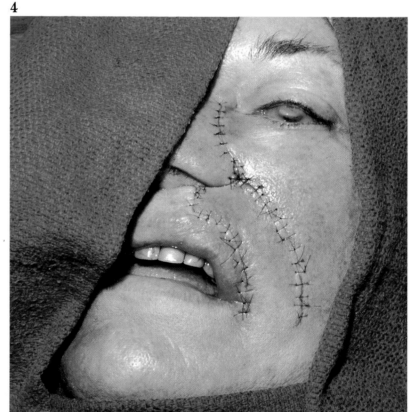

Nasolabial flap repair for the upper lip

Defects of the skin of the upper lip and those resulting from excision of the skin and underlying musculature are most amenable to reconstruction using an inferiorly based nasolabial flap. The latter is a highly reliable, axial skin flap which provides skin coverage and enough soft tissue replacement for the excised portion of the upper lip. However, one distinct disadvantage of this flap is that it does not restore muscular action of the upper lip, and thus there is functional deficit which persists although, esthetically, the defect can be safely closed. Thus, nasolabial flap repair would be unsatisfactory for full-thickness resection of upper lip defects.

The patient shown in (1) has a recurrent basal cell carcinoma of the skin of the upper lip on its lateral aspect. This lesion was previously electrodesiccated and curetted out prior to presentation for treatment. The lesion involves underlying soft tissues but does not infiltrate through the musculature of the upper lip. The inferior margin of the lesion approaches the vermilion border and, medially, the lesion reaches the alar groove.

The extent of surgical excision necessary for adequate removal of this tumor and intended outline for the nasolabial flap are shown in (2). The nasolabial flap is elevated longer than its anticipated length so that the re-

pair can be accomplished without tension and the donor site defect closed with little distortion of the facial features.

The surgical defect following excision of this lesion shows the musculature of the upper lip in the depth of the defect (3). The nasolabial flap has been elevated, and it will now be rotated inferiorly and medially to fill the surgical defect. It is important to trim the tip of the nasolabial flap so that it fits the surgical defect satisfactorily. The donor site defect is primarily closed by mobilization of the skin of the cheek. A two-layered closure is performed using 3-0 chromic catgut interrupted sutures for subcutaneous tissues and 5-0 nylon for skin.

The patient's appearance following closure of the skin incision on the operating table is shown in (4). Note that the upper lip appears to be everted and drawn upwards near the commissure on the left side.

The same patient's appearance approximately 1 year later (5) shows very gratifying result with the use of the nasolabial flap for repair of the skin defect of the upper lip. The donor site defect is barely perceptible and the contour of the lips and vermilion border appears essentially normal.

5

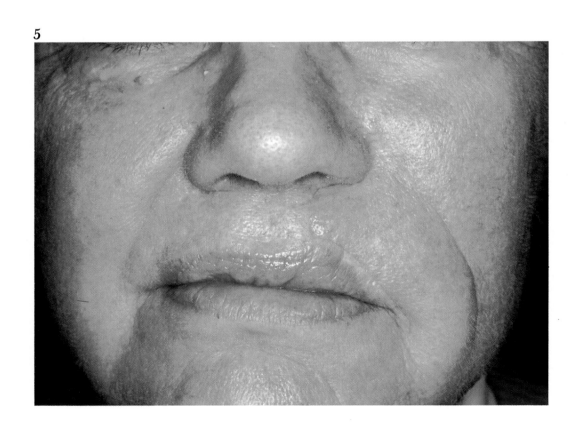

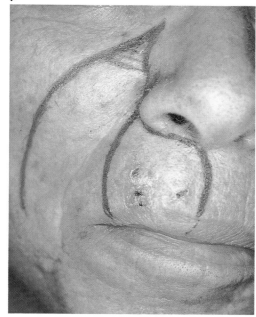

7

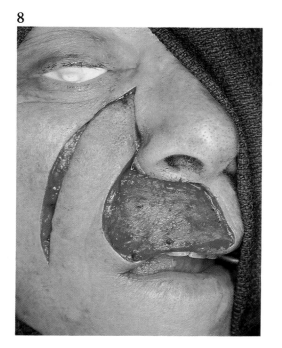

8

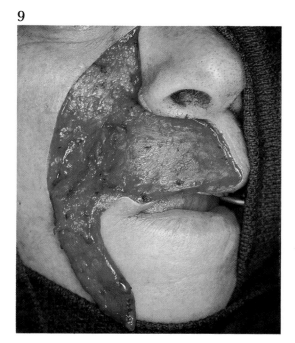

9

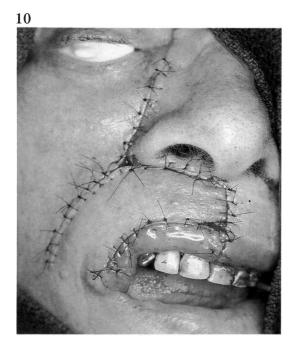

10

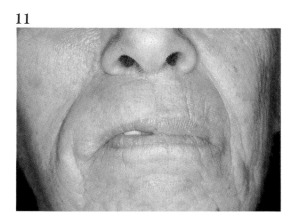

11

Another patient with a multifocal recurrent basal cell carcinoma involving the skin of the upper lip adjacent to the vermilion border is shown in **(6)**. The extent of surgical excision and the proposed outline of the naso-labial flap are marked out.

The surgical defect with excision of the skin of the upper lip exposing the underlying musculature with sac-rifice of the vermilion border to ensure adequacy of re-section is shown in **(7)**. The nasolabial flap should be elevated well up to the commissure so that when rotated it does not form kinking and a 'dog ear' deformity at the commissure of the mouth **(8)**.

In order to restore the vermilion border, the mucosa of the upper lip is released as a bipedicled flap by a transverse incision in the gingivolabial sulcus **(9)**. The labial mucosa is then elevated in a submucosal plane keeping it as a bipedicled flap, everted and rolled out to form the new vermilion border. The nasolabial flap is now rotated and sutured to this everted mucosa to re-store the new vermilion surface. Appropriate trimming of the tip of the skin flap is necessary so that it fits the surgical defect.

The same patient's appearance approximately 1 year later **(10)** shows satisfactory restoration of the upper lip and the vermilion mucosa. Although the latter is re-stored, it does not match the normal vermilion border of the upper lip on the left side. This is largely due to the following factors: the everted labial mucosa is pinker in color and is moister compared to the normal vermil-ion; it also lacks the direct muscular support necessary to maintain the normal substance and configuration of the vermilion border. Thus, if restoration of the vermil-ion is undertaken for only half the lip, a contrasting de-formity is bound to occur since the normal half of the lip is present for direct comparison.

Reconstruction of the oral commissure

Full-thickness resection of the cheek including the oral commissure presents a significant functional and esthetic deformity for the patient. A variety of reconstructive techniques are available for restoration of the full-thickness of the cheek, including: a folded forehead flap; a forehead flap with a skin graft; a forehead flap with tongue flap; and either a deltopectoral or pectoralis myoocutaneous flap with skin graft or any combination of the above. None of these reconstructive methods, however, restore the competency of the oral commissure, and drooling because of lack of competency of the oral cavity remains a problem. However, a modification of the Estlander flap, described by Converse as the 'over-and-out technique', can be used satisfactorily.

The patient shown in (1) had recurrent carcinoma of the cheek mucosa, which had previously failed radiation therapy. A through-and-through resection of the cheek including the oral commissure was performed, and the cheek was reconstructed using a folded forehead flap, which was then used to provide inner lining as well as

outer coverage. The patient's appearance approximately 3 months after forehead flap reconstruction shows restoration of the cheek and closure of the surgical defect, but lack of oral competency due to the absence of the oral commissure (1).

The proposed outlines for both the Abbe–Estlander flap as well as excision of the skin in the flap to create a space for insertion of the Estlander flap is shown in (2).

The Estlander flap is elevated in the usual fashion keeping its pedicle on the left side (3). The blood supply is derived from the superior labial artery. It is a full-thickness through-and-through flap providing skin coverage as well as mucosa and vermilion surface. The flap is rotated 180° demonstrating its very thin pedicle (4), and then further rotated 90° to a total rotation of 270° (5), and inserted in the space created between the two layers of the forehead flap by excising the skin edge as shown in (4). The Estlander flap is now sutured in two layers leaving a transient bridge between the upper lip

1

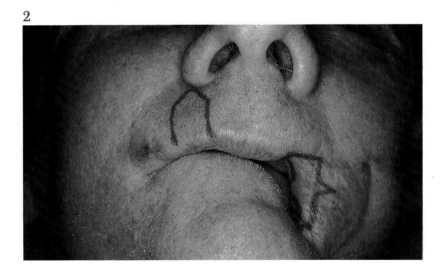

2

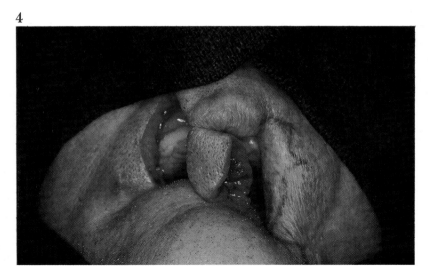

3

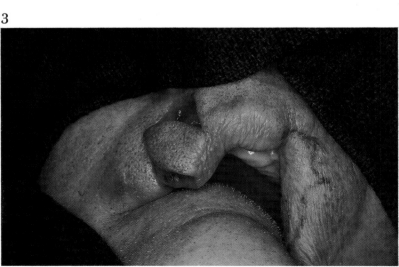

4

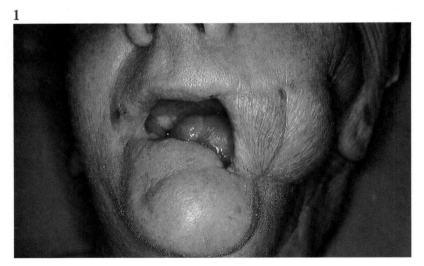

5

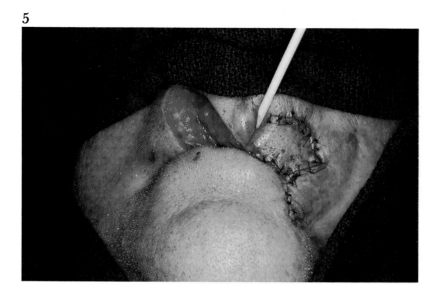

6

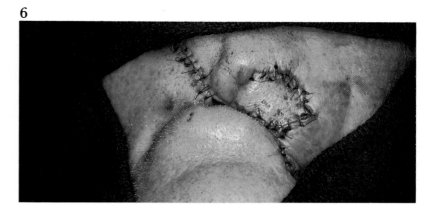

7

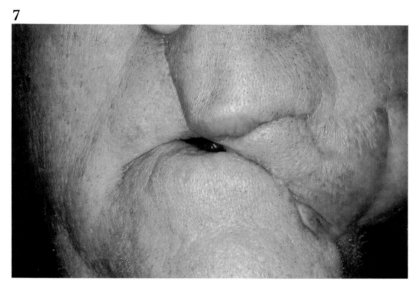

8

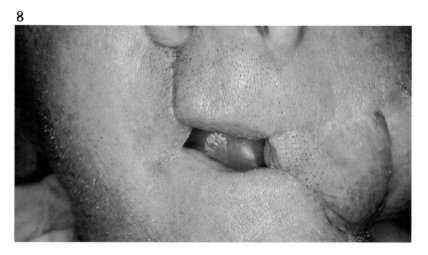

9

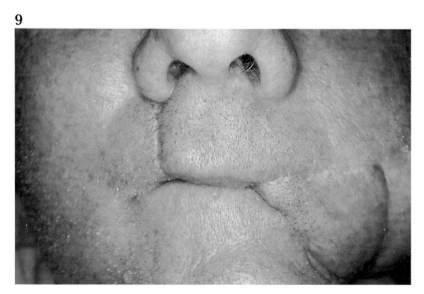

and the commissure on the left side. The surgical defect in the upper lip at the donor site of the Estlander flap is visible in (5). A wooden stick is inserted through the opening in the upper lip between the bridge of the Estlander flap and the reconstructed commissure demonstrating the pedicle of the flap.

The final closure of the surgical defect at the donor site demonstrates the immediate appearance of the patient on the operating table (6). The bridge of the pedicle divides the oral cavity into two separate openings.

The same patient's appearance approximately 3 weeks after this operative procedure shows the small bridged flap still attached through its pedicle to the upper lip (7). The pedicle of the flap is divided, and the configuration of the commissure is achieved by suturing the apex of the mucosa of the Estlander flap to the inner lining of the cheek, as in a V–Y plasty, pulling the mucosa and creating a horizontal crease in the pedicle.

Following completion of restoration of the commissure, the patient's appearance with the open oral cavity is shown giving acceptable size with complete competency of the reconstructed commissure (8).

The same patient is shown in (9) with the mouth closed giving an acceptable esthetic appearance with reconstruction of the commissure and restoration of full competency of the oral cavity.

5: The Scalp and Calvarium

Introduction

The scalp is a unique adaptation of the epithelial covering of the body. Anatomical variations present in the scalp modify both tumor behavior and the treatment of tumors in this area. The hair-bearing area of the scalp consists of a thick padding of hair follicles, sweat glands, fat, fibrous tissue and lymphatics that are interspersed with numerous arteries and veins (1). This thick padding is supported by a tough aponeurotic layer that is fused in the anterior region with the frontalis muscle, and in the posterior region with the occipital muscle. This inelastic layer rests loosely on the periosteum of the skull creating a potential subaponeurotic space. Laterally, the temporalis muscle provides an additional barrier between the galea and the periosteum.

Three principal arteries provide a rich blood supply to each side of the scalp. Two of these, the superficial temporal and occipital, are branches of the external carotid artery, while the supraorbital artery is a branch of the internal carotid artery. The lymphatic network of the scalp is also different in that there are no lymph barriers in the scalp, which contains many medium-caliber channels both subdermally and subcutaneously. The lymphatics drain towards the parotid gland, the preauricular area, the upper neck and the occipital region.

Surgical excision of scalp tumors thus depends largely upon the depth of infiltration. Excision through partial thickness of the scalp can be carried out for superficial tumors while excision through the entire thickness of the scalp including the periosteum may be necessary in deeply infiltrating tumors. On the other hand, tumors that are adherent to or involve the underlying cranium must have removal of the outer table of skull, or a through-and-through resection up to and often including the dura, if necessary. Hypothetical situations where the depth of infiltration of tumor is related to the type of surgical procedure that would be satisfactory for tumors of the scalp are shown in (2), (3), and (4).

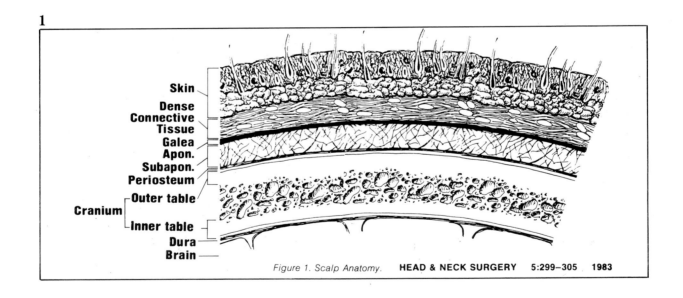

Figure 1. Scalp Anatomy.   **HEAD & NECK SURGERY   5:299–305   1983**

Note: Pictures **1** to **4** reproduced with permission from Lang, N.P. *et al "Head and Neck Surgery"* **5:**299-305, 1983.

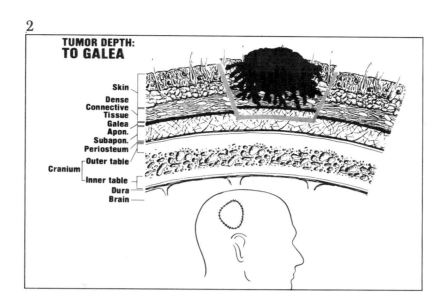

2

TUMOR DEPTH: TO GALEA

Skin
Dense Connective Tissue
Galea Apon.
Subapon.
Periosteum
Cranium — Outer table
Inner table
Dura
Brain

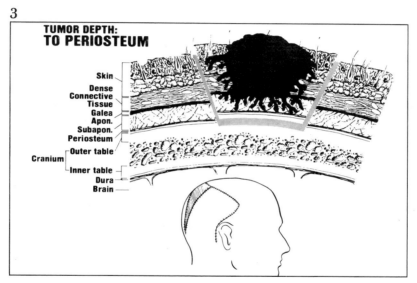

3

TUMOR DEPTH: TO PERIOSTEUM

Skin
Dense Connective Tissue
Galea Apon.
Subapon.
Periosteum
Cranium — Outer table
Inner table
Dura
Brain

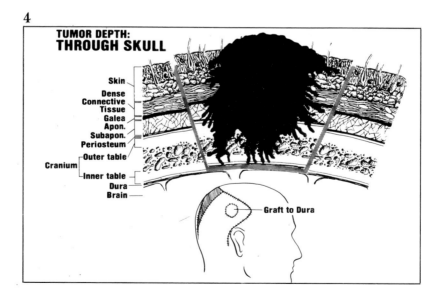

4

TUMOR DEPTH: THROUGH SKULL

Skin
Dense Connective Tissue
Galea Apon.
Subapon.
Periosteum
Cranium — Outer table
Inner table
Dura
Brain

Graft to Dura

78

Excision of scalp tumor and split-thickness skin graft

The patient presented in (1) shows a nodular pigmented basal cell carcinoma of the scalp measuring approximately 2.5 × 4.5 cm. in it's surface dimensions. This skin tumor is freely mobile over the underlying periosteum, so the galea aponeurotica will form the deep margin of the surgical specimen for this tumor.

Although most of the lesion is nodular and protuberant in nature, there is additional intracutaneous component which could only be seen after the scalp was shaved. The surgical procedure is performed under general endotracheal anesthesia. The scalp is shaved enough to expose the area of intended surgical excision (2). The planned area of surgical excision is outlined with a generous margin of normal skin around the visible tumor. Generally, a margin of at least a centimeter on each side of the lesion is desirable. The incision on the scalp is made with a number 15 scalpel. The incision is made obliquely so that the cut edge of the scalp is beveled, with the bevel sloping toward the center of the surgical defect (3). This maneuver is undertaken in order to facilitate subsequent healing of the skin graft and avoiding an indentation between the skin graft and the remaining scar. The incision in the scalp is made circumferentially with a sharp knife, and the rest of the elevation of the specimen and dissection is performed using electrocautery (4). Brisk hemorrhage due to the rich blood supply of the scalp is to be anticipated from the cut edges, but with use of suction with a Frazier suction tip and prompt use of several clamps will minimize blood loss. Major bleeding vessels will need a suture ligature, while fine bleeding points can be safely electrocoagulated. Once the proper plane between the

1

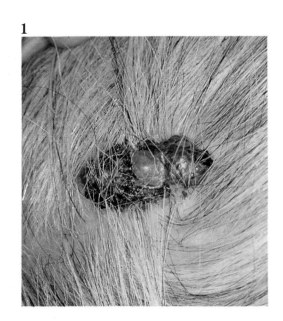

2

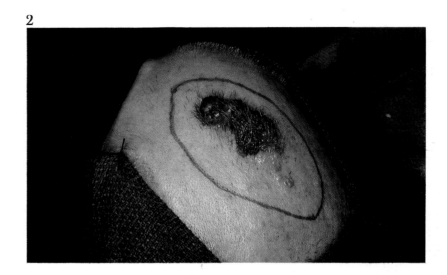

3

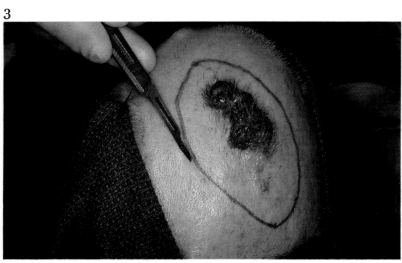

4

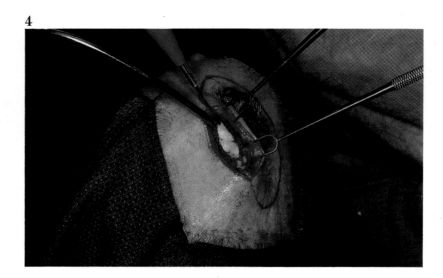

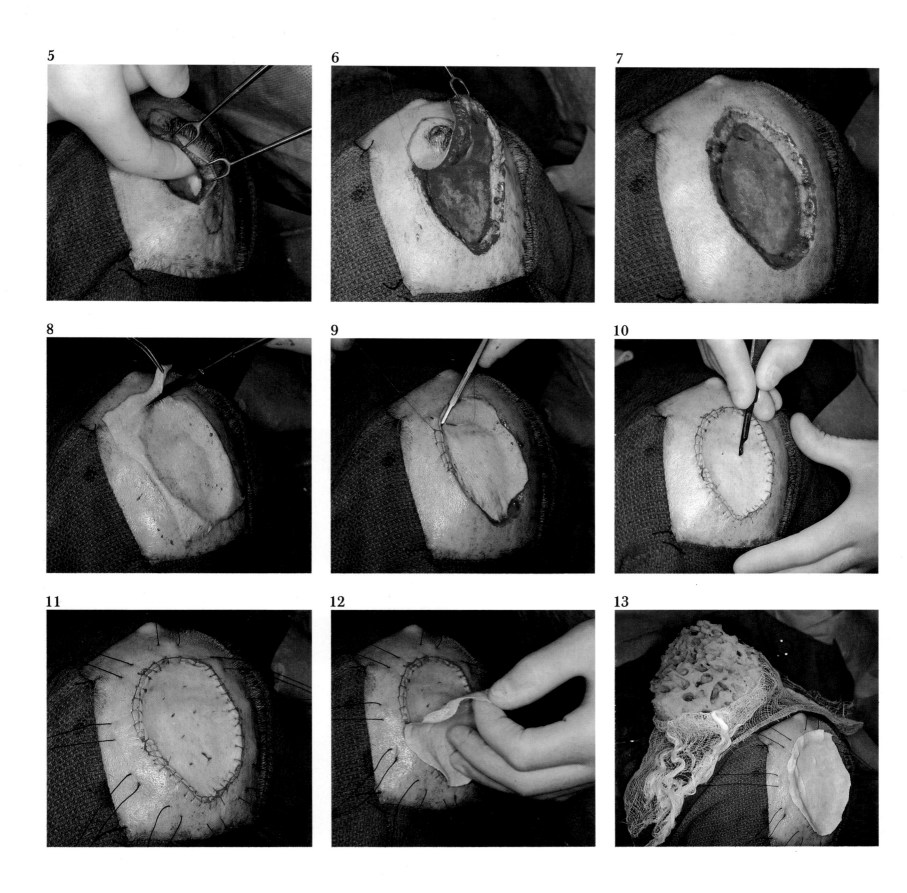

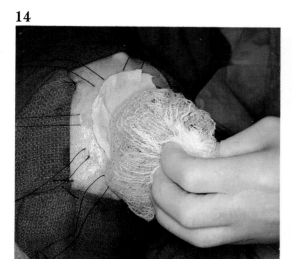
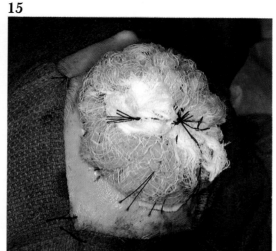
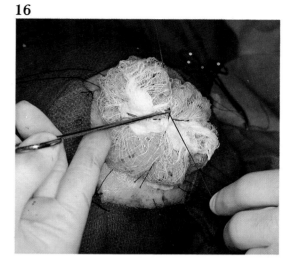

galea aponeurotica and the periosteum of the skull is reached, elevation of the surgical specimen becomes very simple, as the plane consists of loose areolar tissue (**5**). This mobilization is best accomplished digitally. Once the undersurface of the surgical specimen is completely mobilized, remaining circumferential incision is completed through its full thickness (**6**), and the surgical specimen is removed.

Complete hemostasis is secured by ligating, suture ligating, or electrocoagulating the bleeding points from the cut edges of the scalp. The surgical defect is shown in (**7**). The depth of the surgical defect shows periosteum of the scalp, which will be the bed to receive a split-thickness skin graft. Previously harvested split-thickness skin graft is now brought into the field and laid over the surgical defect. A fairly thick split-thickness skin graft (1/18000″) is desirable to avoid ulceration and trauma on the scalp. Thin split-thickness skin grafts give a very tight and shiny appearance and are prone to frequent ulceration. The skin graft is appropriately positioned and excess is trimmed off (**8**). The skin graft is sutured to the edges of the surgical defect using continuous interlocking absorbable suture material (**9**).

Continuous interlocking sutures provide hemostasis, and secure the graft in proper position. Several buttonholes are made with a number 15 scalpel in the center of the graft to provide for drainage of serous material from beneath the graft. This maneuver is often called "pie crusting" (**10**). The skin graft is further secured tightly and apposed against the periosteum using xeroform gauze and a pressure dressing with a sea sponge bolster secured with silk sutures taken on the scalp at the periphery of the surgical defect (**11**). A layer of xeroform gauze is applied to the skin graft (**12**). A sea sponge is now trimmed to the required size and is wrapped in a 4×8″ gauze piece (**13**). The assembly of sea sponge wrapped in gauze is now placed over the xeroform gauze dressing and is properly positioned to exert even pressure to all areas of the skin graft (**14**). The silk sutures taken at the periphery of the surgical defect are now tied over the bolster of sea sponge (**15**).

The dressing is now completely secured in position providing adequate and even pressure over the skin graft, which remains apposed to the periosteum of the skull (**16**). This dressing is left in position for one week, at which point the pressure dressing is removed.

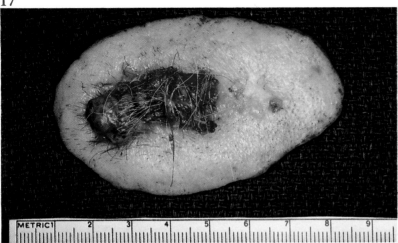

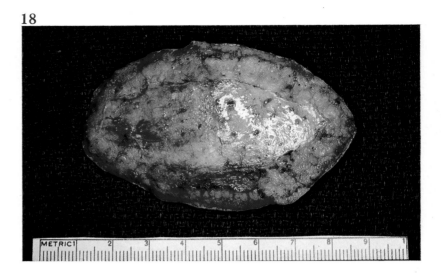

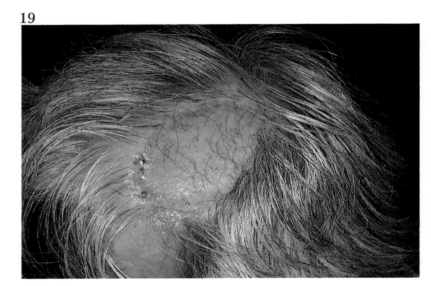

17

Surgical specimen of the excised tumor shows a generous portion of normal skin around the tumor, and the deep surface of the specimen shows galea aponeurotica which is grossly uninvolved by tumor (**17** and **18**).

When the bolster dressing is removed, trimming of crust and clots at the edges of the surgical defect is necessary to keep it clean until full maturation of the grafted area takes place. Patient should be instructed in avoiding direct trauma or injury to this area.

The post-operative appearance of the patient approximately three months following surgery shows 100% take of the skin graft at the site of the surgical excision (**19**). Split-thickness skin graft in the hair bearing area of the scalp is a very satisfactory procedure for immediate coverage of the surgical defect resulting from excision of tumor where the periosteum can be preserved.

Excision of scalp tumor with advancement rotation flap

Surgical excision of tumors in the non-hair-bearing areas of the scalp requires coverage of the surgical defect with tissues that resemble the normal tissues in the area for a satisfactory esthetic appearance. Although split-thickness skin graft can be used to cover such surgical defects, its esthetic appearance is unacceptable. Advancement rotation scalp flaps provide a very satisfactory method of closure of medium-size surgical defects. The defect is covered with the adjacent scalp while the donor site deformity is transferred posteriorly in the hair-bearing area of the scalp which may be either closed primarily or, on occasion, be covered with a split-thickness skin graft.

When surgical excision of a scalp tumor requires excision of the underlying periosteum, then bare bones of the calvarium are exposed. Scalp flaps are the ideal method of coverage of such surgical defects.

The patient shown in (1) had recurrent basal cell carcinoma involving the forehead and the hairline area of the scalp on the left side. The intended extent of surgical excision and the outline of the rotation advancement flap are shown. Even though the anticipated surgical defect is relatively small, a large area of the scalp has to be elevated because of its inelasticity to provide sufficient mobilization and coverage. The blood supply of this scalp flap is through both the superficial temporal as well as the occipital artery. The flap is advanced anteriorly and rotated inferiorly to cover the surgical defect. Meticulous attention should be paid in the outline of the flap by appropriate measuring of the surgical defect and the rotated scalp flap, keeping the pivot point in mind. Ideally, a 4 × 8 gauze piece is taken, one end being held at the pivot near the external ear and the other brought up to the apex of the surgical defect inferomedially. Using that length as a radius, the scalp flap is outlined all the way up to the occiput, and posteriorly it is cut from the posterior edge of the incision anteriorly towards the pivot point. Thus, if proper measurements are taken, the flap will satisfactorily rotate and cover the surgical defect. The skin tumor is excised in the usual fashion through full thickness of the scalp (2). The scalp flap is now elevated through the subgaleal plane. There will be brisk hemorrhage from the cut edges of the scalp, which should be promptly controlled. Elevation of the flap through the subgaleal plane remaining superficial to the periosteum is very easy; then complete hemostasis is obtained by suture ligating or electrocoagulating the bleeders from the cut edges on both sides.

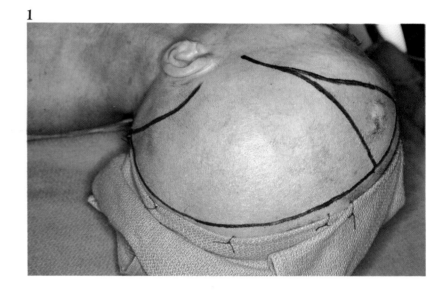

1

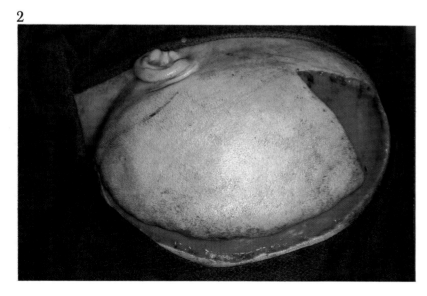

2

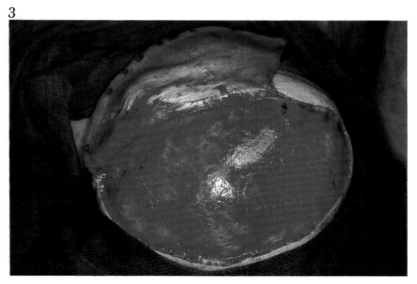

3

4

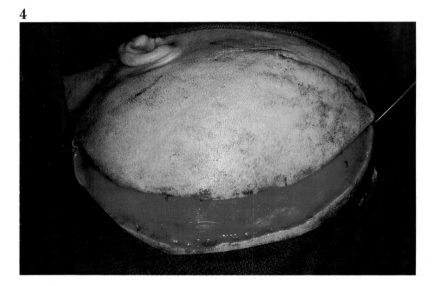

5

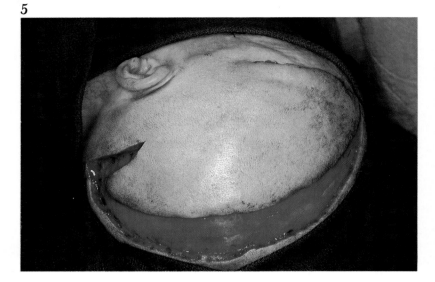

6

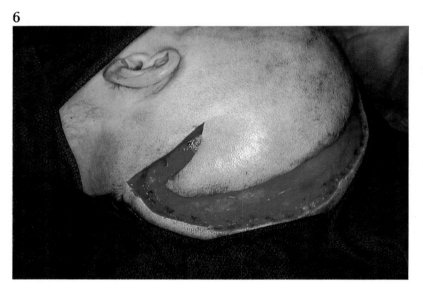

7

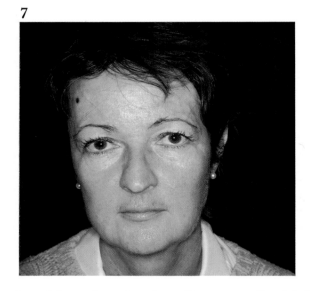

The flap in **(3)** is reflected downwards showing its proximal mobilization up to the vascular pedicle near the pinna. Meticulous attention should be paid to preserve the feeding vessels carefully—that is, the superficial temporal artery and the posterior auricular artery, a branch of the occipital artery. The periosteum of the entire scalp is kept intact. The flap is now rotated both anteriorly and inferiorly to cover the surgical defect **(4)**. The anterior end of the scalp flap should be adequate to match the lower border of the surgical defect. Closure is performed first with 3-0 chromic catgut interrupted subcutaneous sutures. Once the lower border of the surgical defect is completely closed, the rest of the scalp on the right side is mobilized, and appropriate spacing sutures placed to match the convex medial edge of the scalp flap to the concave edge of the remaining scalp. These sutures are bound to be under some tension, but the scalp is vascular enough to handle this with little difficulty.

The posterior edge of this rotated scalp flap will now leave a donor site defect in the occipital scalp that can be either closed primarily or a split-thickness skin graft applied **(5, 6)**. Most surgical defects of this nature and size are easily closed in a V–Y way. A suction drain is placed beneath the scalp flap and is brought out through a separate stab incision. Pressure dressings are applied over the entire head. Minimal drainage is to anticipated and the drainage tube can be removed in approximately 48–72 hours. Sutures from the scalp are left for approximately 10 days and then removed in several stages to avoid disruption of the wound which may have been closed under tension.

The postoperative appearance of the patient approximately 8 months following surgery is shown in **(7)**. There is excellent restoration of the surgical defect near the hairline without any significant functional or esthetic deformity.

Advancement rotation scalp flaps are very satisfactory for most defects of the anterior scalp. However, if these defects are of significant size, then primary closure of the donor site is not possible and a split-thickness skin graft would be necessary in the occipital region.

En bloc resection for tumor of the scalp and cranium

Tumors of the scalp which involve the entire thickness of the scalp with extension to the cranium require a through-and-through resection often including the underlying dura. Primary tumors of the scalp, and primary or metastatic tumors of the cranium, warrant this type of surgical resection.

The radiographs of the patient presented here show a lytic lesion involving the cranial vault in the parieto-oc-cipital region on the right side (1). This lesion, on needle aspiration biopsy, confirmed the diagnosis of a metastatic renal cell carcinoma (2). The tumor was adherent to the overlying scalp and had invaded the underlying dura. CT scans of the patient clearly demonstrate the extent of the lesion involving the overlying scalp and with extension through the cranium to involve the underlying dura (3) and (4). This was a solitary metastasis.

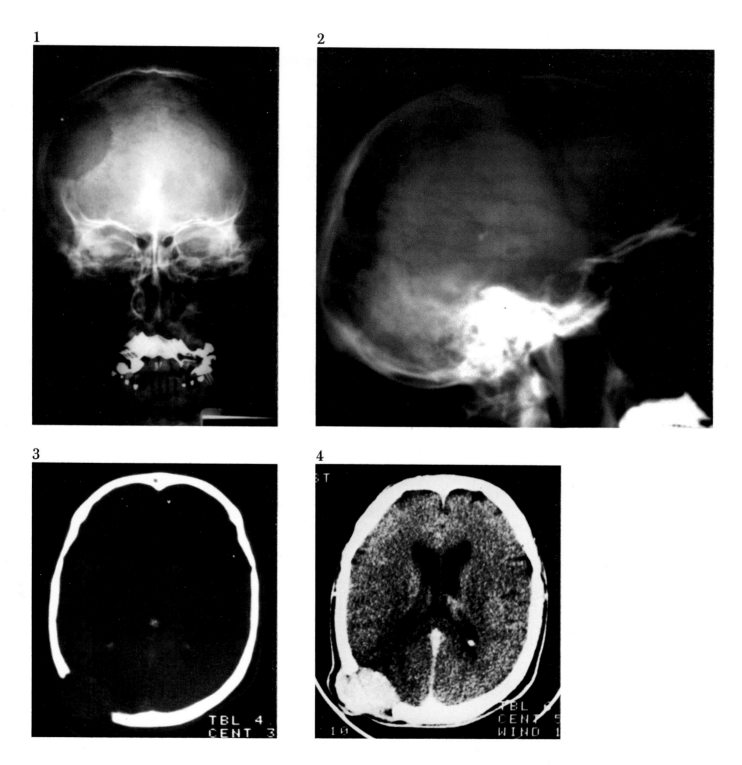

5

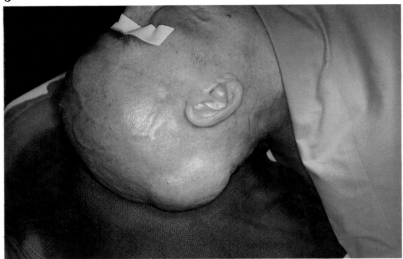

6

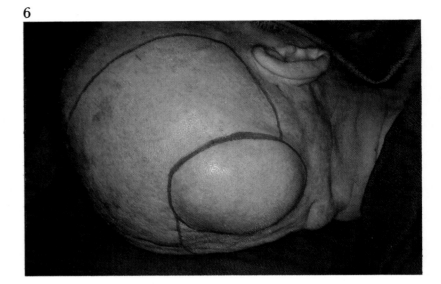

7

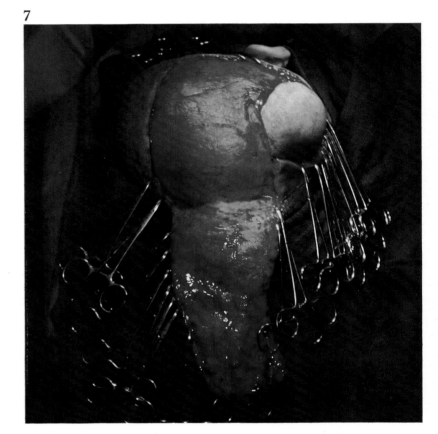

The patient is placed under general endotracheal anesthesia in the supine position on the operating table with the head resting on the left parietal region on a standard U-shaped head-rest (5). After shaving the entire scalp, the gross dimensions of the lesion become clearly apparent. An indwelling spinal catheter is placed to both monitor cerebrospinal fluid pressure and facilitate withdrawal of cerebrospinal fluid to slacken the brain if necessary.

The incisions are outlined on the scalp. The extent of scalp that would have to be sacrificed with resection of the tumor is shown in (6). A parietal scalp flap is outlined, which would be based on the left side with the entire scalp elevated from the pinna of the ear on the right side up to that on the left side. The vascular supply of this flap is derived from the superficial temporal and occipital arteries of the left side. The scalp flap is elevated first in a subgaleal plane remaining superficial to the periosteum of the skull, all the way on the left side up to the pinna of the ear and the mastoid process (7). The periosteum on the skull is preserved for subsequent use. A circumferential incision is now made through the periosteum remaining at least 1½–2 cm away from the edges of the scalp to be sacrificed with the specimen. The skull is now exposed subperiosteally in a circumferential way around the tumor (8). Multiple burr holes are now made, and with a craniotome a circumferential craniectomy is completed around the gross tumor. The plane of dissection is still extradural. Care and caution must be exercised during the making of burr holes to stay well away from gross tumor in order to avoid compromising the adequacy of resection. Using a dural dissector, an attempt is made to elevate the dura from the undersurface of the parietal bone, but this is not possible, the dura being adherent to and involved by the tumor.

As shown in (9), the dura is entered by making an incision with a sharp knife. Using sharp scissors, the dura is incised circumferentially around the tumor to facilitate a monobloc resection, and the surgical specimen becomes more mobile allowing external rotation to further facilitate exposure of the remaining dural attachments and division.

The surgical specimen is now reflected posteriorly with the dura attached to the tumor and exposing the underlying brain (10). During this phase of the operation, it is necessary to withdraw approximately 30 to 40 cc's of cerebrospinal fluid to slacken the brain and prevent unnecessary cerebrospinal fluid leakage. Bleeding from dural vessels is easily controlled with a bipolar cautery.

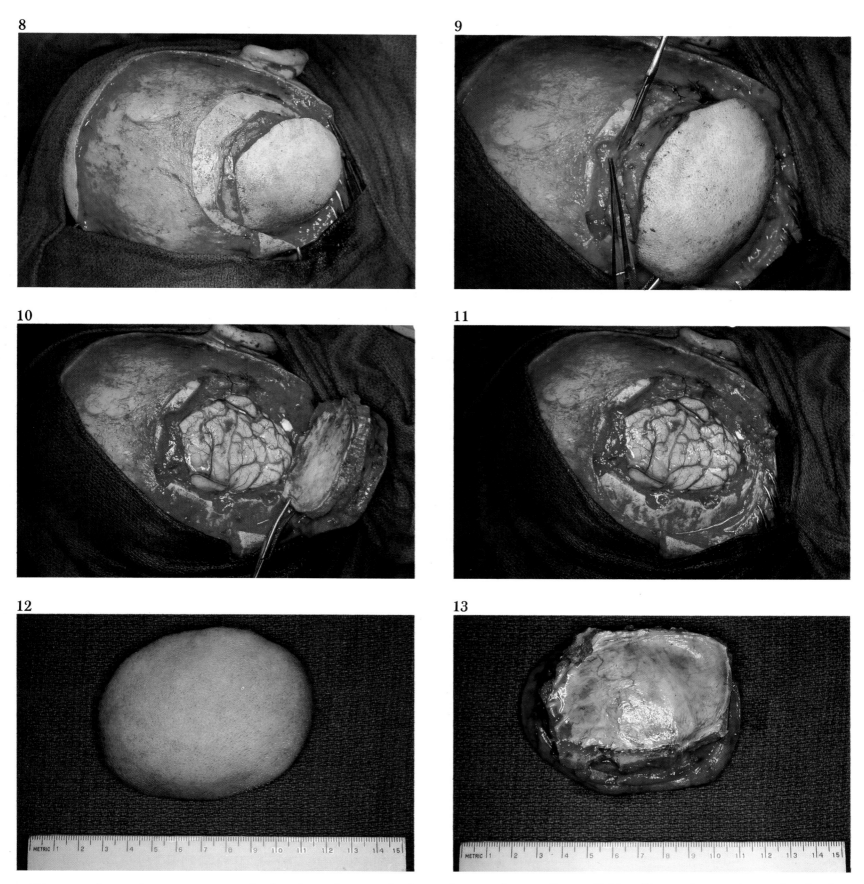

8

9

10

11

12

13

The specimen is now removed showing the surgical defect (11–13). The brain is exposed because the dura was sacrificed with the craniectomy in a monobloc way to resect the tumor. Complete hemostasis at this point is mandatory from all bleeding points prior to beginning of closure of the dural defect. Bleeding from the edges of the craniectomy defect is controlled using bone wax.

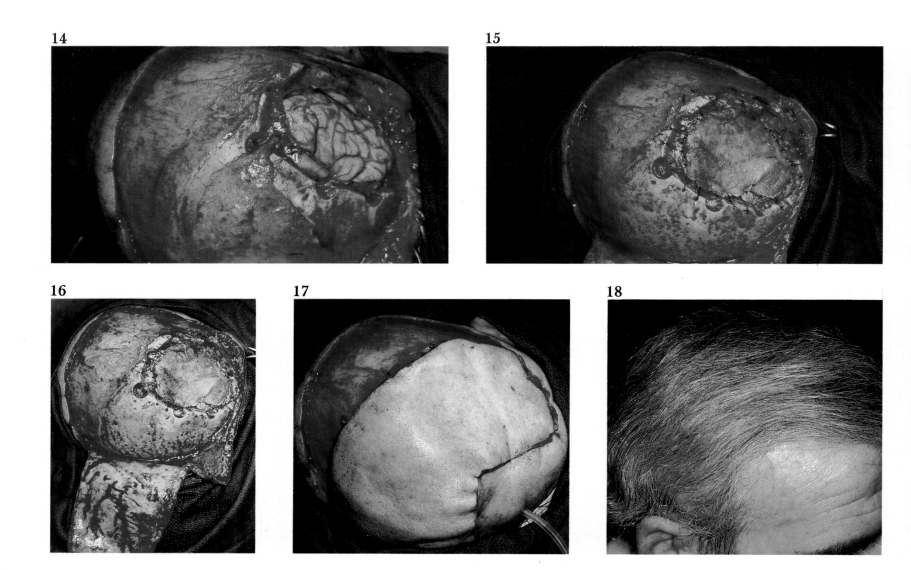

The previously elevated scalp flap is now elevated further posteriorly to expose the left occipital region (14), exposing the periosteum covering the skull in the occipital region on the left side. A generous portion is now available for use as a free graft for repair of the dural defect. No attempt is made to remove the periosteum from the right parietal region since it will be necessary to support the skin graft. Sufficient periosteal graft should be obtained to fill the dural defect, and the graft is sutured to the edges of the dura with number 4-0 neurolon sutures (15). A watertight closure must be obtained to prevent cerebrospinal fluid leakage. Previously withdrawn cerebrospinal fluid is now reintroduced slowly.

After satisfactory coverage of the dural defect, the sharp edges of the craniectomy defect are smoothed out (16). The previously elevated scalp flap is now rotated posteriorly to cover the craniectomy defect. Closure of the scalp edges is performed in two layers using interrupted chromic catgut subcutaneous sutures and 3-0 nylon sutures for the skin. The donor site defect in the scalp of the right parietal region still has its periosteum intact (17). Split-thickness skin graft harvested from the thigh is now applied to the exposed periosteum. The skin graft is secured with continuous, absorbable sutures to the edge of the scalp, and retained in position with a sea sponge bolster dressing. A suction drainage is placed beneath the rotated scalp flap. Appropriate dressings are applied and patient is transferred to the recovery room following withdrawal of the lumbar puncture catheter. Pressure dressing on the skin graft is retained for 1 week when it is removed together with sutures from the scalp.

The postoperative appearance of the patient approximately 9 months after surgery (18) shows satisfactory restoration of the scalp defect. Although there is no bony support at the site of the craniectomy, the defect is covered with full-thickness scalp while the split-thickness skin graft covers the donor site. This kind of rotated scalp flap provides a very satisfactory coverage for craniectomy defects following resection of primary or metastatic tumors of the calvarium.

Excision of carcinoma of the temple with craniectomy and orbital exenteration

Tumors of the scalp and the skin of the forehead which involve the underlying bone and extend to the orbit require *en bloc* resection including exenteration of the orbit if the tumor extends into the orbit to displace and/or involve the globe.

The patient shown here (1) has recurrent squamous cell carcinoma which was treated initially by wide excision and split-thickness skin graft. Local recurrence at the margin of the previous surgical excision was treated by external irradiation with failure to control the tumor. At the time of presentation and treatment, he had diplopia secondary to displacement of the globe medially and inferiorly; he was also in constant pain, and had a fungating, foul-smelling ulceration.

Computerized transaxial tomography through the orbits show the presence of recurrent tumor invading the superolateral wall of the orbit, with extension of tumor into the orbit to involve the orbital process of the frontal bone (2, 3). The tumor was fixed to the underlying frontal bone, but there was no demonstrable extension of it intracranially.

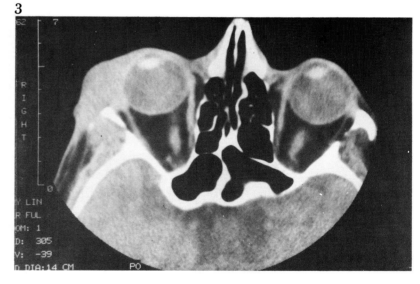

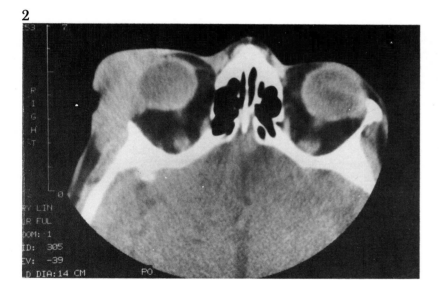

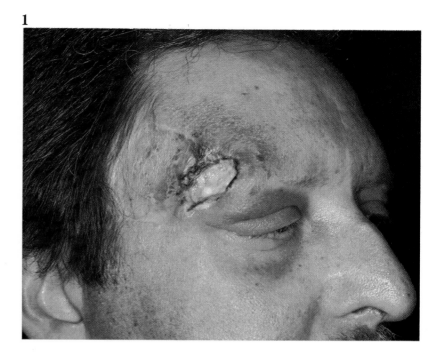

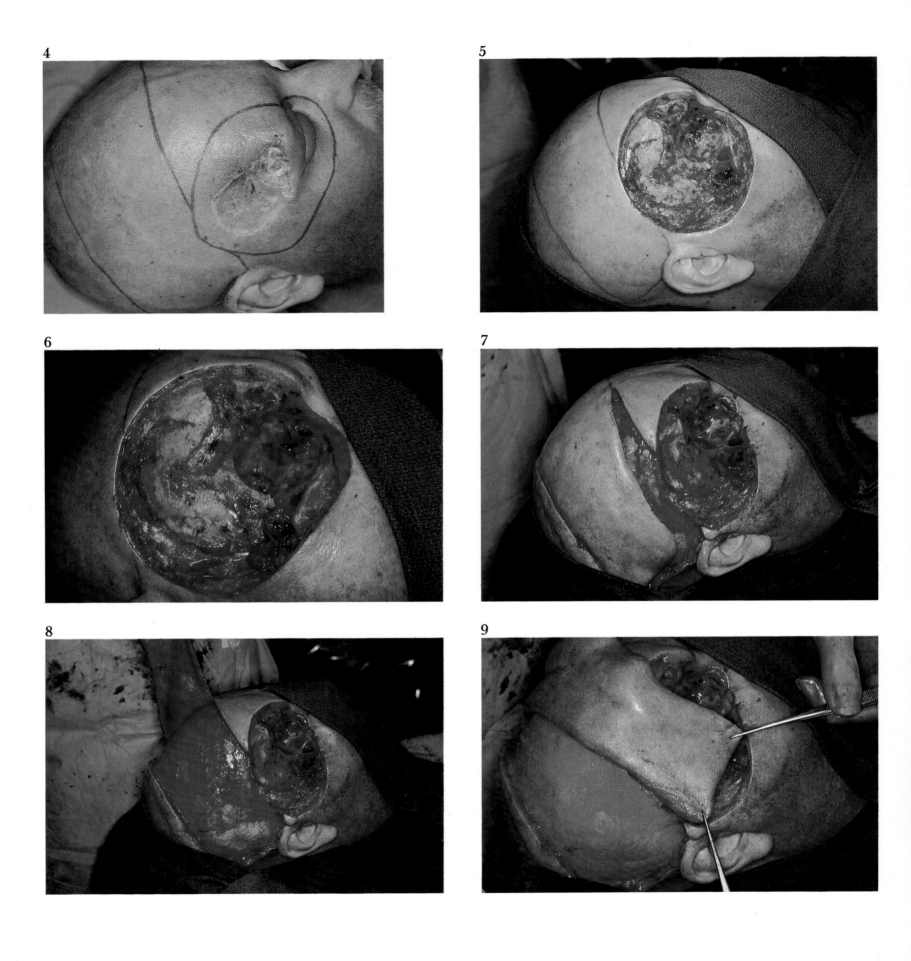

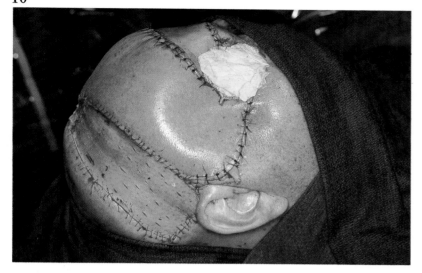

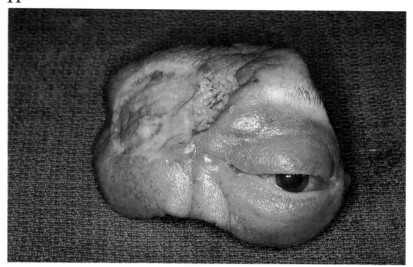

The proposed plan of surgical excision and repair using a scalp flap is outlined here (4). The surgical excision would be taken through and through with underlying frontal bone and the contents of the orbit. The scalp flap is based on the superficial temporal and occipital vessels of the left side; on the right side, the flap extends to the upper part of the pinna and well into the occipitoparietal region.

The surgical excision required full-thickness resection of the scalp with excision of the underlying frontal bone as the deep margin of the surgical specimen (5). The dura on the undersurface of the frontal bone was easily dissected away from the bone since it was not involved, and the entire dissection remained extradural. Multiple burr holes are made with the craniotome. With appropriate dural dissectors, the dura is very carefully dissected free from the undersurface of the frontal bone at the site of the burr holes. A guide strip for the gigli saw is then passed from one burr hole to the other to protect the dura. The saw is passed then through two burr holes, dividing the intervening bone, a maneuver continued circumferentially around the proposed site of excision. Once this is accomplished, the dural dissectors are used to separate the dura attached to the undersurface of the frontal bone. Again this dissection is very meticulously and slowly performed to avoid entry into or unnecessary tears in the dura. The entire excision of the frontal bone is performed extradurally without any leakage of cerebrospinal fluid.

Exenteration of the orbit is performed in a subperiosteal plane. In this patient, the orbit was entered from the roof, but the periosteum of the orbit was kept intact. A periosteal elevator is used to lift the orbital periosteum in its medial half. No attempt is made to disturb the periosteum of the orbit in its upper outer quadrant in the vicinity of the tumor where it is kept in continuity *en bloc* with the surgical specimen. The orbital process of

the zygomatic bone is divided next, followed by the zygomatic process. Then a heavy Mixter clamp is used to clamp the extraocular muscles, the optic nerve with its central retinal artery at the apex of the orbit, and these are transected using heavy Mayo scissors. The rest of the specimen attached through the lateral wall of the orbit is then divided using a small osteotome and heavy Mayo scissors. The surgical defect is shown here (5) following complete monobloc excision of the tumor.

Closeup of the surgical defect (6) shows the exposed dura, the transected edges of the frontal bone, and the cut edge of the orbital process of the zygomatic bone, the ethmoid air cells in the medial aspect of the orbit, and the temporalis muscle seen in the upper part of the surgical defect where it was transected to remove the specimen. Complete hemostasis is obtained by ligating and/or coagulating the bleeding points as they are encountered. The stumps of the extraocular muscles and optic nerve are suture-ligated with 2-0 chromic catgut suture.

The scalp flap is now elevated in the usual fashion in the subgaleal plane (7). The scalp flap is elevated all the way to the left side carefully preserving the periosteum over the cranium (8). Basically, the purpose of this flap is to protect the exposed dura and provide support to it where the frontal bone is resected. The flap is now rotated both anteriorly and inferiorly to provide coverage for the roof of the orbit which has been excised *in toto* (9). The medial wall of the orbit is covered with a split-thickness skin graft which is retained in position with xeroform packing. The scalp flap is sutured to the rest of the edges of the surgical defect with interrupted nonabsorbable suture material. A split-thickness skin graft is applied to the donor site defect on the parietal scalp on the right side, retained in position with sea sponge bolster dressing (10).

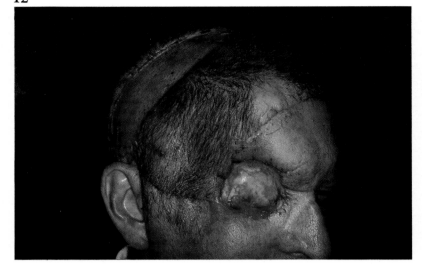

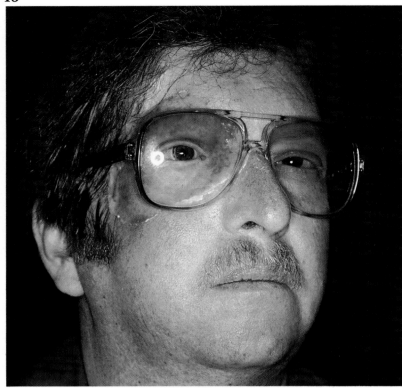

The surgical specimen in **(11)** shows the excised recurrent tumor together with excision of the site of previous surgery and skin graft, and including resection of the contents of the orbit and the underlying frontal bone.

The postoperative appearance of the patient approximately 1 month after surgery **(12)** shows the scalp flap healed per primum with a satisfactory take of the split-thickness skin graft in the orbit and on the scalp. An orbital prosthesis is fabricated to enhance the patient's esthetic appearance **(13)**.

Craniofacial resection for sarcoma of the frontal bone

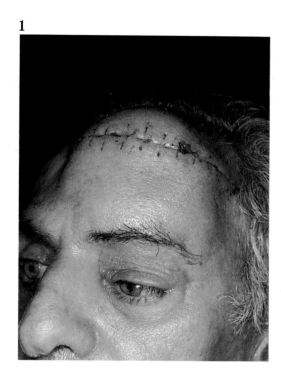

1

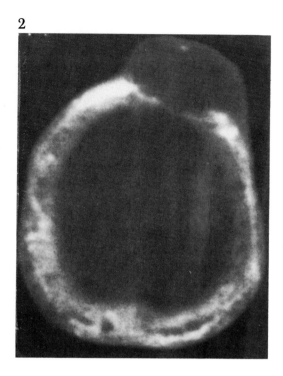

2

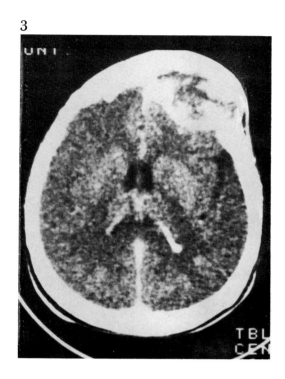

3

Malignant tumors of the calvarium, adherent to the overlying scalp and underlying dura, require through-and-through monobloc resection. However, when these tumors involve the anterior cranial fossa, a craniofacial resection is necessary. If the tumor involves one orbit, then orbital exenteration in conjunction with formal craniectomy and *en bloc* excision are indicated.

The patient presented here has an osteogenic sarcoma arising in the calvarium involved by Paget's disease (1). The patient presented to a local surgeon with an enlarging mass in the forehead of approximately 6 months' duration. A generous open biopsy was performed with a transverse incision in the skin of the forehead which confirmed the diagnosis of osteogenic sarcoma. At that point the patient was referred for appropriate surgical treatment.

The CT scan of the head through a bone window shows that the entire skull is involved with Paget's disease (2). The tumor is in the left-side of the frontal bone with extension of disease to the right-side. There is significant soft tissue extension extracranially. Soft tissue windows show significant intracranial extension of disease with displacement and/or involvement of the frontal lobe on the left side (3).

Coronal cut through the orbits show direct extension of the tumor from the frontal region through the roof of the orbit into the orbital socket displacing the globe inferiorly and laterally (4). The tumor does not involve the contents of the nasal cavity.

4

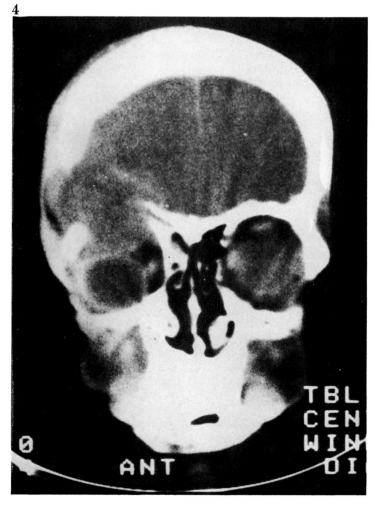

5

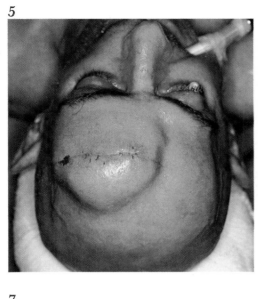

6

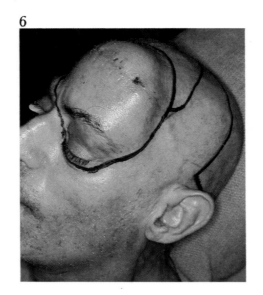

7

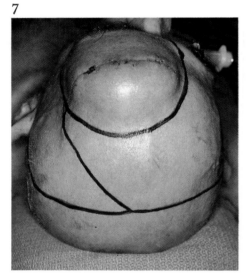

8

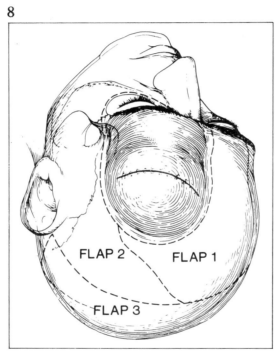

FLAP 2   FLAP 1

FLAP 3

9

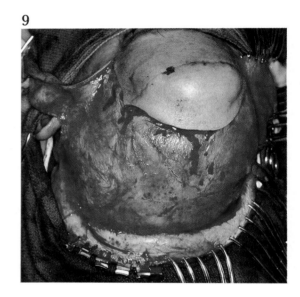

10

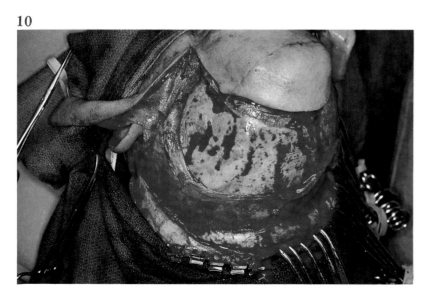

11

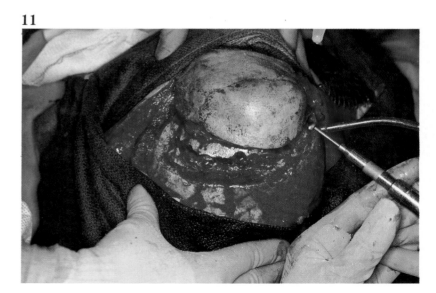

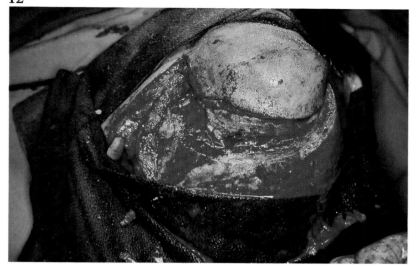

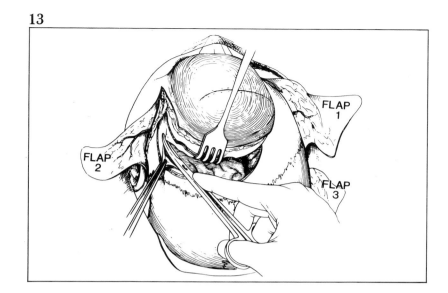

The operative procedure in this clinical setting necessitates two surgical teams: a neurosurgical team who begin with the craniotomy aspect of the operation; and the head and neck team who accomplish the facial aspect of the procedure and reconstruction of the surgical defect with appropriate scalp flaps (5). The patient is positioned supine on the operating table with an indwelling, spinal catheter to monitor cerebrospinal fluid pressure. The head is allowed to rest free on a U-shaped headrest. General anesthesia is induced with the endotracheal tube passed through the oral cavity. The right eye is protected with a corneal shield.

The incisions are marked out demonstrating the extent of sacrifice of the skin of the forehead, scalp and the eyelids with the surgical specimen (6). Appropriate scalp flaps are also outlined to assist in resurfacing the craniectomy and orbital exenteration defect to support the brain. Three scalp flaps are outlined in (7).

Basically, this is a modification of bipedicled parietal flap which would be divided just to the left of the midline to provide satisfactory exposure for craniotomy. The third flap is based on the left side, but rotated anteriorly to cover the defect created by the first two flaps. The scalp incisions are taken to elevate the first two flaps. On the left side, the anterior incision is taken up to the zygomatic process, and the posterior incision is taken up to the apex of the pinna of the ear. A similar incision on the right side is taken up to the supraorbital ridge anteriorly and up to the pinna of the ear posteriorly. This bipedicled scalp flap is divided in the middle, as shown in (8), obliquely to create flaps 1 and 2. These

flaps would be then used to cover the surgical defect later on. Both flaps 1 and 2 are now retracted laterally to expose the parieto-occipital region. The posterior scalp is retracted posteriorly to expose the cranial surface covered by the periosteum (9). The latter is divided now around the excised part of the skin leaving a cuff of at least 1 cm around the periphery of the specimen. Elevation of the periosteum on the skull, in this instance, causes significant bleeding because of the increased vascularity of the cranial bones involved by Paget's disease (10).

The exposed skull is now prepared for multiple burr holes, which are made along the proposed site of excision of the frontal bone remaining posterior to the scalp incision. The burr holes are connected after elevation of the underlying dura using a gigli saw with a guide strip. Brisk hemorrhage due to the hypervascularity of the Paget's bone occurs from the transected edges of the bone, and is controlled using bone wax. Sharp spicules of the bones are smoothed out using a rongeur, which is also used to further divide the frontal bone up to the left-sided supraorbital ridge. All sharp edges of the bone on the patient side are smoothed out with a drill using a fine diamond drill bit (11).

Since there is intracranial extension of the tumor, the dura is to be sacrificed, and is therefore opened on the left of the midline remaining well posterior to the tumor (12). Using sharp tenotomy scissors, the dura is incised along the proposed site of excision of the specimen towards the right side (13). Brisk hemorrhage from the dura is to be expected because of increased vascularity

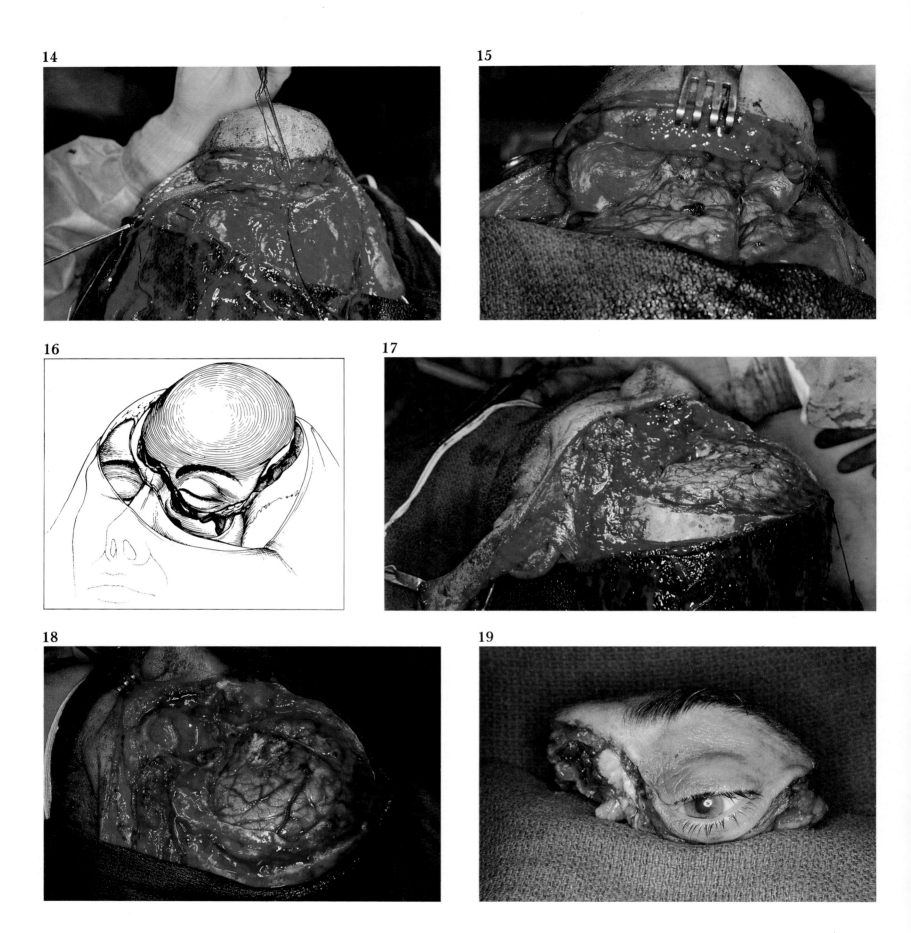

14

15

16

17

18

19

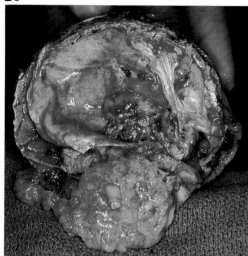
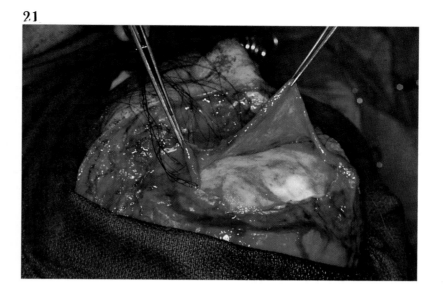

due to tumor. As the incision in the dura approaches midline, the sagittal sinus is suture-ligated and divided **(14)**. Division of the dura on the right of the midline continues along the circumference of the proposed specimen.

Once the division of the dura is completed up to the anteroinferior aspect of the proposed surgical specimen, it can be lifted up with the use of a sharp rake retractor. This brings into view the extension of the tumor involving a portion of the frontal lobe which will have to be sacrificed along with the specimen **(15)**. The cortical aspects of the frontal lobe are divided using a bipolar cautery and sharp scissors. On the right side, entry is made into the ethmoid air cells at the base of the skull through the cribriform plate. Continued division of the dural attachments in the midline further facilitates mobilization of the specimen.

The head and neck surgical team now scrubs in and continues the incision along the proposed surgical specimen through the medial aspect of the orbit and the lower eyelid up to the lateral canthus, meeting the lateral incision of the scalp **(16)**. A periosteal elevator is used to lift the periosteum of the lower half of the orbit, retaining its contents in continuity with the tumor. Transection of the orbital process of zygoma is completed to facilitate lateral mobilization of the specimen. Using heavy Mayo scissors, the ethmoid air cells on the left side are divided, and the bony cut through the frontal bone and the ethmoid air cells through the region of the crista galli, is completed. Rongeurs and heavy scissors are used during mobilization of the specimen in

this area to facilitate complete division of the bony, dural and soft tissue attachments. Using a heavy Mixter clamp, the contents at the cone of the orbit are clamped and the extraocular muscles and optic nerve are divided. Finally, the bony roof of the orbit is divided to totally mobilize the specimen.

The surgical defect, thus created, is continuous with the lower half of the orbital socket and the contents of the frontal fossa with exposed brain in that region **(17)**. A closeup of the surgical defect shows the exposed brain of the left frontal lobe with a large segment of missing dura which was resected with the specimen **(18)**. Laterally, the stumps of the temporalis muscle are visible in the temporal region.

The surgical specimen with the orbit, frontal bone and the tumor excised in a monobloc fashion is shown in **(19)**. The posterior view **(20)** shows the contents of the orbit in the lower part, with the frontal region dura showing the tumor perforating through it into the frontal fossa in the upper part. On the right-hand side, the crista galli and the cribriform plate region can be seen. A satisfactory monobloc resection of the osteogenic sarcoma of the frontal bone is accomplished via a craniofacial approach.

A large segment of the periosteum from the posterior aspect of the skull is now excised and used as a free graft to repair the defect in the dura **(21)**. The periosteum is sutured to the dura with 4-0 neurolon sutures, with a watertight closure to prevent any cerebrospinal fluid leakage.

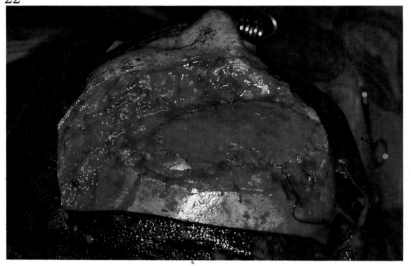

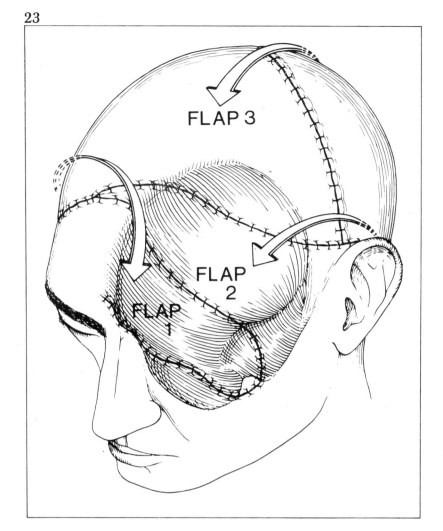

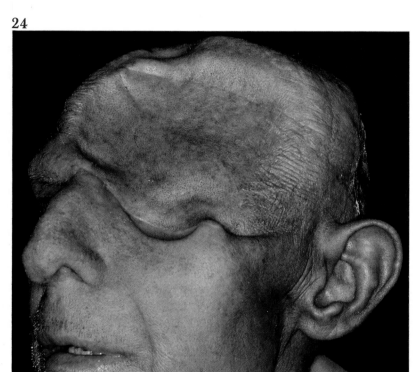

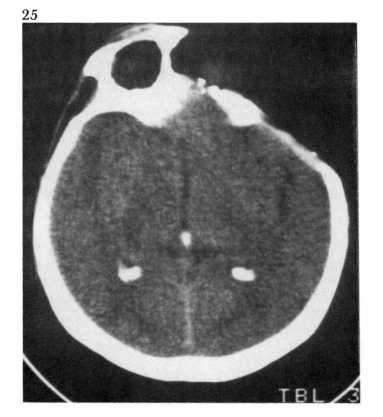

Following complete closure of the dura, the suture line is inspected for leakage of cerebrospinal fluid (22); if so additional sutures are taken to ensure a watertight closure. At this point, the previously withdrawn cerebrospinal fluid is slowly reintroduced through the spinal catheter. All bleeding points are rechecked to ensure complete hemostasis. Suction drains are inserted through separate stab incisions in the scalp, to remain over both the skull and the defect.

The previously elevated scalp flaps are now brought back into the surgical defect (23). Flap 1 from the right side is brought into the orbital socket to cover the medial aspect and the floor of the orbit; flap 2 covers the superiolateral aspect and the roof of the orbit; flap 3 covers the defect created by the first two flaps. Split-thickness skin graft is applied in the occipital region to cover the scalp defect created by flap 3. The scalp flaps must be trimmed appropriately in order to fit the surgical defect.

The postoperative appearance of the patient approximately 3 months after surgery (24) shows primary healing of all the suture lines and the scalp flaps. An esthetic prosthesis will be now fabricated for a better external appearance.

A postoperative CT scan of the patient demonstrates total excision of the tumor of the frontal region with satisfactory margins (25).

6: The Eyelids

Introduction

The eyelids are a complex set of paired, anatomical structures that protect the eye. Cross-sectional anatomy of the eyelids reveal that their exterior is covered by skin while the inner surface is covered by conjunctiva. In between is the tarsal plate with the orbicularis oculi muscle, the hair follicles of the eyelashes, and the meibomian glands. Most of the motion of the eyelids is performed by the upper eyelid, with the lower eyelid being relatively less mobile.

Excision of basal cell carcinoma of the skin of the lower eyelid

Skin carcinomas involving the lower eyelid are easily managed by wide excision and closure by mobilizing skin locally from the lateral aspect of the cheek and the temporal region. When excision of a skin lesion of the lower eyelid is performed in a transverse axis with primary closure of the defect, ectropion will often result; so whenever feasible, the surgical excision is planned in such a manner that a lateral advancement flap is brought in to close the surgical defect, thus avoiding ectropion. The patient presented here (1) has a basal cell carcinoma involving the skin of the lower eyelid. The lesion does not reach the tarsal margin and is not infiltrating the underlying musculature or cartilage.

The plan of surgical excision is outlined here (2). The surgical defect resulting from excision will be of a triangular shape with lateral extension of the upper transverse skin incision along the lateral canthus into the temporal region, advancing the skin from the temporal region into the surgical defect. This allows an essentially oblique closure between the two edges of the surgical defect. Adequate mobilization of the lateral skin is necessary to avoid tension on the suture line and secondary pull on the lower eyelid.

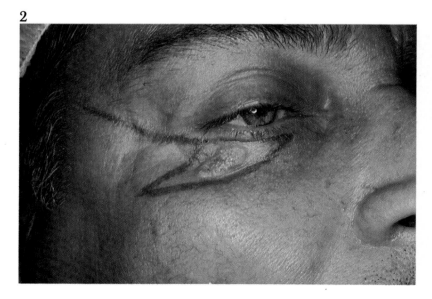

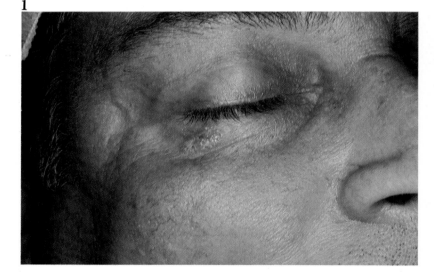

100

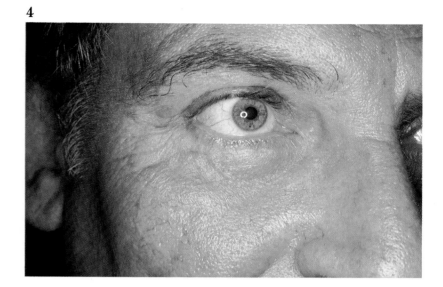

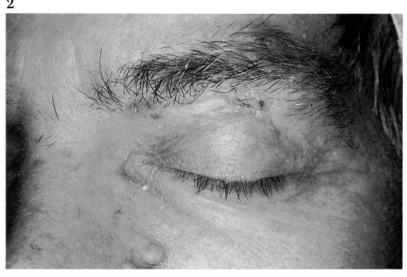

The completed surgical closure shows skin sutures with 6-0 nylon in place (3). Note that the skin sutures beneath the lower eyelid are left long, and their ends are taped to the skin of the cheek so that the suture stumps would not rub against the cornea postoperatively. No dressings are necessary, but Bacitracin ophthalmic ointment is applied to the suture line.

The postoperative appearance of the patient approximately 8 weeks after surgery is shown in (4). Note that the scar of the surgical excision is almost imperceptible and the disposition of the lower eyelid remains within normal limits without any ectropion. Surgical excision of skin lesions in the lower eyelid are thus best managed where the surgical defect is closed by advancing skin from the cheek laterally.

Excision of carcinoma involving the skin of the upper eyelid

Unlike the lower eyelid, the upper eyelid has a generous amount of lax skin available, making primary closure of surgical defects following excision of even large skin carcinomas possible. The patient presented here (1) has a superficially infiltrating squamous cell carcinoma involving the skin of the upper eyelid, and extending into the eyebrow. On palpation, the lesion is confined to the skin and does not infiltrate into either the underlying musculature or the tarsal plate.

On closure of the eyelid, the extent of the lesion becomes clearly manifest (2), involving a significant portion of the skin of the upper eyelid with extension into the hair-bearing area of the eyebrow skin.

Wide excision of this lesion will mean sacrifice of a considerable portion of the skin of the upper eyelid including some of that containing the eyebrows. It is essential that the eyebrow be maintained in its normal shape while surgical excision is contemplated. Thus, in

1

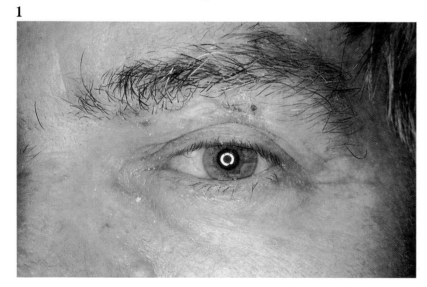

2

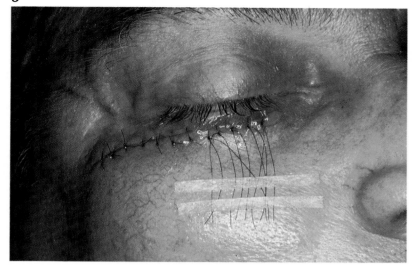

order to maintain the continuity of the eyebrow, surgical excision here will have to be oriented vertically, while excision of the upper eyelid skin will have to be oriented transversely—in fact, like an inverted letter 'T.'

The surgical defect following excision of the lesion is as described above (3). Frozen sections must be obtained from the margins of the surgical defect to ensure adequacy of excision, and care taken to avoid sacrifice of undue amounts of underlying musculature. After achieving satisfactory hemostasis, the skin edges are undermined on the lateral aspects of the upper portion of the surgical defect. Closure of the upper part of the surgical defect is accomplished vertically using interrupted 3-0 chromic catgut sutures to restore the continuity of the eyebrow between its medial and lateral parts. The rest of the surgical defect in the skin of the upper eyelid is closed transversely in two layers, the completely closed wound resembling an inverted letter (T).

The postoperative appearance of the patient approximately 8 weeks after surgery is shown in (4). Note that the eyebrow is reconstructed in its normal disposition, and that the upper eyelid has essentially no disfigurement because closure of the surgical defect is transverse. Because of the generous amount of skin available in the upper eyelid, the resultant scar is most satisfactory.

3

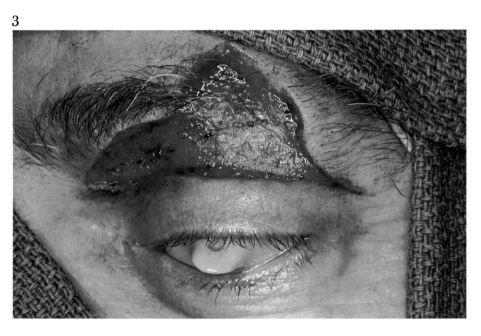

4

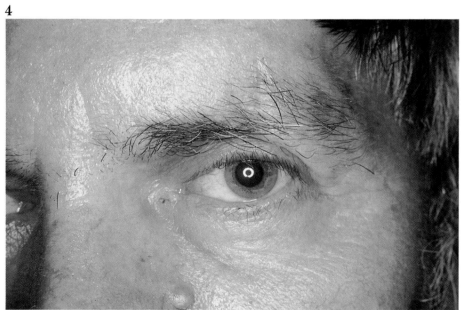

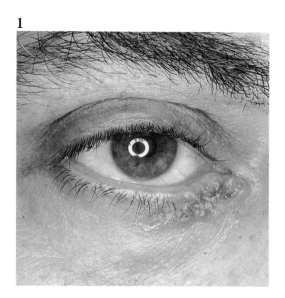

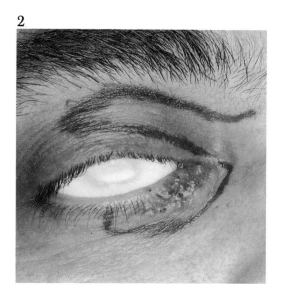

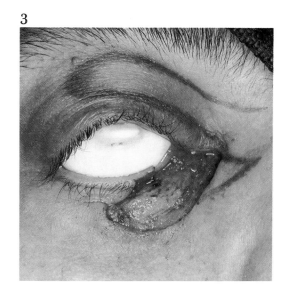

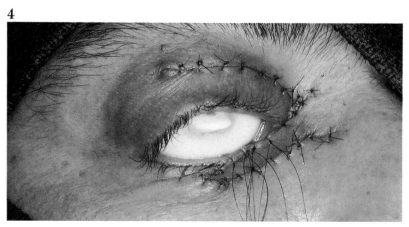

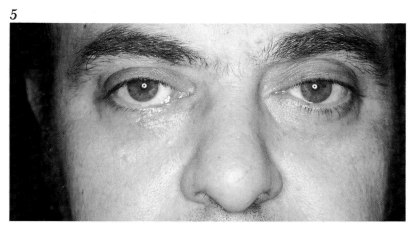

Excision and repair of skin lesion of the medial of the lower eyelid

Skin lesions of the medial half of the lower eyelid which involve the tarsal margin or are in close proximity to it present a significant problem for the reconstructive surgeon. Advancing skin from the lateral aspect of the cheek in this setting is not satisfactory for repair, as the line of tension will draw the medial canthus downwards and laterally causing ectropion and epiphora. Skin lesions requiring a limited extent of resection, therefore, are best repaired using a medially based skin flap from the upper eyelid. The patient shown in (1) has a basal cell carcinoma involving the skin of the lower eyelid, with involvement of the tarsal margin near the medial canthus.

The plan of surgical excision is outlined as shown in (2). The tarsal plate will be taken with the surgical specimen in the medial third of the tarsal margin. A medially based skin flap from the upper eyelid is elevated and rotated downwards to fill the surgical defect.

Surgical excision has been completed (3). Frozen sections are obtained from the margins of the conjunctiva as well as a skin margin on the cheek and these are reported to be negative. The medially based random skin flap from the upper eyelid, as outlined, will now be elevated.

The skin flap is transferred to fill the surgical defect and the donor site defect is closed primarily (4). Meticulous attention should be paid to delicate handling of this skin flap since the skin in this area is very thin and it would tear easily with rough handling. The skin closure is performed with 6-0 nylon sutures, the ends of the sutures being left long and taped onto the skin of the cheek to avoid trauma from the sutures to the cornea. No dressings are necessary but ophthalmic antibiotic ointment is applied to the sutures.

The postoperative appearance of the patient 8 weeks after surgery shows very satisfactory repair of the surgical defect in the region of the medial canthus of the lower eyelid (5). The patient has no functional disability and the esthetic result is quite pleasing.

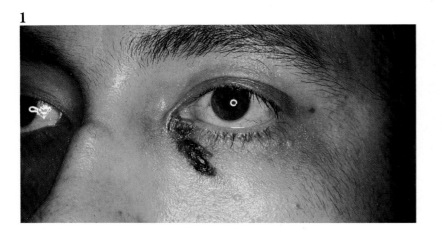

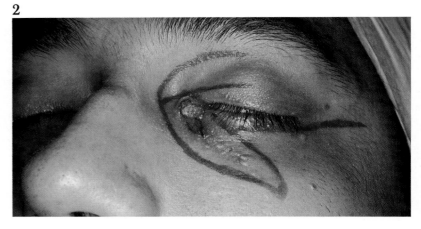

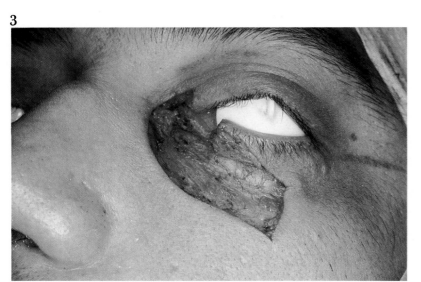

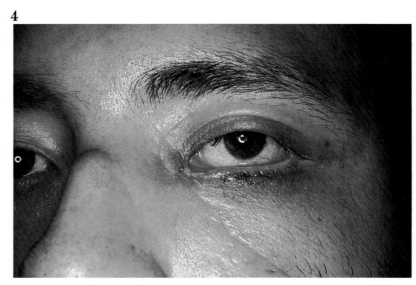

Excision and reconstruction of skin lesion involving the medial canthus

Skin lesions involving the medial canthus of the lower eyelid can be excised and repaired with a medially based skin flap from the upper eyelid as described in the previous operative procedure. However, if the extent of surgical excision reaches the base of the medially based upper eyelid skin flap then that particular method of reconstruction is not applicable. The patient shown in (1) has a pigmented basal cell carcinoma involving the skin of the lower eyelid and the medial canthus. Because of the extent of surgical excision that would be necessary in this patient, the medially based upper eyelid skin flap is not applicable here. So the plan of surgical excision and reconstruction would include a laterally based upper eyelid skin flap which would be rotated inferiorly and medially to reach the region of the medial canthus, and medial advancement of skin of the cheek from the lateral aspect allows repair of the resultant surgical defect in the skin of the lower eyelid.

Skin incisions are marked out for both the planned surgical excision and the anticipated skin flaps to be elevated following excision (2).

Surgical resection is completed here showing adequate excision of the skin cancer with resection of the medial canthus and a generous portion of skin around the primary lesion (3). Frozen section must be obtained from several margins of the surgical defect to ensure adequacy of excision. Laterally based skin flaps are elevated as previously outlined; a flap from the upper eyelid is rotated inferiorly and medially, and the cheek flap is advanced medially.

The postoperative appearance of the patient approximately 3 months following surgery is shown in (4). Note that the patient does not have ectropion. Since eyelashes in the medial part of the reconstructed lower eyelid are missing, there is some esthetic deformity but, functionally, patient has no other problems. Thus, combination of medial advancement of skin of the lateral aspect of the cheek and advancement rotation flap from the skin of the upper eyelid prove to be a satisfactory combination for reconstruction of surgical defects in the region of the medial canthus.

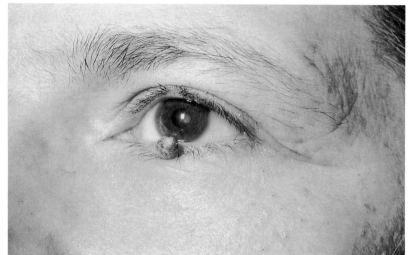

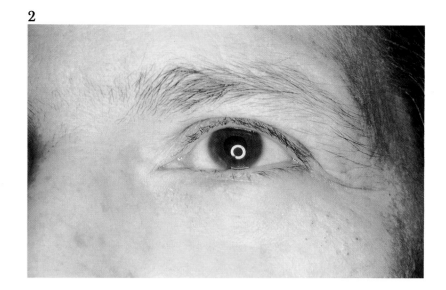

V excision of the lower eyelid

When skin lesions involving the lower eyelid in the region of the tarsal margin demand the need for full-thickness resection, a V excision is most satisfactory if the extent of surgical resection is limited. Up to one-third of the lower eyelid can be resected in a wedge excision with primary repair.

The patient shown here (1) has a nodular basal cell carcinoma involving the tarsal margin of the lower eyelid. A through-and-through wedge excision of the lower eyelid is performed including the skin, the tarsal plate, and the conjunctiva. Frozen sections are obtained from the margins of the surgical defect to ensure adequacy of resection. Reconstruction of the surgical defect requires reapproximation of the tarsal plate which is accomplished using a non-absorbable suture material. The suture begins at the gray line of the tarsal edge, entering through the tarsal margin and the underlying tarsal plate; it then exits through the transected edge of the tarsal plate on one side, re-enters the transected edge of the tarsal plate on the opposite side, and exits from the

tarsal margin at the opposite end of the surgical defect. This suture is snugly tied to reapproximate the tarsal plate, and the remaining surgical defect is closed in two layers using 6-0 silk sutures for the conjunctiva and 6-0 nylon sutures for the skin of the lower eyelid. Meticulous attention should be paid to accurate reapproximation of the tarsal cartilage defect, otherwise indentation at the site of the surgical closure will cause an unpleasing esthetic appearance.

The postoperative appearance of the patient at 3 months after surgery is shown in (2). Note that the tarsal margin is accurately reapproximated without any indentation, leaving no functional or esthetic deformity at the surgical excision site. Wedge excision of the lower eyelid is a very satisfactory operative procedure, if only a limited amount of lower eyelid has to be sacrificed. This operative procedure is, therefore, best suited for lesions which need through-and-through resection of limited portions of the lower eyelid.

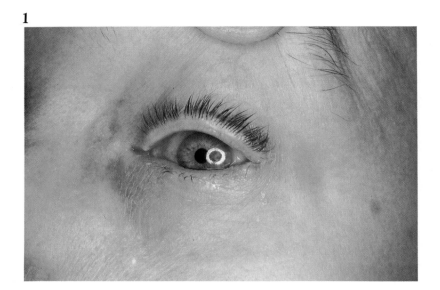

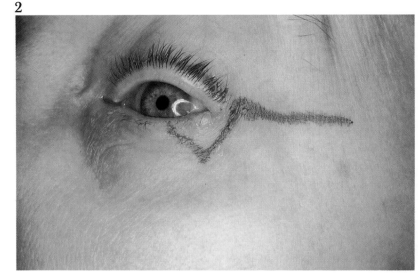

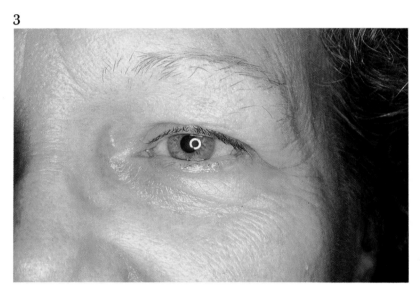

Full-thickness resection of the lateral aspect of the lower eyelid

Lesions involving the tarsal margin in the lateral third of the lower eyelid require an excision to reach the lateral canthus. These lesions are, therefore, not suitable for primary closure and require an advancement flap of skin from the lateral aspect of the surgical defect. The patient shown here (1) has a squamous cell carcinoma involving the tarsal margin of the lower eyelid near the lateral canthus.

The plan of surgical excision is outlined as shown (2). The primary tumor is resected in a wedge fashion, the lateral aspect of the wedge including the lateral canthus. A transverse skin incision is taken along the skin crease near the lateral canthus, well into the temporal region. The skin in the lower part of the cheek is undermined and mobilized to allow its medial advancement for repair of the lower eyelid. No special attention is neces-

sary for the resected edge of the tarsal plate in this situation. The skin with the underlying soft tissues is advanced medially and accurately approximated to the skin edge at the medial margin of the surgical defect. The upper edge of the advanced skin flap is sutured to the transected margin of the conjunctiva with 6-0 silk sutures.

The postoperative appearance of the patient at 3 months after surgery is shown in (3). Note that the reconstructed lower eyelid leaves no esthetic deformity. There is no indentation at the transected margin of the tarsal plate and the advanced skin flap provides enough substance to the lateral aspect of the lower eyelid for restoration of the soft tissues of the lower eyelid. The donor site scar is virtually imperceptible.

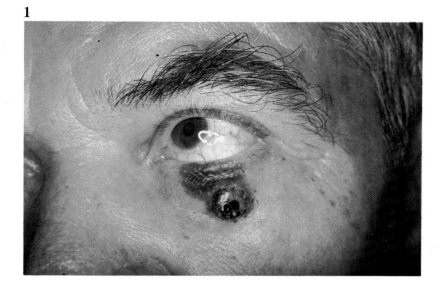

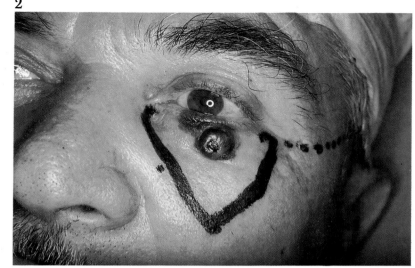

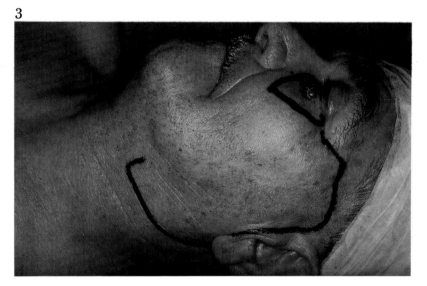

Note: Pictures **1** to **7** in this sequence courtesy of Ronald Spiro, MD.

Radical excision of the lower eyelid and reconstruction with a Mustardé flap

When the entire lower eyelid has to be resected due to malignant lesions, the reconstruction becomes a significant problem. The patient presented here (1) has a nodular melanoma involving the skin and the tarsal margin of the lower eyelid.

The plan of surgical excision for the primary tumor is outlined as shown in (2). The entire lower eyelid is resected along with a generous portion of the skin of the cheek as shown here. A portion of the palpebral conjunctiva is excised but the bulbar conjunctiva remains intact.

The skin incision necessary for elevation and ad-

vancement rotation for the Mustardé flap is shown here (3). Note that the skin incision for the Mustardé flap must be taken higher than the lateral canthus in the temporal region to prevent ectropion. The skin incision in the temporal region is taken high and then turned inferiorly towards the preauricular skin crease continuing on into the upper part of the neck where it curves anteriorly to permit satisfactory elevation and rotation of the skin flap. The latter is elevated superficially to the terminal branches of the facial nerve to prevent any injury to them.

4

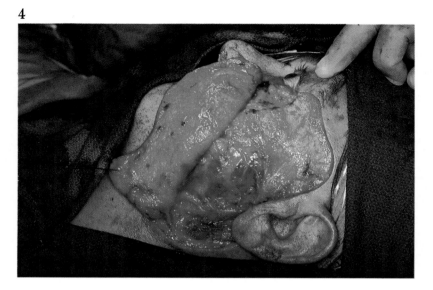

5

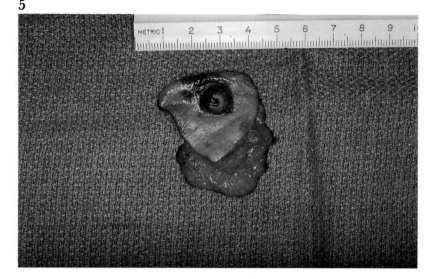

6

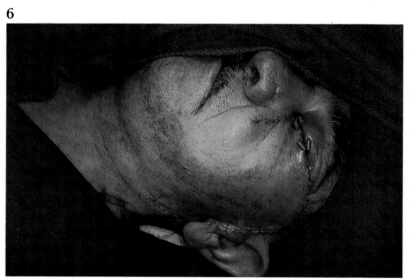

7

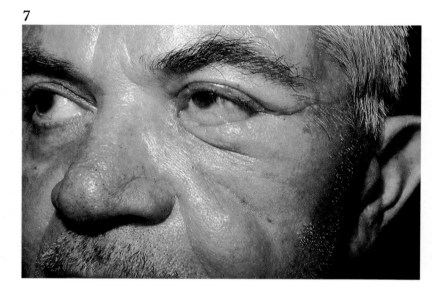

The surgical defect following superficial parotidectomy and upper neck dissection with elevation of the Mustardé flap is shown in (4). Note that the entire lower eyelid is resected to encompass the primary tumor.

The surgical specimen showing full-thickness resection of the lower eyelid with the underlying soft tissues is shown in (5). The appearance of the patient on the operating table following complete closure of the surgical defect with the Mustardé flap is shown in (6). The flap is advanced medially and rotated inferiorly to fill the surgical defect.

The postoperative appearance of the patient at 2 months after surgery is shown in (7). Note that because of the lack of tarsal plate and the support necessary for the lower eyelid, some degree of ectropion is present, and there is eversion of the conjunctival mucosa. The absence of eyelashes also impairs the esthetic restoration of the lower eyelid, but functionally patient has no trouble with the eye; he does have minimal epiphora due to eversion of the palpebral conjunctiva, but the cornea is fully protected. The Mustardé advancement rotation flap provides an excellent choice for reconstruction of a full-thickness defect following resection of the entire lower eyelid.

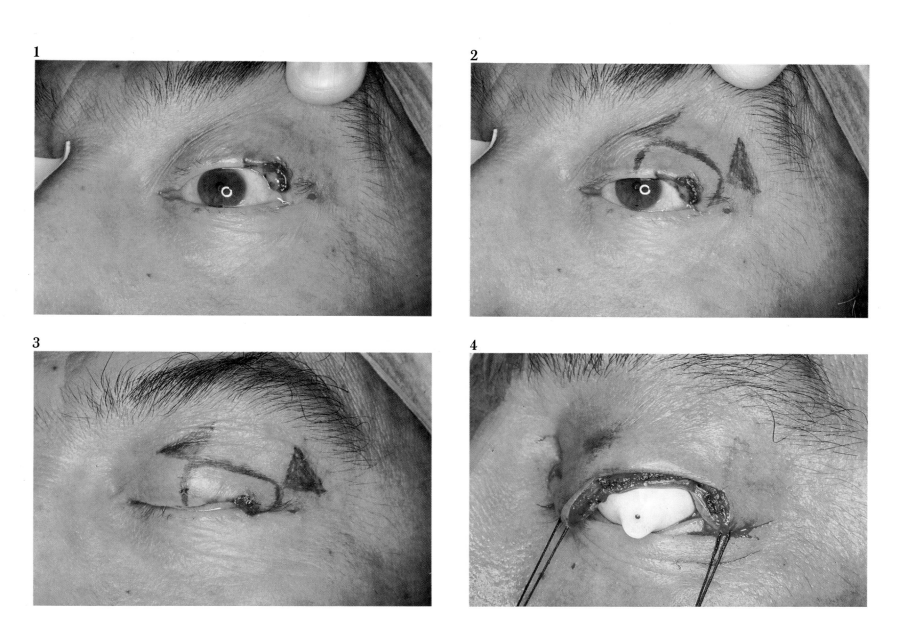

Full-thickness resection and reconstruction of the upper eyelid

Full-thickness resection of any portion of the upper eyelid poses a significant reconstructive problem, unlike the lower eyelid which is relatively easy to repair. Since the upper eyelid provides most of the lubricating function and protection to the cornea and globe, its accurate reconstruction is extremely important to prevent any subsequent injury to the cornea. The patient presented here has a pigmented basal cell carcinoma involving two-thirds of the width of the upper eyelid, the tarsal margin and the adjacent conjunctiva, as seen clearly in (1). Surgical excision of the lesion will require a full-thickness through-and-through resection of that part of the upper eyelid with immediate, appropriate repair.

The plan of surgical excision is outlined as shown here (2). A rectangular portion of the full thickness of the upper eyelid will be resected. The triangular-shaded

areas at the two upper corners of the rectangular excision are wedges of skin which will have to be excised to permit advancement of the skin of the upper eyelid for reconstruction (3). A ceramic corneal shield is inserted to protect the cornea. Two heavy, silk sutures are taken through the full thickness of the tarsal margin of the upper eyelid on the periphery of the intended site of excision; these stay sutures are held with hemostats to stabilize the eyelid during excision.

Through-and-through resection of the upper eyelid along the previously outlined area of rectangular excision is completed (4). Note that the surgical excision is just medial to the stay sutures which help stabilize the cut edges of the surgical defect. Complete hemostasis is obtained by ligating and/or coagulating the bleeding points during the excision. Similar heavy, silk stay su-

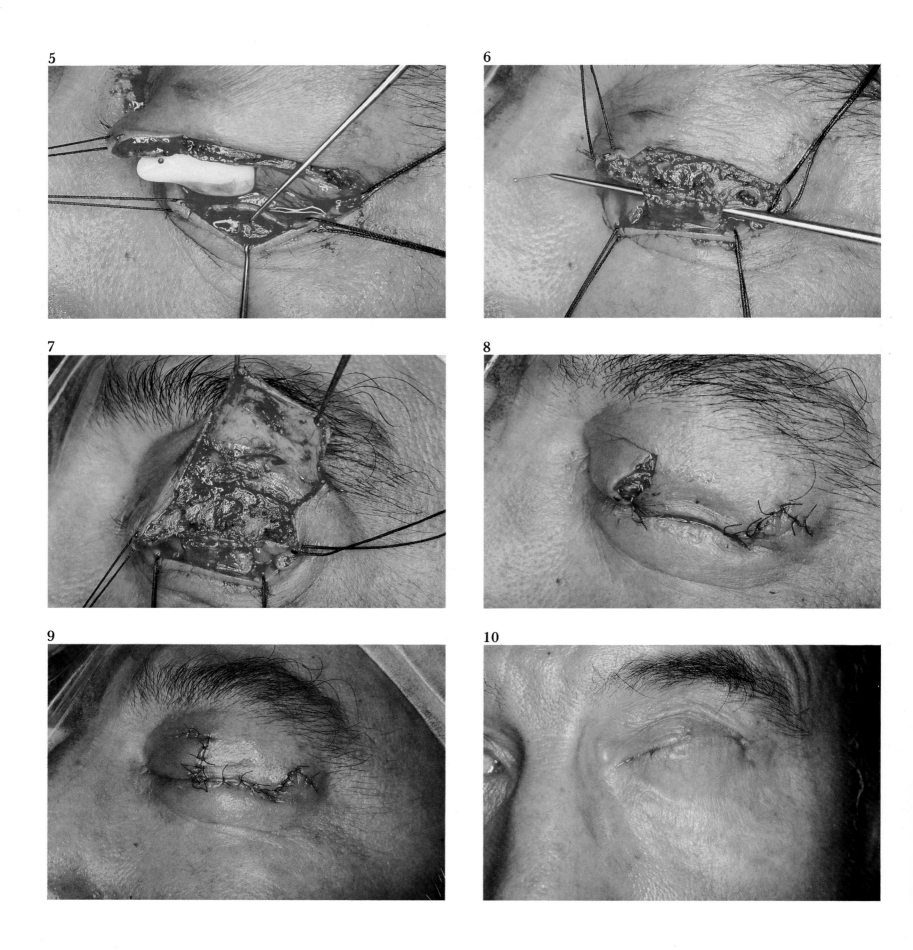

11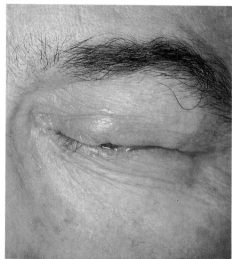

12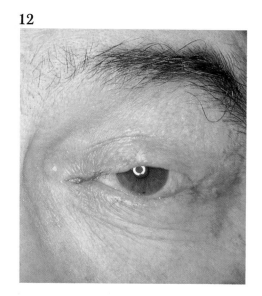

13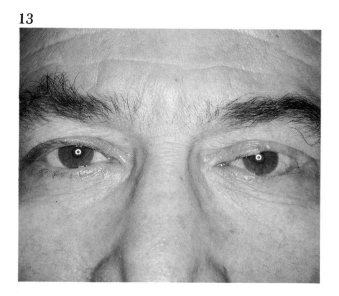

tures are applied to the tarsal margin of the lower eyelid **(5)**, and an incision is now made through the gray line of the tarsal margin of the lower eyelid between the two stay sutures. The skin is retracted inferiorly to expose the tarsal plate. Using a sharp, fine knife, the tarsal plate is divided in a coronal plane through its thickness in order to retain the inner aspect of the tarsal plate attached to the palpebral conjunctiva, while its outer aspect remains continuous with the rest of the tarsal plate. Using sharp scissors two incisions are made in the palpebral conjunctiva with the attached, split tarsal plate to match the surgical defect of the upper eyelid, and the incision is taken down to its reflection over the globe. This will, therefore, provide a composite conjunctival flap containing a portion of the split tarsal plate from the lower eyelid, which is then advanced cephalad and sutured to the horizontal cut edge of the conjunctiva of the upper eyelid in the rectangular surgical defect **(6)**. The conjunctival sutures are taken with 6-0 plain catgut sutures. Several interrupted sutures are applied and the knots are kept outside to be buried in the soft tissues.

Once this bridged conjunctival repair is completed, skin incisions are made in the upper eyelid further cephalad from the rectangular defect to match the previously outlined triangular areas of skin to be sacrificed, and then the previously marked triangular wedges of skin are excised **(7)**. This allows downward displacement of the skin flap from the upper eyelid which is sutured to the cut edge on the skin side of the tarsal margin of the lower eyelid, using 6-0 nylon sutures for approximation of the skin edges of the upper eyelid skin flap and the skin margin of the lower eyelid **(8)**. The remaining skin closure is completed along the lateral aspect of the skin flap and then transversely through the region of the excised wedges of the skin; this is the first stage of reconstruction of the upper eyelid **(9)**. At the conclusion of the operation, the upper and lower eyelids are fused, and remain so for 8 weeks. Skin sutures are removed in approximately 1 week. During fusion, patient is instructed to irrigate the eye and keep the area as clean as possible.

At 8 weeks after the first stage of the operation, the patient is returned to the operating room where the fused eyelids are divided **(10)**, under topical and local anesthesia. Two drops of topical anesthetic are introduced into the conjunctival sac and local anesthetic is infiltrated along the palpebral fissure through the fused eyelids. A fine, lacrimal probe is introduced from the palpebral fissure medial to the bridge of skin, and is brought out through the fissure lateral to the bridge to protect the cornea during division of the fused eyelids. Using sharp, curved scissors, the bridge of the fused eyelids is divided along the line of the palpebral fissure, and full thickness through-and-through division of the bridged reconstruction is performed to separate the reconstructed upper eyelid from the lower eyelid. Minimal bleeding is to be expected from the cut edges of the reconstructed area, but this will stop with slight pressure.

The postoperative appearance of the patient 1 week following division of the bridged lower eyelid flap to reconstruct the upper eyelid is shown in **(11)**. The functional and esthetic restoration is complete, and the final postoperative result is very gratifying **(12, 13)**. Bridged repair of the upper eyelid defects using a split tarsal plate and conjunctival composite flap is a very satisfactory means of immediate reconstruction of sizable defects of the upper eyelid.

7: The Nasal Cavity and Paranasal Sinuses

Introduction

The nasal cavity is the air space communicating with the exterior and the upper aerodigestive tract. It is lined by squamous epithelium which is partly cuboidal and partly celiated. The mucosa lining the nasal cavity also contains mucous glands and minor salivary glands as well as neuroepithelial cells, the so-called olfactory neuroblasts responsible for the sense of smell. The nasal cavity is divided on two sides by the nasal septum which is covered on each side by the nasal mucosa, and comprises the vomer bone and the septal cartilage. Laterally, the nasal cavity contains the nasal conchae, the inferior concha being part of the nasal cavity, and the superior and middle conchae being composite parts of the ethmoid complex. The nasal cavity is surrounded by air containing bony spaces, the so-called paranasal sinuses, the largest of which, the maxillary antrum, is present on each side. The ethmoid air cells occupy the superior aspect of the nasal cavity, and separate it from the anterior skull base at the level of the cribriform plate. Superoanteriorly, the frontal sinus contained within the frontal bone forms a biloculated or multiloculated pneumatic space within the frontal bone. The sphenoid sinus in the upper part of the nasal cavity in the roof of the nasopharynx is the only single sinus which can also be loculated by a median septum. The most frequent site of tumors in this area is in the maxillary antrum followed by the nasal cavity, and the ethmoid air cells. One rarely sees tumors arising primarily in the frontal or sphenoid sinuses.

Ohngren described a hypothetical line joining the medial canthus of the eye and the angle of the mandible dividing the maxillary antrum into two halves (**1**). The inferior and anterior half is called the 'infrastructure', while the posterosuperior half is called the 'suprastructure'. Satisfactory surgical resection is usually possible for tumors of the infrastructure. On the other hand, tumors of the suprastructure which involve the pterygoid fossa or skull base do not offer satisfactory margins in spite of the most aggressive surgical resection. The cure rate is better for tumors of the nasal cavity and infrastructure, while more extensive tumors and those arising in the suprastructure have an unfavorable prognosis.

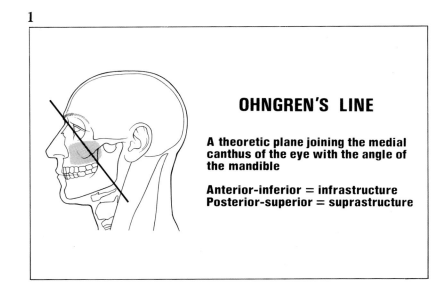

OHNGREN'S LINE

A theoretic plane joining the medial canthus of the eye with the angle of the mandible

Anterior-inferior = infrastructure
Posterior-superior = suprastructure

Radiographic evaluation

Adequate radiographic evaluation must be performed to better prepare the surgeon for assessing the extent of the tumor prior to the surgical procedure. Basic information can be obtained by plain X-rays, as well as coronal and sagittal conventional tomograms, of the paranasal sinuses. However, CT scan and magnetic resonance imaging of the nasal cavity provide a better resolution of the anatomy of the bony structures and the soft tissues, and is preferable over conventional tomograms in most instances. Preoperatively, the crucial areas that need thorough evaluation are the pterygoid plates, pterygomaxillary fossa, infratemporal fossa, floor of the orbit, ethmoid air cells, cribriform plate and the base of the skull. When CT scan is requested, both transverse as well as coronal cuts should be obtained to assess more accurately the extent of the tumor. For patients in whom extension of disease into the soft tissues is suspected, CT scan with intravenous contrast provides a more accurate definition of the extent of the tumor. Interpretation of radiographic findings should always be correlated with clinical findings and the patient's symptoms.

Preoperative dental preparation

Dental evaluation of the patient for assessment of oral hygiene and appropriate preoperative dental care is mandatory. Grossly septic teeth are attended to promptly. However, loose teeth in the tumor-bearing alveolus are best not disturbed preoperatively. Dental impressions are obtained for the preparation of immediate surgical and subsequent, definitive palatal obturator, the design of which is influenced by the anticipated surgical defect. The fabrication of an adequate, immediate obturator is facilitated by proper communication between the surgeon and the prosthodontist who should be available in the operating room for its insertion. The surgeon marks the extent of resection of the palate on the preoperative dental cast model. If a portion of the soft palate is to be resected, the prothesis generally requires posterior extension to avoid nasal regurgitation. The availability of the immediate dental obturator aids postoperative recovery in terms of restoration of swallowing and retention of packing, and also maintenance of pulmonary toilet by the patient's ability to cough effectively. Thus, a tracheostomy is generally avoided when an immediate dental obturator is applied following surgery for tumors of the paranasal sinuses. A bacteriological culture of the contents of the nasal cavity should be obtained preoperatively, and prophylactic antibiotics to combat bacterial infection in the surgical wound are recommended.

Anesthesia and position

General endotracheal anesthesia with satisfactory muscle relaxation is essential for adequate exposure of the oral cavity to provide access and ease of instrumentation during surgery. Either nasotracheal or orotracheal intubation is employed. It is, however, vital for the skin incision to be marked prior to intubation and taping of the endotracheal tube to avoid distortion of facial skin lines.

The patient is placed in a supine position, the upper half of the body is elevated 30°, and the neck is extended and slightly rotated to the ipsilateral side. Since the eye on the side of surgery may be in the surgical field, protection of the cornea with a ceramic corneal shield is desirable. Alternatively, the eyelids can be sutured together. Draping of the patient's head is done so that movement of the head during operation avoids contamination of the sterile field. A transparent plastic head drape provides isolation of the anesthetic tubings and offers clear visibility of patient's eyes, nose and endotracheal tubes to both surgeon and anesthesiologist. If the need for split-thickness skin graft to cover the surgical defect is anticipated, then it is obtained from a suitable donor site prior to beginning of the surgical procedure, usually from the thigh.

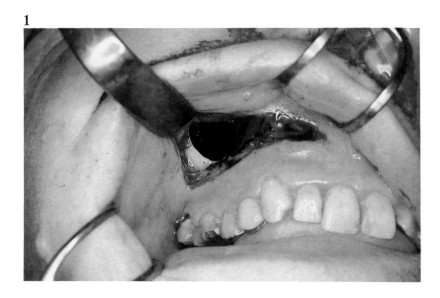

Caldwell–Luc antrostomy

Caldwell–Luc antrostomy is an operative procedure which can be diagnostic as well as therapeutic in certain cases. The procedure in itself provides limited access to the maxillary antrum and is therapeutic in patients with chronic maxillary sinusitis where effective drainage is provided for a chronically inflamed and infected antrum. On the other hand, when a tumor is suspected, the operative procedure is only diagnostic. It provides access to the maxillary antrum for obtaining adequate tissue sampling prior to definitive treatment. It is, however, recommended that Caldwell–Luc antrostomy be avoided as a diagnostic procedure where a tumor in the maxillary antrum is suspected. Breaking through the anterior bony wall of the maxillary antrum containing the tumor is ill-advised. It will cause contamination of the anterior soft tissues of the cheek leading to an unsatisfactory subsequent definitive therapeutic operation. It will also allow leakage and/or permeation of tumor cells into the anterior soft tissues requiring sacrifice of considerable anterior soft tissue at the time of definitive treatment. Thus, Caldwell–Luc antrostomy should be avoided at all times when a tumor is suspected. In that clinical setting, histological diagnosis can be obtained by needle aspiration tissue sampling through the medial wall of the maxillary antrum via the nasal cavity. The so-called nasal antrostomy is much more safe and desirable for obtaining tissue for diagnosis where tumors are suspected in the maxillary antrum.

The Caldwell-Luc operation is done through the oral cavity. The upper lip and oral commissure are retracted to expose the gingivolabial sulcus. An incision is made in the gingivolabial sulcus using needlepoint electrocautery in the region of the canine fossa. The mucosal incision is deepened up to the bone of the anterior wall of the maxillary antrum. A periosteal elevator is then used, and the periosteum of the anterior wall of the maxilla is elevated as far up as possible to gain wide exposure. However, care must be exercised to avoid injury to the infraorbital nerve as it exits through the infraorbital foramen.

A Richardson retractor is used next and all the soft tissues of the cheek, including the elevated periosteum, are retracted cephalad. An antrostomy is made either using a small osteotome and a mallet, or preferably a high speed drill with a round drill bit (1). If inspection and drainage is the only purpose for the antrostomy, then the opening in the antrum is made at the most dependent portion near the socket of the canine tooth. The opening is enlarged with a high speed drill to provide wide exposure of the interior of the maxillary antrum for visual inspection and instrumentation. After inspection of the interior of the maxillary antrum, any fluid contents are irrigated out. The mucosa is inspected for any abnormalities, and if the process is only inflammatory, then using appropriate, straight and curved curettes, the entire mucosa of the maxillary antrum is curetted out and sent for histopathological evaluation. The maxillary antrum is again irrigated with antibiotic solution (Bacitracin 1 g in 1000 ml of saline). A loose packing is inserted into the maxillary antrum and brought out through the antrostomy. The mucosal incision is now partly closed, with interrupted 3-0 chromic catgut sutures, leaving enough room for removal of the packing and to provide satisfactory drainage. The retractors are withdrawn and the patient is awakened.

Minimal postoperative care is necessary except for continued administration of antibiotics and occasional use of warm compresses on the cheek on the side of surgery to avoid undue discomfort and swelling.

Lateral rhinotomy and excision of nasal tumor

Small, localized tumors of the nasal cavity, either benign or malignant, which are inaccessible through the nasal vestibule are best approached via a lateral rhinotomy. The operative procedure causes minimal functional and/or esthetic deformity and provides excellent exposure of the lower part of the nasal cavity and nasal septum. Tumors which are best managed via this approach are papillomas, inverted papillomas, and malignant tumors of limited extent arising on the septum or the lateral and inferior wall of the nasal cavity.

The patient is placed in the supine position on the operating table under general endotracheal anesthesia with the endotracheal tube inserted through the oral cavity. An incision line is marked out prior to insertion and taping of the endotracheal tube to avoid distortion of skin lines for choosing the line of incision. In (1), the intended line of incision is marked out, beginning at the philtrum of the upper lip and extending around the vestibule of the nose and the ala of the nasal cavity to the nasolabial crease.

Using a nasal speculum, the extent of the tumor is inspected; the lower part is visualized here (2). This lesion proved to be an inverted papilloma on biopsy prior to surgical excision. It is, however, important to assess the extent of the lesion adequately before taking a lateral rhinotomy approach for excision of the tumor.

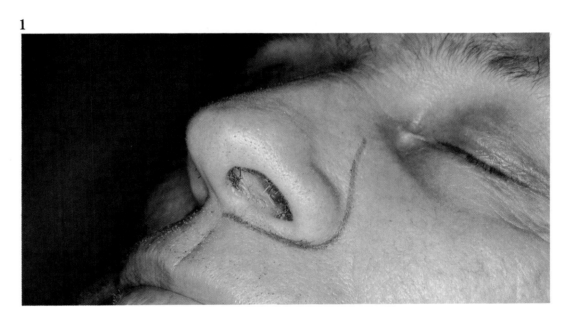

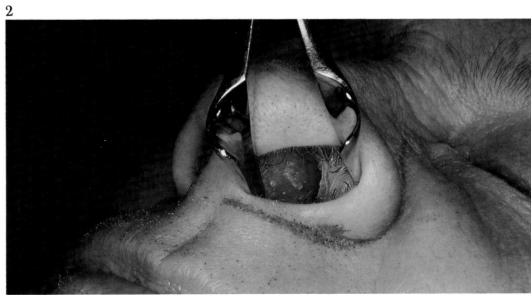

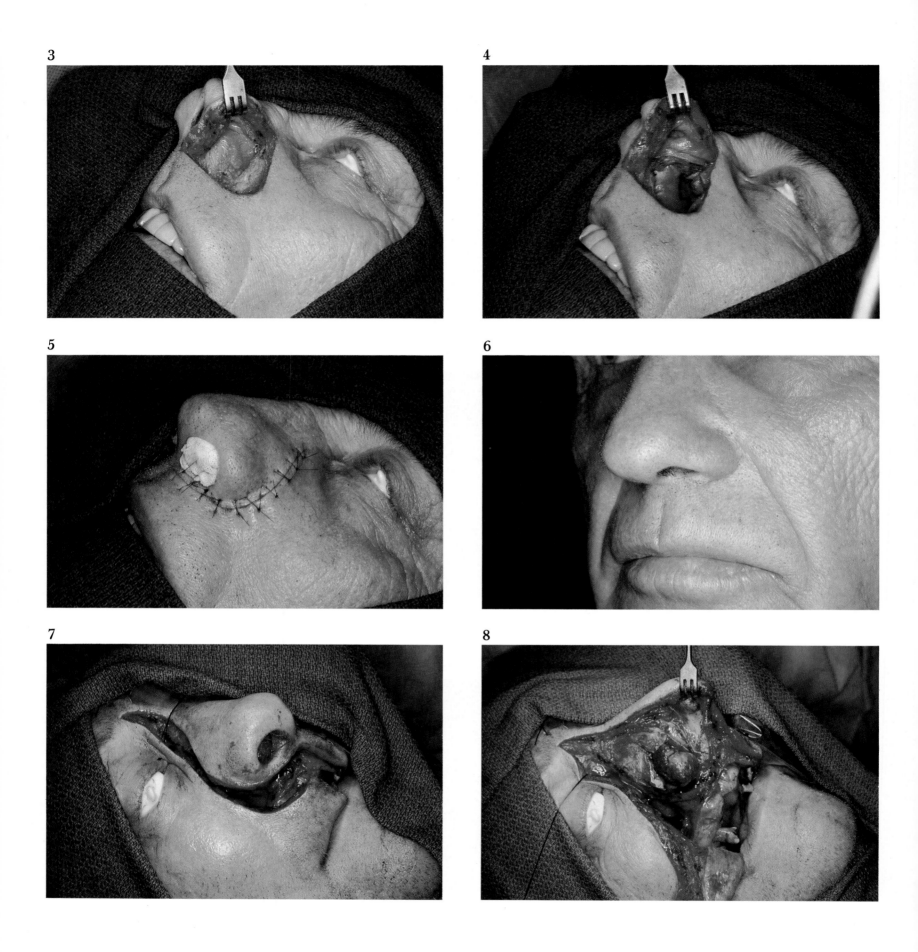

The skin incision is deepened through the adjacent soft tissues to gain entry into the nasal cavity. Musculature of the face and the nasolabial skin crease will have to be divided all the way up to the nasal process of maxilla, laterally, and through the mucosa of the lateral wall of the nasal cavity to gain entry into the nasal cavity (3). A rake retractor is now used to retract the ala of the nostril to the right side to provide wide exposure of the lower part of the interior of the left nasal cavity. The tumor arising from the mucosa of the nasal septum is widely exposed here. Using needlepoint electrocautery, an incision is made in the mucosa of the nasal septum around the primary tumor giving generous margins of the adjacent mucosa. Electrocautery is used to transect the nasal septal cartilage through the area of the mucosal incision to obtain a through-and-through resection. Once the cartilage is incised circumferentially through the line of mucosal incision, a periosteal elevator (and suction with Frazier suction tip to keep the field dry) is used to elevate the mucosa of the right side of the nasal cavity over the septum to separate the mucosa on the opposite side and keep it intact. Once circumferential elevation of the cartilage is obtained, the surgical specimen which contains the tumor presenting on the left side of the mucosa of the nasal septum is delivered, along with the adjacent, generous margins of the septal mucosa and underlying septal cartilage.

The surgical defect in (4) shows the raw area of the septal mucosa of the right nasal cavity with a septal cartilage defect created by resection of the tumor of the left nasal cavity. Hemostasis is usually obtained by electrocoagulation of fine bleeding points from the margins of the surgical defect, and no specific measures are necessary for its closure; the nasal cavity is then irrigated with Bacitracin solution.

A xeroform gauze is placed in the nasal cavity to cover the area of the surgical resection and avoid hemorrhage and/or crusting (5). The skin incision is closed in layers paying meticulous attention to facial skin lines and appropriate approximation of the skin edges. The packing in the nasal cavity is removed in 48 hours and the patient is taught nasal irrigation to keep the area clean. Epithelization of the raw areas will take place in approximately 10 days to 2 weeks, and the patient will then have normal nasal function.

The postoperative appearance of the patient approximately 3 months after surgery (6) shows satisfactory healing of the wound with essentially no distortion in the facial skin lines secondary to a lateral rhinotomy.

A limited rhinotomy, as described in the above operative procedure, can be extended to obtain wider access for tumors that arise in the nasal septum. As shown in (7), the lateral rhinotomy is extended cephalad to take the incision all the way up to the medial aspect of the eyebrow, and inferiorly it is taken down to split the upper lip providing wide access to the lateral wall and contents of the right nasal cavity.

This patient presented with a malignant melanoma arising on the nasal septum requiring exenteration of the nasal cavity which could be performed via the extended lateral rhinotomy approach (8). In this situation, excision of part of the nasal process of maxilla, as well as the right nasal bone, will have to be performed to provide adequate resection of the melanoma arising from the mucosa of the nasal septum. Even though no part of the maxilla needs to be resected in this patient, access to the nasal cavity is improved by extension of the lateral rhinotomy incision, both cephalad and caudad, with division of the upper lip in the midline for elevation of the upper cheek flap to provide wide access to the interior of the nasal cavity.

Partial maxillectomy

Malignant tumors of limited extent arising in the maxilla can be adequately excised by partial maxillectomy. Tumors of the upper gum, hard palate or floor of the maxillary antrum are best suited for this procedure, which requires removal of the lower half of the maxilla.

The patient shown here (1) presented with 3 months' history of an enlarging, submucosal mass on the hard palate. Although the lesion was painless, he did experience discomfort in mastication, and the presence of a mass in the hard palate.

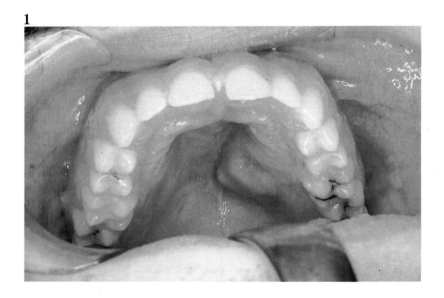

1

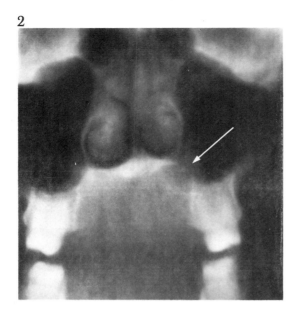

2

A coronal tomogram performed through the hard palate shows the presence of a submucosal tumor mass destroying the bony floor of the maxillary antrum with presence of the tumor in the maxillary sinus (2). The tumor, however, does not involve the hard palate beyond the midline neither does it encroach upon the medial wall, the lateral wall or roof of the maxillary antrum, and is confined to the infrastructure of the maxillary antrum. Biopsy of this mass confirmed it to be an intermediate-grade mucoepidermoid carcinoma. The clinical presentation and radiographic findings are suggestive of a carcinoma arising from minor salivary glands of the hard palate with secondary extension into the maxillary antrum through the hard palate.

The patient is placed on the operating table under general anesthesia maintained through an orotracheal tube. The proposed incision is marked, beginning in the midline of the upper lip through the philtrum up to the columella of the nasal cavity, curving around the nasal vestibule and ala of the nostril up to the nasolabial crease, and then along the nasolabial crease up to the region of the medial canthus of the left eye (3). The dotted lines show two possible extensions of this incision which can be employed for additional exposure if necessary. The extension, cephalad, up to medial edge of the eyebrow is called the Lynch extension, and is best suited for a medial maxillectomy. The extension along the tarsal margin of the lower eyelid up to the lateral canthus is called the Diffenbach extension, which provides exposure to the lateral and posterolateral aspect of the maxilla, and is best employed when a total maxillectomy is necessary. This extension is, however, often avoided since it leaves a less than desirable esthetic scar and occasionally leads to ectropion which is difficult to correct; but it does provide excellent exposure of the pterygomaxillary fossa.

Once the skin incision is made with a scalpel, use of electrocautery for the elevation of the cheek flap provides excellent hemostasis. The upper lip is divided through its full thickness up to the gingivolabial sulcus (4). Brisk hemorrhage from the superior labial artery requires ligation of that vessel. To elevate the upper cheek flap, an incision is now made into the mucosa of the upper gingivobuccal sulcus remaining close to the gingiva; it is elevated full thickness remaining right over the periosteum of the maxilla until its posterolateral aspect is exposed.

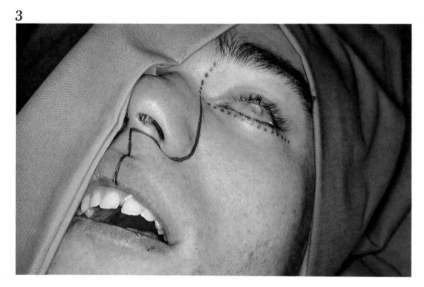

3

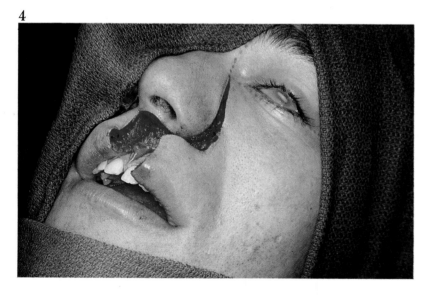

4

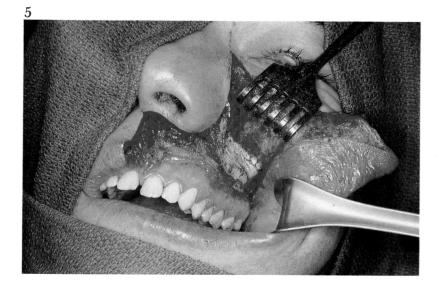

5

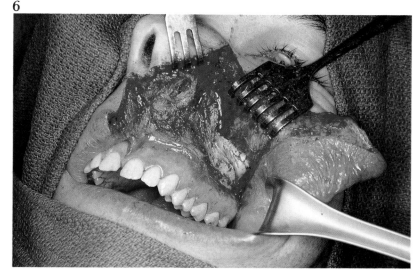

6

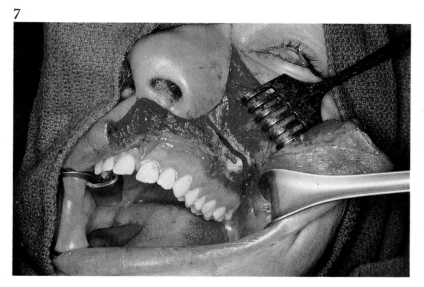

7

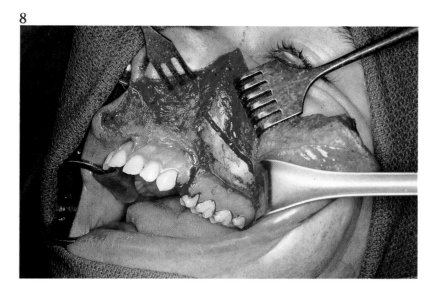

8

Elevation of the cheek flap in its upper part will expose the exit of the infraorbital nerve and its entry into the soft tissues of the cheek (5). If only the lower half of the maxilla is to be resected, then the infraorbital nerve should be preserved, thus retaining the cutaneous sensations of the cheek. It is important to elevate the cheek flap as far back as the posterolateral surface of the maxilla exposing the undersurface of the zygoma in order to gain access to the pterygomaxillary fissure.

Entry is made into the nasal cavity by dividing the soft tissues along the ala of the nose until the mucosa of the lateral wall of the nasal cavity is completely divided (6). Once entry is made into the nasal cavity under direct vision, the ala of the nostril is retracted medially, and the rest of the mucosa of the floor of the nasal cavity and the lateral wall of the nasal cavity up to the nasal bone is incised, providing satisfactory exposure.

A mouth gag is now introduced on the opposite side and the oral cavity is opened as wide as possible to provide adequate exposure of the alveolar process and the hard palate (7). Using a high speed drill and very fine drill bit, entry is now made into the maxillary antrum, approximately midway between the infraorbital foramen and the alveolar process. The line of entry is extended anteriorly and posteriorly to create a proposed line of transection through the anterior wall of the maxillary antrum to allow division of the lower half of the maxilla as the surgical specimen. The high speed drill is used to carry on the line of transection, anteriorly, through the nasal process of maxilla and, posteriorly, up to the zygomatic process of maxilla and around the posterolateral surface.

The proposed line of transection through the alveolar process is now examined (8). If there is space between two teeth the line of fracture is carried between them;

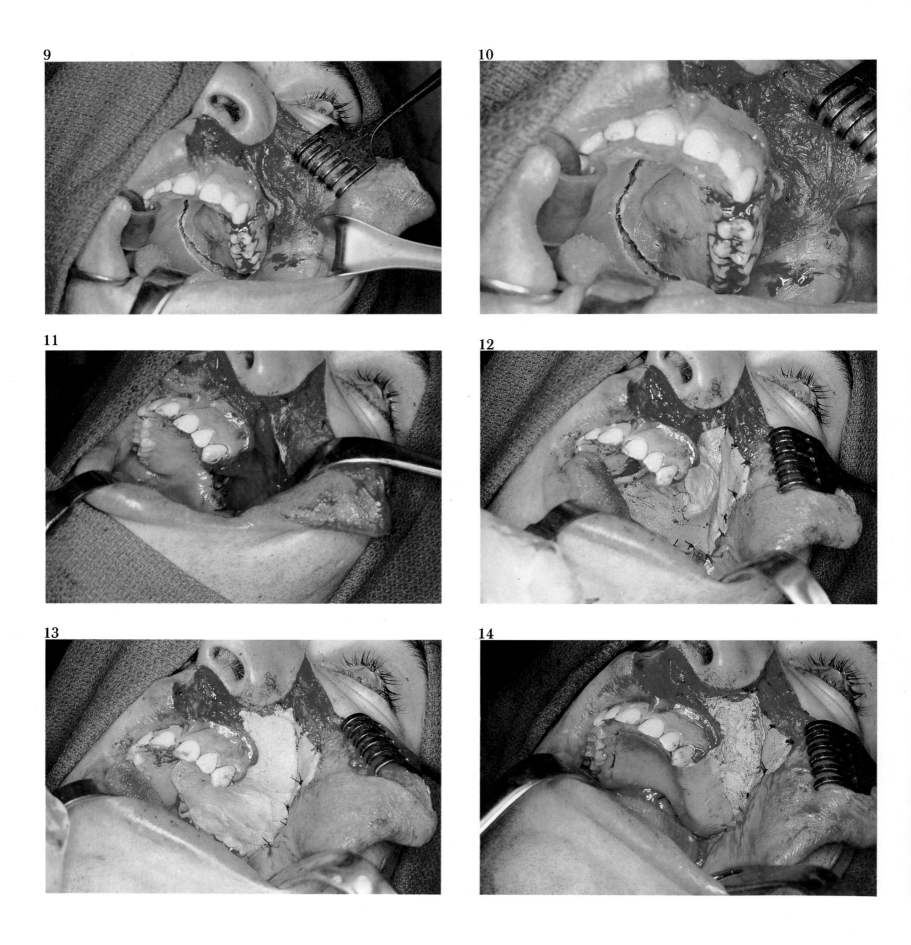

but if the teeth are compact it is quite likely that the last tooth on the remaining alveolar process will become loose and may be lost, so it is advisable to extract one tooth at the proposed line of transection of the alveolar process as was done in this patient. The high speed drill is used again, and the bone cut between the previously created transverse line of transection and the alveolar process is connected. Using a high speed drill with a fine drill bit gives a very precise line of transection through the maxilla for the proposed specimen.

Attention is now focussed on the mucosa of the hard palate, and with the mouth wide open a tongue depressor is used to give adequate visualization and access (9). Using needlepoint electrocautery an incision is made into the mucosa of the hard palate around the primary tumor keeping satisfactory mucosal margins in all directions. Posteriorly, the incision begins at the maxillary tubercle and then it curves medially, and anteriorly to the left around the anterior aspect of the tumor remaining posterior to the alveolar process containing the incisor and canine teeth on the left side. This mucosal incision meets the socket of the extracted first molar tooth to complete circumferential mobilization of the specimen. The mucosal incision in the hard palate is deepened through the mucoperiosteum all the way up to the bone throughout its length.

A close-up view of the incised mucosa and mucoperiosteum of the hard palate, as well as a portion of the soft palate posteriorly mobilizing the surgical specimen, is shown in (10). Using the high speed drill as before, the hard palate is divided through the line of mucosal incision; alternatively, a right-angled or, preferably, a sagittal saw can be used. Brisk bleeding during this part of the operation is encountered due to hemorrhage from the palatine vessels and the branches of the internal maxillary artery coming through the posterior wall and pterygoid fossa into the maxilla. Attempts at control of this bleeding are unsuccessful until the surgical specimen is removed. Therefore, it is essential to expedite this step of the operation.

Once all the bony cuts are made with the high speed drill or an appropriate saw, an osteotome is used to connect the fracture lines permitting the specimen to be rocked over the soft tissue attachments (11). Using either electrocautery or heavy Mayo scissors, the posterior soft tissues of the specimen (pterygoid muscles) are divided and the surgical specimen of the lower half of the maxilla is delivered.

Bleeding at this point is usually from the branches of the internal maxillary artery, the sphenopalatine artery and smaller blood vessels of the soft palate. Hemorrhage from the internal maxillary artery is controlled by ligation of that vessel, or alternatively a chromic catgut suture ligature is placed through the stumps of the pter-

ygoid muscles. However, bleeding from the sphenopalatine artery is rarely amenable to control by ligation; the stump of this vessel is usually in a bony crevice and hemostasis is best achieved by electrocoagulation.

The surgical defect now shows the upper half of the maxillary antrum which is lined by mucous-secreting epithelium. The mucosa of the maxillary antrum should be curetted out completely if it shows chronic inflammatory changes. This will provide a specimen for histological analysis of the mucosal lining of the maxillary antrum and leave the bony remnant of the antrum clean. If inflamed mucosa is left behind chronic edema in it will lead to pseudopolyp formation with excessive amounts of mucus which drains directly into the oral cavity, giving a salty taste. However, if the antral mucosa appears normal and does not show any inflammation, it may be left alone. All sharp spicules on the bony edges are now smoothed out with a burr. The cut edges of the mucosa of the anterior and posterior wall of the soft palate are approximated with interrupted chromic catgut sutures. The entire wound is irrigated with Bacitracin solution and blood clots are evacuated.

A split-thickness skin graft is now used to line the undersurface of the cheek flap as well as the bare, bony wall of the maxillary antrum, and approximated to the cheek flap using interrupted 3-0 chromic catgut sutures (12). The lower edge of the skin graft is sutured to the mucosa of the cheek. Superiorly, the skin graft is not sutured but merely applied to the bare, bony surface of the upper half of the antrum, and retained in that position using xeroform gauze packing, which fits snugly into the maxillary defect. Once the complete skin graft is sutured and anchored appropriately, packing begins from the roof of the antrum using the xeroform gauze which is applied into the defect digitally and retained in that position by gentle digital pressure to conform to the crevices and corners of the maxillary antrum.

Packing of the rest of the defect continues until it is completely filled with the packing that conforms to the excised surgical specimen (13). It also stretches the skin graft to fit snugly over the raw areas of the cheek and the maxillary antrum. Once the packing is completed, the patient is ready for the dental team to scrub in and apply the immediate, surgical, dental obturator previously fabricated.

The dental obturator is wired to the remaining teeth to replace the excised portion of the hard palate (14), but if the patient is edentulous, it is wired to the remaining alveolus via drill holes. Once the obturator is applied, additional xeroform gauze packing is used to keep the skin graft over the cheek flap in position with a moderate degree of pressure. Installation of the dental obturator replaces the lost portion of the hard palate and allows the patient to swallow liquids and soft diet

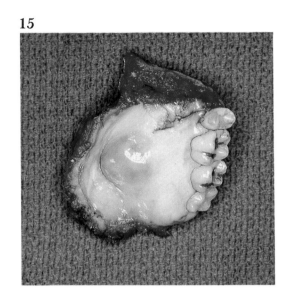

15

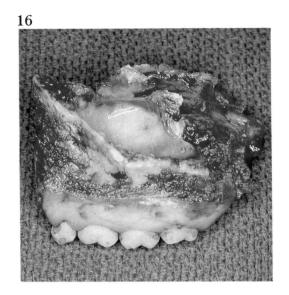

16

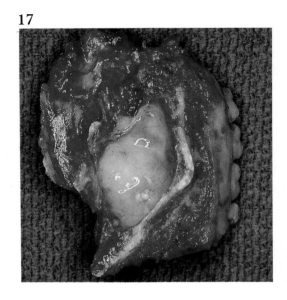

17

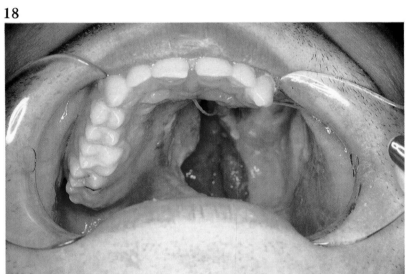

18

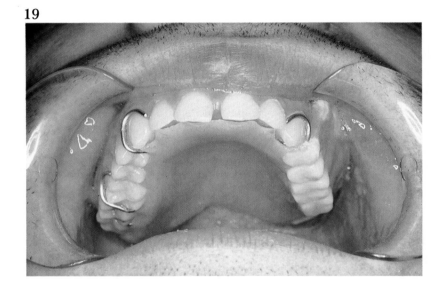

19

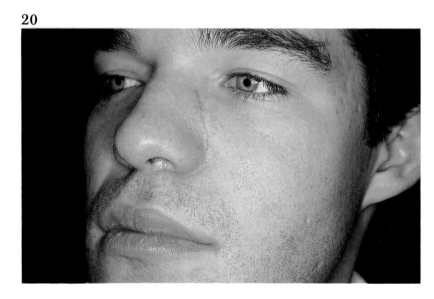

20

122

immediately postoperatively without much difficulty. If for any reason a palatal obturator is not available, the packing is held in place by silk sutures tied over the packing from each edge of the defect. However, as it is difficult to maintain good oral hygiene in such cases the patient should have a nasogastric feeding tube inserted.

The skin incision is now closed in two layers using chromic catgut interrupted sutures for subcutaneous tissues and nylon for skin. Meticulous attention is paid to accurate approximation of the skin edges since the eventual esthetic result of the surgical scar will depend on the proper approximation of the edges. The corneal shield from the eye is removed. A fine coating of Bacitracin ointment is applied to the incision. A pressure dressing is usually not necessary. Blood loss during this operation is minimal. The patient is awakened soon from anesthesia and the endotracheal tube is removed promptly. A moderate degree of swelling of the lower eyelid and the cheek is apparent on the day after surgery, but this is transient and usually resolves within 2–3 days without any specific measures. Most patients are able to tolerate a liquid or soft diet within a day after surgery.

The surgical specimen in (15) shows the palatal aspect of the excised portion of maxilla. Note that the tumor mass presenting submucosally is well within the center of the excised hard palate with sufficient mucosal and bony margins in all three dimensions.

The lateral view of the surgical specimen in (16) shows the excised lateral wall of the maxilla with a submucosal tumor mass presenting in the floor of the antrum with adequate margins in all directions.

A superior view of the surgical specimen shows the nasal process and anterior wall of the maxilla in its lower part with the tumor mass contained well within the floor of the antrum (17). Posteriorly and medially, as seen on the left side and in the upper aspect of (17), the surgical specimen provides adequate bony and soft tissue margins.

The postoperative appearance of the surgical defect approximately 3 months after surgery shows a clean maxillary defect with the lost portion of the alveolus and hard palate on the left side (18). The skin graft covers the raw areas of the cheek on the left side. The inner aspect of the cheek is soft, supple and clean.

The permanent dental obturator is clasped onto the remaining teeth providing complete replacement of the excised hard palate and lost dentition (19). This permanent obturator will allow the patient to speak normally and eat all kinds of foods.

Postoperative care

Postoperative care of the patient following partial maxillectomy centers around the maintenance of optimal oral hygiene and care of the facial wound until sutures are removed. Meticulous attention is paid to removal of all clots and crusts over the suture line, as they provide a nidus for infection and may lead to suture line sepsis with occasional wound separation. Use of warm compresses over the cheek is occasionally necessary if there is persistent swelling and/or inflammatory reaction.

On the second postoperative day, the patient is taught to irrigate and rinse his oral cavity every 3–4 hours with a solution of baking soda and salt in warm water to keep the mouth clean of all debris and secretions. This is done with a plastic bag and rubber tubing with water flowing through the tube into the oral cavity via gravity feed. Mechanical cleaning of the oral cavity with a power spray of half-strength hydrogen peroxide and saline is desirable at least once a day.

The postoperative appearance of the patient in (20) shows a well-healed skin incision with essentially no esthetic or functional deformity.

After 7 days, the patient is seen by both surgeon and prosthodontist for removal of the immediate obturator, by cutting the wires; then the packing is soaked with saline and carefully removed. The skin graft in the surgical defect is inspected, and any excess shreds of the graft are trimmed off and the surgical defect is adequately debrided to keep it clean. An interim obturator is now made using soft, Silastic mold material, and retained with clasps on the remaining teeth. Retention of a prosthesis in edentulous patients is difficult and often initially unsatisfactory. Oral and nasal irrigations, as well as sprays, continue until the patient is discharged from the hospital with instruction that he should continue oral irrigations at least after every meal while the surgical defect is still healing. It may take several weeks for it to heal completely, scar down and organize, at which time the permanent dental obturator is fabricated.

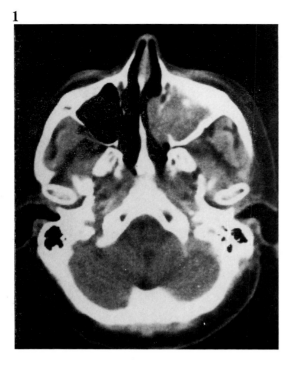

1

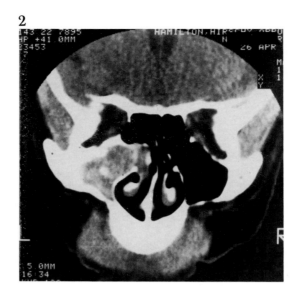

2

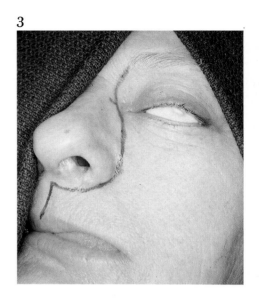

3

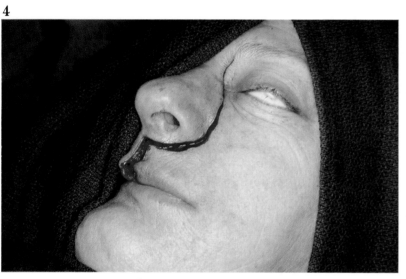

4

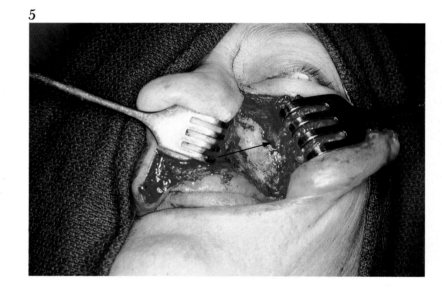

5

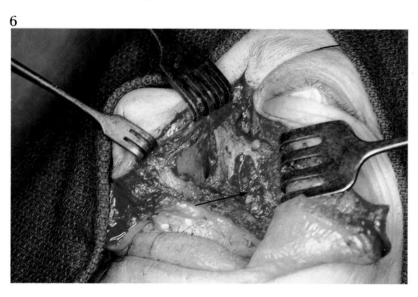

6

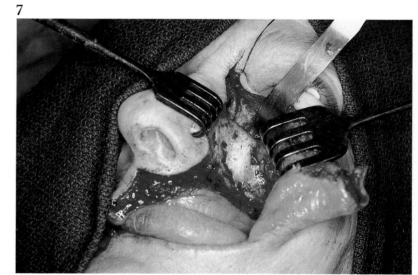

7

Medial maxillectomy

This operation is indicated for well-differentiated malignant tumors, inverted papilloma and other tumors of limited extent on the lateral wall of the nasal cavity or medial wall of the maxillary antrum. The surgical approach remains essentially the same, but technically it is often difficult to remove the surgical specimen *en bloc*. Because of the fragile nature of ethmoid air cells, mobilization of an ethmoid tumor should be handled with extreme delicacy.

Computerized tomograms of the patient shown in this procedure (1, 2) demonstrate a tumor mass arising on the medial wall of the maxillary antrum with extension into the nasal cavity and obstruction of the remaining maxillary antrum. In the transverse cut, note that the medial wall of the maxilla is destroyed by the tumor, but the lateral and anterior walls are intact (1). The tumor extends into the nasal cavity in the region of the inferior turbinate. On coronal cut, the tumor appears to arise in the region of the medial wall of the maxillary antrum superior to the lower turbinate (2). However, it does not extend into the orbit since the orbital plate of the maxilla is intact. Biopsy done through the nasal cavity showed this lesion to be an inverted papilloma.

The incision for exposing tumors arising in the medial wall of the maxillary antrum is similar to that described previously, a Weber–Ferguson approach (3). For a medial maxillectomy, however, the Lynch extension of

8

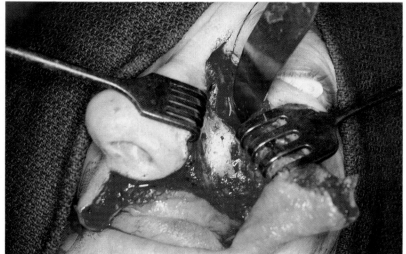

this incision is necessary taking it up to the medial end of the eyebrow. A corneal shield is placed on the eyeball. The skin incision is deepened through the soft tissues and the musculature of the upper lip and cheek up to the anterior bony wall of the maxilla (4). Superiorly, the incision is extended through the soft tissues up to the bony margin of the orbit. The intended area of resection is the entire medial wall of the maxillary antrum along with the inferior turbinate and ethmoid air cells with the lamina papyracea on that side *en bloc*. As the cheek flap is elevated, the infraorbital nerve near the orbital rim is carefully preserved (5).

Entry into the maxillary antrum is now made with a high speed drill and a burr. Use of the high speed drill permits enlargement of the anterior wall antrostomy in a precise manner. A good portion of the anterior wall of the maxillary antrum is burred out to allow digital access in the maxillary antrum (6). The interior of the maxillary antrum is carefully examined to assess the extent of the tumor in the antrum.

If medial maxillectomy is feasible, then the periosteum of the medial wall of the orbit is incised along the medial orbital rim, using a periosteal elevator to separate it from the lamina papyracea. During this maneuver, the medial canthal ligament is detached and retracted with orbital periosteum laterally. Note that in (7) a silk suture is shown through the detached medial canthal ligament for identification, and left long for subsequent reapproximation to the nasal bone. Meticulous attention is paid to preserve continuity and contour of the bony rim of the inferior and inferomedial margin of the orbit. A malleable retractor is used to retract the periosteum and the contents of the orbit laterally to aid dissection in the inferomedial quadrant of the orbit. Both the lacrimal sac and duct will now have to be elevated from the lacrimal fossa.

Using a fine periosteal elevator facilitates dissection of the lacrimal sac and lacrimal duct from the lacrimal fossa (8). The lacrimal duct is transected flush with the rim of the orbit, and dissection of the medial orbital periosteum is taken posteriorly as far back as possible. This way the anterior ethmoidal artery, as it exits from the lamina papyracea, will have to be transected and ligated or electrocoagulated. Once adequate mobilization of the orbital contents is performed in an extraperiosteal plane, a dry gauze is inserted between the orbital contents and the lamina papyracea for hemostasis.

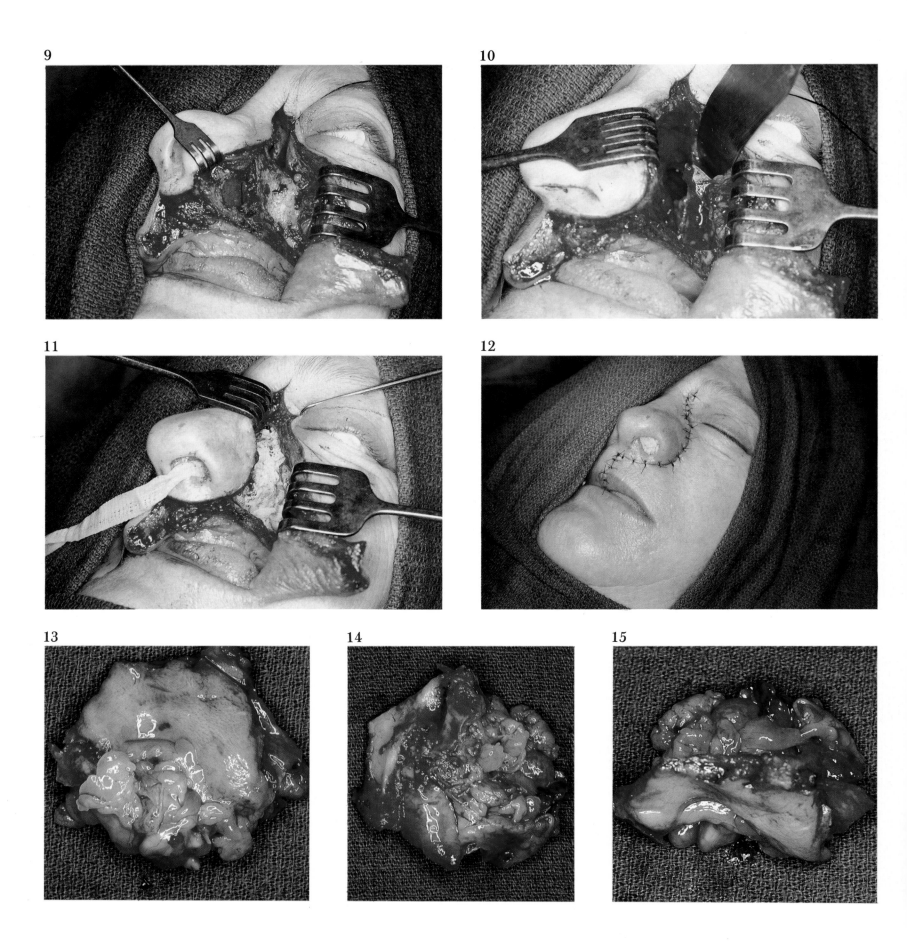

16

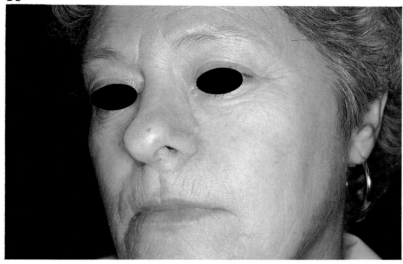

Attention is now focussed on dissection of the ala of the nose and its retraction medially (9), allowing entry into the nasal cavity. A curved osteotome is used to divide the medial wall of the maxillary antrum in a horizontal plane. This is accomplished with gentle strokes using a mallet over the osteotome until the posterior margin of the maxillary antrum is reached, as seen through the anterior wall antrostomy. Similarly, the bony cut of the medial wall is extended, cephalad, up to the medial wall of the orbit using the same instruments. In some patients, the ipsilateral nasal bone may have to be removed to give a satisfactory *en bloc* resection.

Once the medial wall of the maxillary antrum is adequately mobilized, the index finger of one hand is inserted into the maxillary antrum, and the index finger of the other into the nasal cavity thus providing bimanual palpation of the surgical specimen which is gently rocked from side to side. This will facilitate fracture of the superior and posterior ethmoid air cells. An osteotome may also be used to fracture the lamina papyracea from the orbital surface of maxilla, the nasal bone, as well as the orbital surface of the frontal bone.

Finally, using angled scissors, the posterior attachment of the surgical specimen near the posterior choana is transected and the entire surgical specimen containing the inferior turbinate, and the middle turbinate with the lower ethmoid air cells is delivered (10). Hemostasis is obtained by electrocoagulation of the bleeding points over the cut bony surfaces.

The wound is now irrigated. A ribbon roll of xeroform gauze packing is used to pack the maxillary antrum and the nasal cavity, and the packing is brought out through the anterior naris (11). Before packing is inserted, it is extremely important to smooth out all the bony spicules since access to the surgical defect for removal of the packing is only from the nostril.

During closure of the surgical incision, it is important to pay attention to realignment of the medial canthal ligament which is sutured back to a drill hole made in the nasal bone using non-absorbable suture material (11). The medial canthus is brought to exactly the same level as the contralateral medial canthus restoring the normal disposition of the orbital contents. A skin graft is usually not indicated since the nasal mucosa re-epithelizes satisfactorily, and it would make postoperative care extremely difficult since access to the graft site is limited. The remaining incision is closed in two layers using absorbable interrupted sutures for the soft tissues and nylon for skin (12). Blood loss during the procedure should be minimal, and most patients will not need blood transfusion.

The surgical specimen in (13) is seen laterally, and shows the medial wall of the maxillary antrum with projecting polypoid tumor into the maxillary sinus. Note the normal mucosa of the rest of the medial wall of the maxilla.

A superior view of the surgical specimen shows (14) the projecting tumor into the maxillary antrum on the right-hand side with the medial wall of the maxilla, and the inferior turbinate on the left-hand side of the surgical specimen. The tumor straddles the medial wall of the maxilla presenting in the nasal cavity but with its bulk filling the maxillary antrum.

A medial view of the surgical specimen (15) shows a small part of the tumor presenting into the nasal cavity with the lateral wall of the nasal cavity seen here, and the bulk of the tumor presenting on the other side of the lateral wall of the nasal cavity into the maxillary antrum.

Postoperative care

Since a skin graft is usually not necessary after medial maxillectomy, debridement of the defect is usually not required. However, vigorous nasal irrigation and provision of excess humidity are vital to remove clots and crusts until complete epithelization of the defect is achieved. Since the only access to the maxillary antrum is through the nasal cavity, patients are taught nasal irrigation with a catheter. There is essentially no esthetic deformity and minimal functional disability, although some patients may experience dry crusting due to lack of mucus in the nasal cavity, and some complain of loss of sense of smell.

The postoperative appearance of the patient (16) shows a well-healed scar and essentially no functional or esthetic deformity. Note that the globe is aligned well with the opposite side and patient has normal binocular vision.

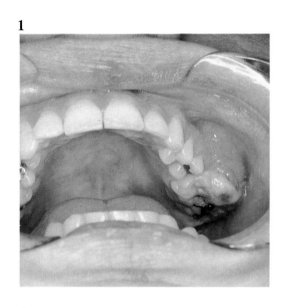

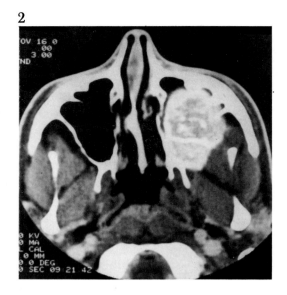

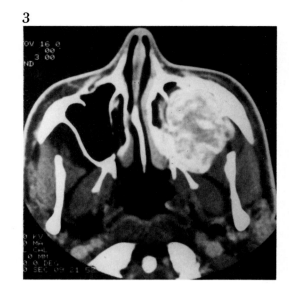

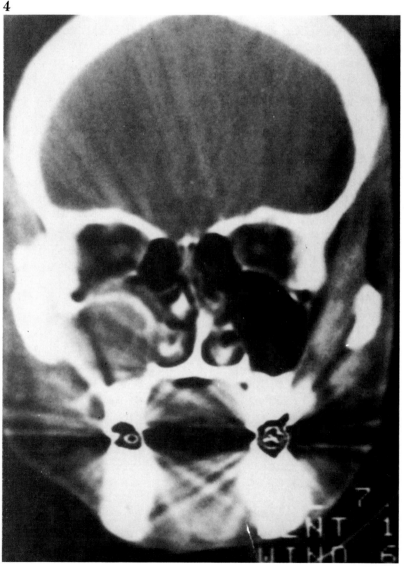

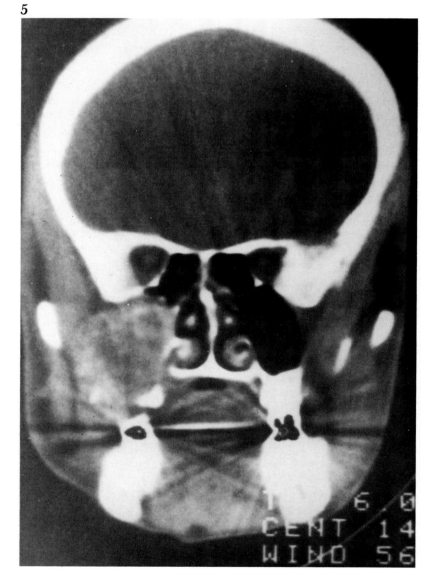

Total maxillectomy

The need for complete removal of the maxilla becomes obvious when a primary tumor arising from the surface lining of the maxillary sinus fills up the entire antrum. Primary mesenchymal tumors arising in the maxilla such as soft tissue and bone sarcomas also need total removal of the maxilla to encompass the entire lesion. Although the surgical approach for total maxillectomy is similar to that used for partial maxillectomy, a much wider exposure is necessary. With proper care and attention to detail, it is usually possible to remove the entire maxilla as a monobloc specimen for total removal of tumors contained within it.

The patient presented here (1) has a primary osteogenic sarcoma of the left maxilla presenting intraorally and posteriorly in the region of the second and third molar teeth through the alveolar process. The intraoral view shows expansion of the alveolus, both medially and laterally, on the left side posteriorly. Radiographic studies (2–5) show the presence of a neoplastic lesion filling up the entire maxilla on the left side and destroying its posterolateral wall. The tumor, however, is contained well within the maxilla both anteriorly and medially. The pterygoid plates appear intact and there is no extension of disease into the soft tissues in the pterygomaxillary space. Coronal cuts show the tumor approaching the orbital plate of maxilla with no extension into the orbit, and patchy calcification can be seen.

The incision for total maxillectomy is essentially the same as described above—the Weber–Ferguson incision with Diffenbach extension along the lower eyelid. Taking this extension provides more exposure of the zygomatic process of maxilla, as well as in the region of the pterygomaxillary fissure for separation of the surgical specimen from the pterygoid plates. This incision extension is also desirable if *en bloc* resection of the maxilla in conjunction with pterygoid plates is undertaken for tumors that break through the anterolateral wall of the maxilla and extend into the soft tissues of the infratemporal fossa or invade the pterygoid plates in a limited way. The upper cheek flap is elevated as usual with a mucosal incision in the upper gingivobuccal sulcus all the way up to the maxillary tubercle posteriorly. It may have to be extended to reach the retromolar trigone for additional exposure. Extreme care and caution must be exercised in placing the lateral skin incision, to avoid a very unsightly and edematous lower eyelid. The incision is placed as close to the eyelashes as possible. There is lack of subcutaneous tissue between the orbicularis oculi muscle and the overlying delicate skin, so extreme care should be taken in elevation of this skin flap without tearing the skin or sacrificing any part of the underlying muscle. The infraorbital nerve is divided at its exit

from the infraorbital foramen. If the tumor is confined within the antrum, then all the soft tissues anterior and lateral to the maxilla can be preserved with the cheek flap. However, if the tumor involves the anterior bony wall of the maxilla or if a previous Caldwell–Luc antrostomy has been done, then a generous amount of soft tissues should be left attached to the specimen while elevating the skin flap through a relatively superficial plane.

The cheek flap, elevated in its entirety, exposes the anterior and anterolateral wall of the maxilla, and can be rapidly elevated with minimal blood loss using electrocautery. Entry into the nasal cavity is obtained by retracting the ala of the nose anteriorly and dividing the soft tissue attachments on the nasal process of the maxilla to provide access. Then the cut edge of the skin incision is retracted medially, elevating the skin over the nose and exposing the nasal bone. Then, using a power saw the nasal process of the maxilla is divided, and a periosteal elevator is used to elevate the periosteum of the orbit from its bony floor. This elevation extends from the medial cut on the maxilla up to the transection margin of the zygomatic process laterally, and is taken as far back as possible on its floor to maintain the orbital surface of the maxilla intact for monobloc resection of the surgical specimen. No attempt is made to elevate the periosteum from the medial and the lateral walls of the orbit since bony attachment of the periosteum on these walls is necessary to prevent inferior displacement of the globe postoperatively.

A power saw is used again to divide the zygomatic process of the maxilla at the level required depending upon the anatomical location of the primary tumor. In order to expose this, extreme lateral retraction of the cheek flap with a rake retractor is necessary. Note that zygomatic process of the maxilla is a sturdy segment of solid bone that requires a deep, bony cut to obtain satisfactory mobilization of the specimen. Complete division of the zygomatic process may require the use of an osteotome since using a power saw in the deeper plane could traumatize the orbital contents or, laterally, the soft tissues of the infratemporal fossa. After this procedure, superior mobilization of the surgical specimen is almost complete. Brisk bleeding is encountered from the cut edges of the zygoma. Electrocautery is then used to divide the soft tissues over the premaxilla in the midline anteriorly giving adequate exposure of the medial margin of the surgical specimen.

The oral cavity is now opened wide using a retractor. An incision is made in the midline of the mucosa of the hard palate up to the junction of the hard and soft palate posteriorly, and extended deeply through the mucoperiosteum up to the bone. Then a lateral mucosal incision is made along the posterior edge of the hard palate at the junction of the hard and soft palate up to the maxillary tubercle, and taken deeply through the musculature of the soft palate, partly to provide soft tissue mobilization posteromedially. The midline of the hard palate is then divided through the floor of the nasal cavity up to the junction of the hard and soft palate using a power saw. The medial mobilization of the surgical specimen by fracturing the hard palate can also be accomplished by using a straight osteotome since the fracture is linear. Bleeding from cut edges of the bone is brisk and immediate hemostasis is not satisfactory, so speed is of the essence during this phase of the operation until the surgical specimen is removed.

The cheek flap is now retracted laterally as far as possible to provide exposure and access to the posterior wall of the maxilla and the pterygomaxillary fissure. The soft tissue attachments in this area, as well as the presence of the buccal fat pad, makes visualization of this area difficult but the pterygomaxillary fissure and the tuberosity of the maxilla can easily be palpated.

A curved osteotome is then used to separate the specimen through the pterygomaxillary fissure. The maxilla is separated from the pterygoid plates by placing the curved osteotome in the fissure, and applying gentle strokes with a mallet. This mobilization again results in brisk hemorrhage from branches of the internal maxillary artery. Once bony separation in this area is achieved, this specimen can be rocked by digital maneuvers. Medial and lateral soft tissue attachments should be divided with the help of electrocautery or heavy, curved Mayo scissors; the final separation of the orbital surface of the maxilla is achieved using Mayo scissors. As the specimen is rocked, soft tissue attachments come into view and they should be divided under direct vision leading to final delivery of the specimen. Extreme care and attention should be paid to gentle handling and division of the soft tissues during this phase of the operation, as rough handling may result in fracture of the specimen and spillage of the tumor.

Once the surgical specimen is removed, several bleeding points can be identified, most of which are from branches of the internal maxillary and the sphenopalatine artery. Following adequate hemostasis, the surgical defect is irrigated with saline. The surgical defect is also inspected to assure the adequacy of surgical resection, and frozen sections from soft tissue margins can be obtained at this time. All sharp, bony spicules are smoothed out with a burr. Every attempt should be made to preserve the integrity of the orbital periosteum since any breech in its wall will cause prolapse of periorbital fat.

The previously obtained split-thickness skin graft is now applied beginning at the superolateral aspect of the surgical defect, the orbital periosteum and the soft tissues in the pterygoid fossa. The undersurface of the cheek flap is also covered with a skin graft, which is usually secured with interrupted 3-0 chromic catgut sutures. A rim of soft tissues is spared at the medial edge of the cheek flap for subcutaneous sutures. Once the skin graft is sutured in position, it is molded into the surgical defect covering all its crevices and corners using xeroform gauze packing, which is placed digitally and under moderate pressure to stretch the skin graft and retain it in position. The previously fabricated immediate dental obturator is now applied to replace the resected portion of the hard palate. If the patient has teeth remaining, the dental obturator is wired to them. But if the patient is edentulous, holes are drilled into the contralateral alveolar process through which wires are passed for retention of the dental obturator. The latter supports the packing and restores the continuity of the roof of the mouth to allow satisfactory swallowing in the immediate postoperative period. The skin incision is next closed as usual in two layers, paying special attention to detail in closure of the lateral extension. An absorbable, continuous subcuticular suture extending from the medial to the lateral canthus is preferred since it avoids any irritation of the eye and provides a very satisfactory approximation of the skin edges. No dressings are necessary. Bacitracin skin ointment is applied to the suture line.

The surgical specimen of total maxillectomy is seen from the inferior or palatal surface (6) and shows removal of half of the hard palate from the midline up to and including a portion of the soft palate anteriorly. The tumor mass presenting in the region of the last molar tooth through the lateral wall is seen under the zygomatic arch, with satisfactory soft tissue and bony margins.

The lateral view of the surgical specimen (7) shows the transected edge of the zygomatic process as well as a generous margin of soft tissues covering the anterolateral wall of the maxilla. Stumps of the pterygoid muscles transected posteriorly are seen at the right-hand side of the surgical specimen.

The medial view of the surgical specimen (8) shows the transected edge of the hard palate with the inferior and middle turbinates resected *en bloc* with the medial wall of the maxilla. The superior surface of the tumor is seen at the very upper part of the maxilla. The superior view of the surgical specimen (9) shows the tumor contained within the antrum with its medial, anterior and anterolateral walls intact removing the entire tumor *en bloc* with the remaining maxilla.

Postoperative care for the total maxillectomy patient is similar to that after partial maxillectomy. Patients are

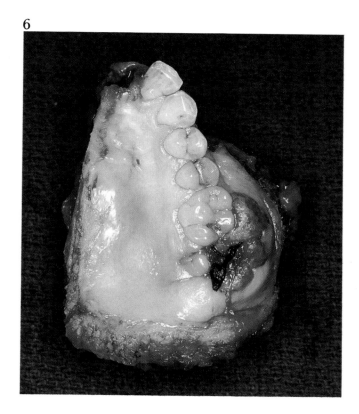

6

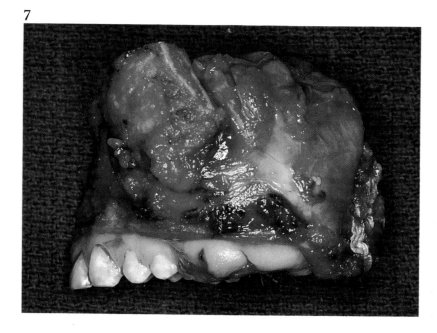

7

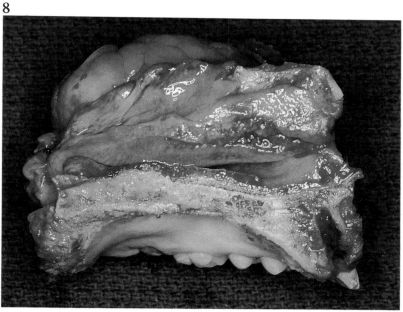

8

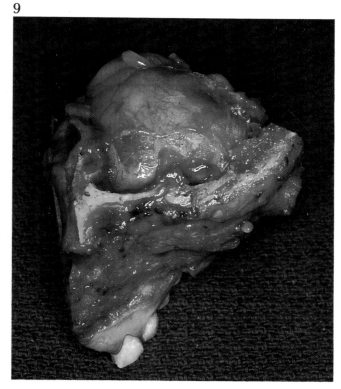

9

encouraged and trained to perform frequent oral irrigation particularly after each meal, and exercises of the jaw to prevent trismus and relieve pain due to fibrosis. Subsequent management of the patient is similar to that described for partial maxillectomy. However, certain aspects deserve special mention: minor bleeding from the raw areas and granulation tissue in the pterygoid fossa

is not uncommon and may require cauterization with silver nitrate; oral exercises are mandatory for several months to prevent trismus; fabrication of the definitive dental obturator should take into consideration obliteration of the air space in the surgical defect to restore satisfactory quality of voice. This is achieved by bolus extension of the dental obturator.

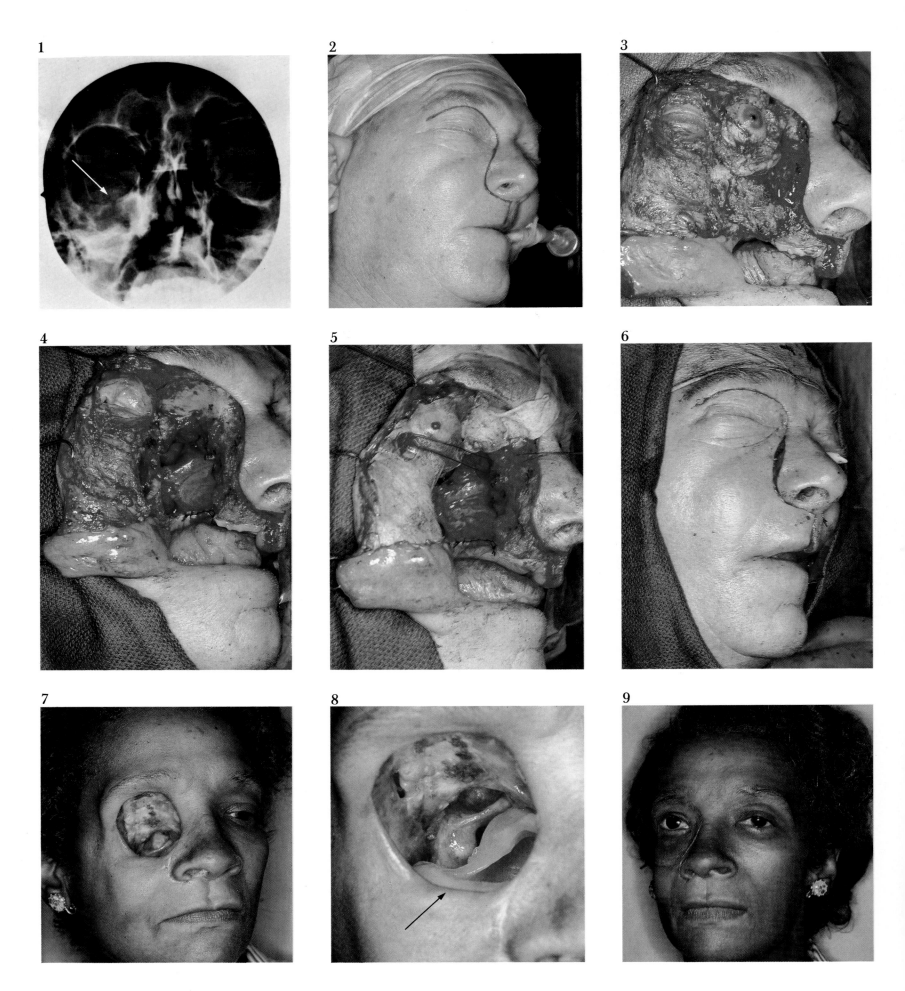

Radical maxillectomy with orbital exenteration preserving eyelids and conjunctival sac

This operation is indicated when primary tumors arising in the maxilla extend through its roof into the orbit (1). Adequate surgical resection is feasible if tumor extends to the anterior aspect of the orbit, but not to the apex of the cone of the orbit through the pterygoid fossa. If tumor extension is present in that location in the orbit, then a satisfactory surgical resection is unlikely. In that setting, orbital exenteration cannot be justified as a palliative measure. Sacrifice of a functioning eye with incomplete removal of tumor is not considered palliation. The skin incision is the Weber–Ferguson incision with Lynch extension up to the medial margin of the eyebrow (2); the skin incision then follows laterally at the lower border of the eyebrow all the way up to the lateral aspect of the eyebrow permitting total reflection of the cheek including both eyelids and palpebral conjunctiva.

The surgical steps for mobilization of the maxilla are essentially the same as that for total maxillectomy as described before (3). However, the skin incisions are modified to include the contents of the orbit. If the eyelids and the tarsal plates are not involved by tumor, they can be spared along with the palpebral conjunctiva for preservation of esthetic appearance of the patient, and to fit the latter with a glass eye. As previously described in medial maxillectomy, the medial canthal ligament is detached and is isolated with a silk suture for subsequent reapproximation. An incision is now made through the reflection of the conjunctival sac over the globe through the upper and lower eyelid. Both the eyelids with the tarsal plates and palpebral conjunctiva are now reflected along with the skin flap. Mobilization of the contents of the orbit now takes place in a subperiosteal plane. The periosteum of the upper half of the orbit is elevated using a periosteal elevator up to the apex of the orbit where the extraocular muscles and optic nerve are divided, under direct vision using angled scissors. The orbital process of the zygomatic bone is fractured throughout the lateral wall of the orbit up to its apex. Similarly, the lamina papyracea at the medial wall of the orbit is divided using a fine osteotome up to the posterior aspect of the orbit. This will complete superior mobilization of the surgical specimen of radical maxillectomy and orbital exenteration. Brisk hemorrhage is encountered from the central retinal artery as well as from smaller vessels through the stumps of the extraocular muscles, and these are ligated or suture-ligated using 3-0 chromic catgut sutures. The rest of the surgical specimen is mobilized as in a total maxillectomy.

The surgical defect is shown (4) after radical maxillectomy and orbital exenteration. The entire cheek flap containing the eyelids is retracted laterally. The surgical defect shows loss of the left half of the hard palate, entire maxilla, contents of the orbit, zygomatic bone, as well as soft tissues of the cheek laterally.

The palpebral conjunctiva of the upper and lower eyelid are sutured to each other, reproducing the conjunctival sac behind the eyelids (5). The skin graft is applied on the posterior aspect of the palpebral conjunctiva to provide support to the conjunctival sac. All sharp, bony spicules are smoothed out prior to application of the skin graft which is applied as described previously and retained in position, by packing with xeroform gauze. The immediate dental obturator is inserted as described before and skin closure is completed. At the time of the closure, however, attention should be paid to reapproximate the medial canthal ligament to the nasal bone (6).

In patients whose eyelids cannot be preserved, the skin incision is modified. A standard Weber-Ferguson incision with a Diffenbach extension is taken up to the lateral canthus of the eye. A second incision is taken from the lateral canthus of the eye along the upper eyelid near its tarsal plate up to the medial canthus. Thus, the cheek flap is elevated in the usual fashion, as is the skin of the upper eyelid to preserve it, but all the contents of the orbit including the eyelids are sacrificed on the surgical specimen. In this setting, however, the patient will not retain the eyelids, and the entire orbital socket will be exposed to the exterior. The latter would be covered with a split-thickness skin graft. These patients require a larger orbital prosthesis with a fixed glass eye for esthetic rehabilitation in addition to dental obturator. Postoperative appearance of a patient who had radical maxillectomy with orbital exenteration (7). These patients require a dental obturator to facilitate mastication and speech. Close-up view of the orbital defect shows the dental obturator in place (8). The orbital prosthesis as seen in (9) restores esthetic appearance.

Postoperative care

Postoperative care and prosthetic management of the patient with radical maxillectomy and orbital exenteration is similar to that described for partial and total maxillectomy. In addition to the dental prosthesis, the patient will require a glass eye for restoration of esthetic appearance of the exenterated eye.

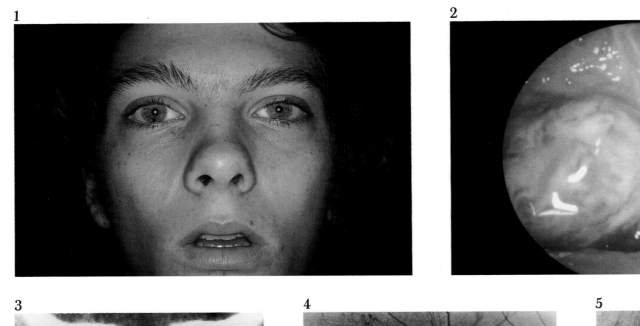

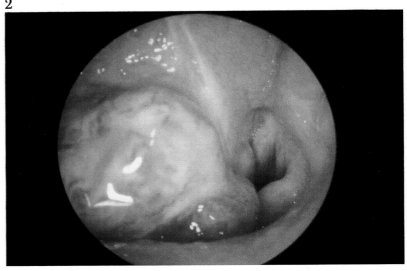

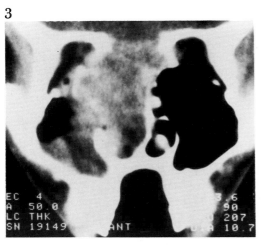

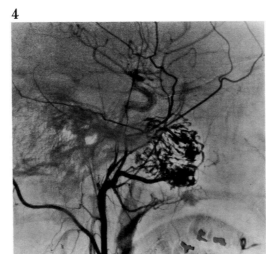

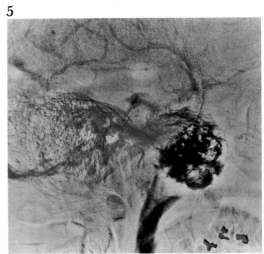

Excision of a Nasopharyngeal Angiofibroma

Nasopharyngeal angiofibromas are highly vascular fibroangiomatous tumors usually presenting in males during the second decade of life. The patient may present with the complaints of nasal obstruction and/or epistaxis. Adequate radiographic documentation of the extent of the lesion with CT scan and angiography is mandatory prior to undertaking surgical excision. Consideration may also be given to arterial embolization of the tumor immediately prior to the surgical procedure to minimize hemorrhage. With adequate exposure and appropriate mobilization of the specimen, it is not difficult to excise these tumors *in toto* with minimal hemorrhage.

The patient shown here (1) is a 16-year-old boy with the history of nasal obstruction and epistaxis of 6 months' duration. Examination of the nasopharynx and posterior choana showed the presence of a tumor projecting from the left posterior choana into the nasopharynx as seen here (2). The posterior choana and the opening of the right nasal cavity is, however, within normal limits. The CT scan in a coronal plane (3) shows a tumor filling up the entire nasal cavity with extension into the nasopharynx and breaking through the medial wall of the maxilla into the left maxillary antrum. Carotid angiography shows this lesion to be a vascular tumor deriving its blood supply mostly from the branches of the external carotid artery including the internal maxillary and sphenopalatine vessels (4). During the venous phase of the angiogram, the true vascular nature of this lesion becomes manifest as seen here (5).

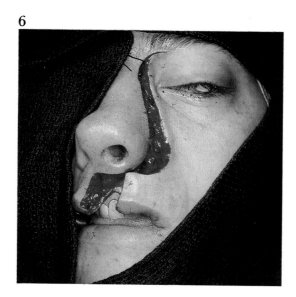

6

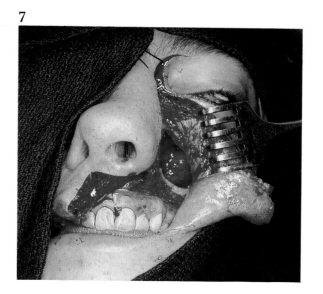

7

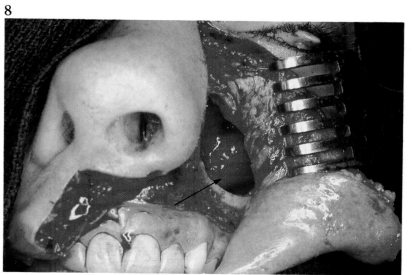

8

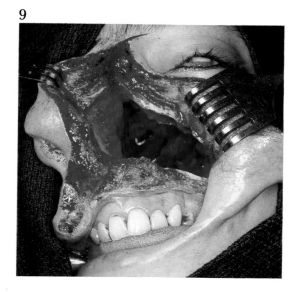

9

The surgical approach to nasopharyngeal angiofibromas presenting in similar locations is via a medial maxillectomy (6). The eye is protected with a corneal shield. A Weber–Ferguson incision with Lynch extension is taken, and extended through the soft tissues of the cheek to expose the anterior wall of the maxilla.

A generous anterior wall antrostomy is made using a high-speed drill with a burr (7). The opening in the anterior wall of the maxilla is made wide enough to provide good digital access to the antrum. Care is taken, however, to prevent injury to the infraorbital nerve which is carefully isolated. The opening in the anterior wall is made up to the nasal process of maxilla.

In a closeup of the exposure obtained so far, the nodular tumor is seen presenting into the maxillary antrum from the nasal cavity (8). Entry is now made into the nasal cavity by retracting the ala of the nostril to the right side and entering the nasal cavity through its lateral wall. Since this is a benign tumor of rubbery consistency, it can be easily mobilized by digital maneuvers

through the antrum, the nasal cavity, and by palpation and mobilization of the tumor through the nasopharynx with a finger behind the soft palate into the nasopharynx. The nasal process of the maxilla is divided, and occasionally it may be necessary to take lower part of the ipsilateral nasal bone, creating a large nasoantral passage. Removing the nasal process of maxilla gives a large opening between the nasal cavity and the maxilla which is now contiguous. Using the appropriate digital maneuvers described above, the angiofibroma is delivered. Meticulous attention should be paid to gradual, smooth complete delivery of all the lobulations of the tumor, as it is easy to fracture the tumor and leave parts of it behind. Brisk hemorrhage is to be anticipated during mobilization and delivery of the specimen. However, as soon as the specimen is delivered, all bleeding can be controlled with packing and electrocoagulation.

The surgical defect after delivery of the specimen (9) shows a large, hollow space in the nasal cavity, nasopharynx and maxillary antrum. All sharp, bony spicules

135

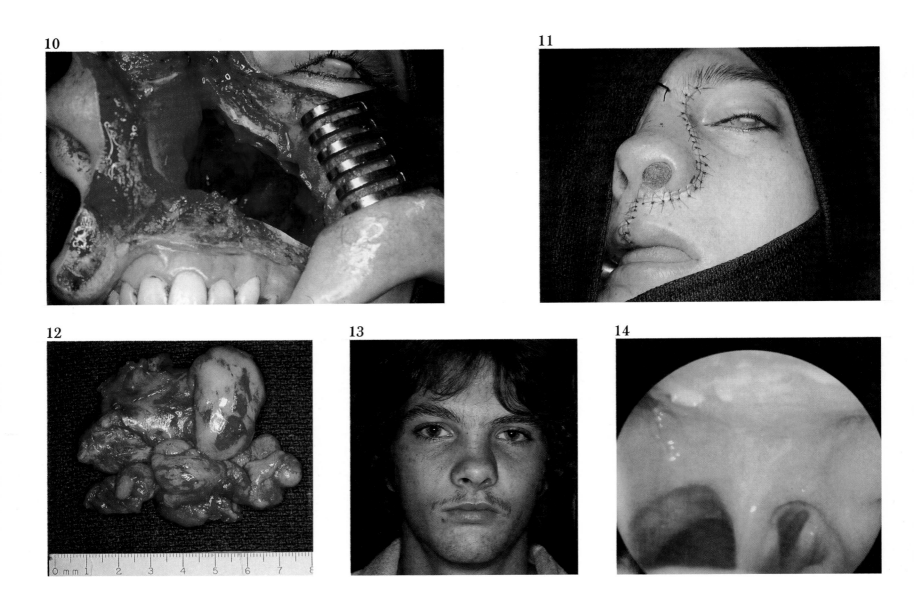

are smoothed out from the edges of the cut bones (**10**). The wound is irrigated with Bacitracin solution, and xeroform packing is used in the surgical defect being brought out through the left nostril. The skin incision is closed in the usual fashion in two layers using 3-0 chromic catgut interrupted sutures for subcutaneous tissues and 5-0 nylon for skin (**11**).

The surgical specimen (**12**) shows multilobulated nasopharyngeal angiofibroma removed from the sphenoid sinus, nasopharynx, nasal cavity and left maxillary antrum.

The postoperative appearance of the patient approxi-

mately 3 months after surgery is shown in (**13**). Note the well-healed, esthetically acceptable scar. The endoscopic view of the nasopharynx shows total removal of tumor with clear choana (**14**). No specific postoperative attention is necessary except for care of the nasal cavity and intranasal wound. Postoperative care is similar to that for medial maxillectomy: the need for frequent nasal irrigations until all crusting has cleared up, the nasal mucosa has epithelized and there is no more bleeding. These patients require excess humidity postoperatively to prevent drying.

8: The Skull Base

Introduction

The complex anatomy of the vital structures at the base of the skull make surgical resection of tumors involving this area extremely difficult. Tumors of the nasal cavity, paranasal sinuses and orbit may extend directly to involve the base of the skull and anterior cranial fossa, and local spread of these tumors can lead to intracranial extension with involvement of the dura or brain. A thorough understanding of the anatomy is, therefore, essential to master complex surgical techniques for operative procedures in this area.

A complete review of the anatomy of the skull base is beyond the scope of this book; however, to recapitulate briefly the anatomical structures at the base of the skull several views of the human skull are presented here.

The sagittal section through the left nasal cavity (1) shows the disposition of the floor of the anterior cranial fossa in relation to the sphenoid sinus, the nasal cavity and the frontal sinus.

The intracranial view of the anterior cranial fossa (2) clearly delineates the anatomical structures located on its floor. The crista galii and cribriform plate as well as the planum sphenoidale are important landmarks to be remembered during surgery of the anterior cranial fossa.

The intracranial view of the middle fossa (3) clearly demonstrates the disposition of the middle meningeal artery over the dura and the petrous portion of the temporal bone along with the sigmoid sinus, so vitally important in surgery of the middle cranial fossa and temporal bone. It is imperative that a skull is reviewed and is available in the operating room when surgical procedures in these areas are undertaken. Review of the anatomy of the petrous portion of the temporal bone in relation to the tumor to be surgically resected is vitally important prior to surgery, and CT scans of the patient should be reviewed with the skull at hand.

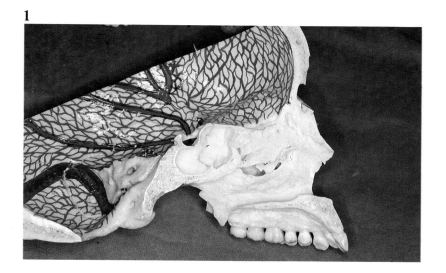

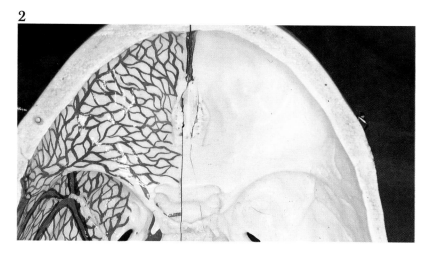

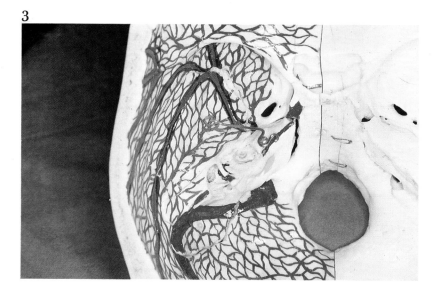

An oblique view of the extracranial aspect of the base of the skull in the middle fossa (4) demonstrates the area of the pterygomaxillary fossa and infratemporal fossa. Tumors presenting here require special attention for exposure and resection, and the complex anatomy in these areas must be reviewed prior to undertaking surgical resection.

The fundamental problem in tumors involving the skull base is that access to these tumors is difficult. If a facial approach alone is taken to these tumors without adequate exposure and control of its intracranial component, one is likely to end up with inadequate resection, cerebrospinal fluid leakage, hemorrhage, infection and its grave sequelae. The principles that must be adhered to in embarking upon craniofacial surgery are: one must obtain adequate exposure of the area of surgical resection; there must be minimal or essentially no brain retraction—the brain can be slackened using either continuous spinal drainage or mannitol-induced diuresis; if the dura is injured or resected, a watertight dural repair must be undertaken, and adequately covered with either a periosteal or a muscle flap.

An appropriate skin graft coverage should be applied to provide for an additional layer of support to the resected skull base. The clearcut advantages of craniofacial surgery are that one gets a clear assessment of the resectability of the tumor. Vital structures are protected, and *en bloc* resection can be achieved. If the dura is involved it can be resected and repaired, and the surgical defect is appropriately reconstructed to support the brain.

For the purpose of classifying operative procedures in various areas of the skull base, a scheme of division of different regions of the skull base is described (5—13). It is preferable to classify those tumors which involve the

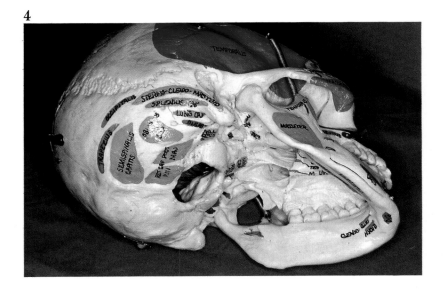

4

midline structures in the floor of the anterior cranial fossa, such as crista galii, cribriform plate and planum sphenoidale as in the anterior fossa cribriform plate region (5). Those tumors involving the floor of the anterior cranial fossa laterally in the region of the roof of the orbit are in the anterior fossa orbit region (6). Those involving the squamous part of the temporal bone, the greater wing of the sphenoid bone and the lower part of the parietal bone are classified as in the middle fossa skull base region (7, 8). Tumors arising in the auditory canal, mastoid process and the petrous portion of the temporal bone are classified as in the temporal bone region (9, 10). Finally, those tumors that secondarily involve the petrous part of the temporal bone, or present posterior to the petrous part of the temporal bone and involve the clivus are called clivus tumors. Tumors that involve the cerebellopontine angle can also present in this location and involve the clivus (11—13).

5

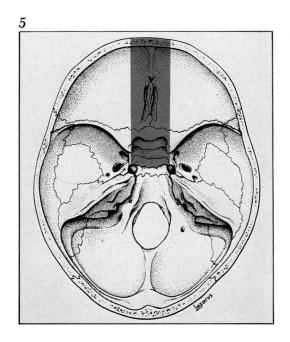

6

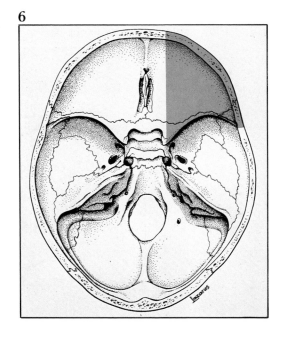

7

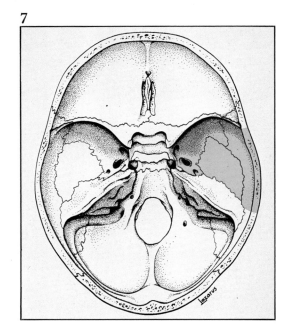

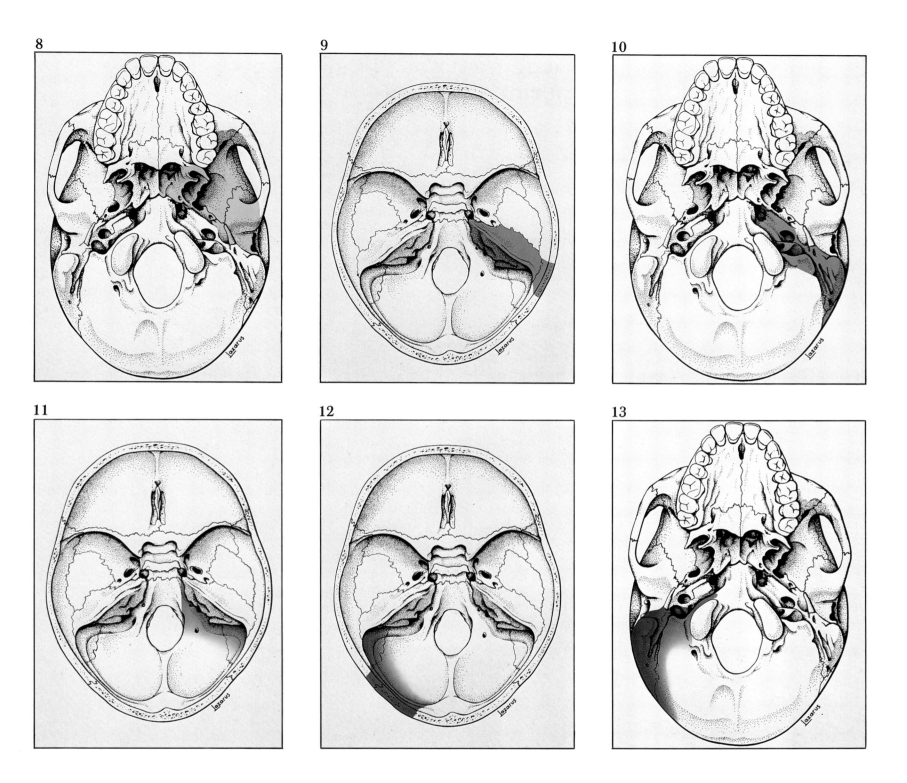

Craniofacial resection for carcinoma of the nasal cavity with invasion of the anterior fossa cribriform plate region

The patient presented in this surgical procedure has a papillary adenocarcinoma of minor salivary gland origin arising in the nasal cavity. He presented with symptoms of nasal obstruction and epistaxis.

A computerized axial tomogram of the ethmoid region shows a primary lesion arising in the ethmoid air cells with extension to involve the anterior wall of sphenoid sinus **(1)**. The tumor appears to be extending right up to the lamina papyracea on the left side. Although there is no bone destruction in the maxillary antrum, there are changes secondary to obstruction in the antrum.

On coronal section of the computerized scan, opacification secondary to the tumor is seen involving the ethmoid complex with extension up to the cribriform plate on the left side **(2)**. The tumor appears to involve the nasal septum with extension to the right side of the nasal cavity, and laterally, approximating the lamina papyracea with secondary obstructive changes in the maxillary antrum. There is, however, no intracranial extension, nor does the tumor extend into the orbit.

The artist's rendering of the extent of the tumor as depicted on the CT scan on coronal section is shown in **(3)**. The dark shadow depicts the radiographic extent of tumor with the proposed area of surgical resection shown in lighter shading. Note that the surgical resection will be a through-and-through excision including cribriform plate.

The extent of both the tumor and the surgical resection are shown in a sagittal plane **(4)**. Both the anterior wall and the floor of the sphenoid sinus will be removed in conjunction with the ethmoid tumor and contents of the nasal cavity on the left side.

A split-thickness skin graft is obtained initially prior to beginning the surgical procedure for resection of the tumor **(5)**; the anterolateral aspect of the thigh is the most suitable donor site.

The patient is then placed in the lateral position and a lumbar puncture performed **(6)**. An indwelling spinal drainage catheter is introduced through the lumbar puncture needle for continuous spinal drainage and monitoring of the cerebrospinal fluid pressure during the operative procedure. The spinal catheter is appropriately positioned and connected to a 50 cc syringe for closed drainage system.

The patient's head is appropriately positioned on the operating table **(7)**, and may be held with neurosurgical tongs as is shown here or, alternatively, the head may be positioned on a U-shaped head rest, and maintained in a neutral position with slight flexion at the atlanto-occipital joint.

The proposed lines of incisions are shown in **(8)**. A bicoronal incision is planned along the hairline extending from the tragus of one ear to that of the other, to provide a wide exposure for the bifrontal craniotomy. The facial exposure is usually obtained through a Weber–Ferguson incision with Lynch extension. The incision splits the upper lip in the midline, follows the curve of the nostril along the nasolabial fold and extends up to the medial end of the eyebrow.

1

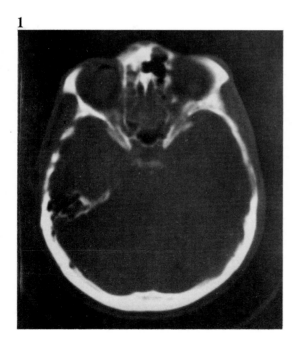

2

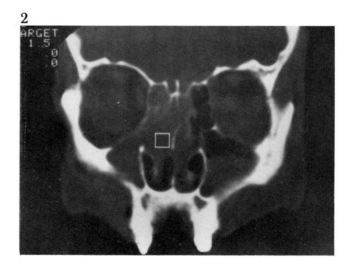

3

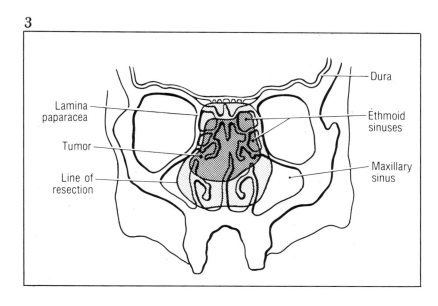

Dura

Lamina
paparacea

Ethmoid
sinuses

Tumor

Maxillary
sinus

Line of
resection

4

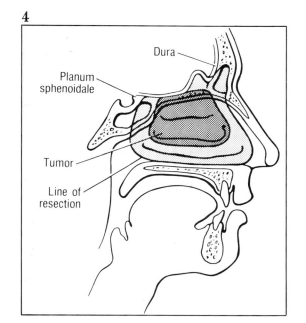

Dura

Planum
sphenoidale

Tumor

Line of
resection

5

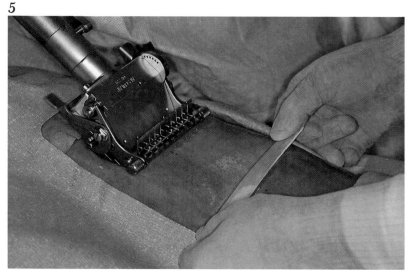

6

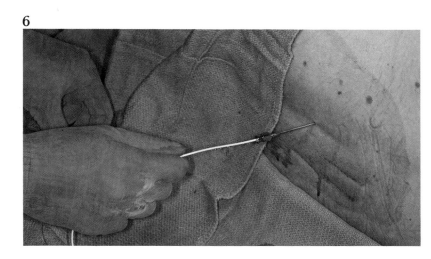

7

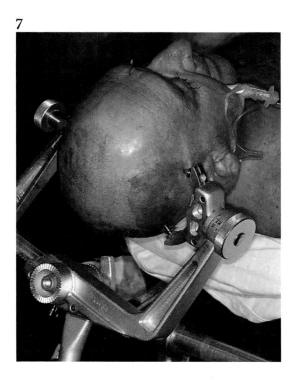

8

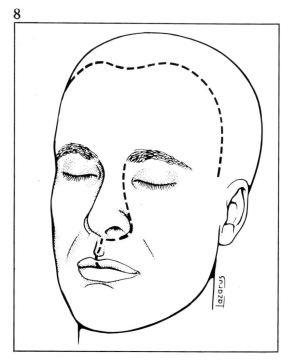

9

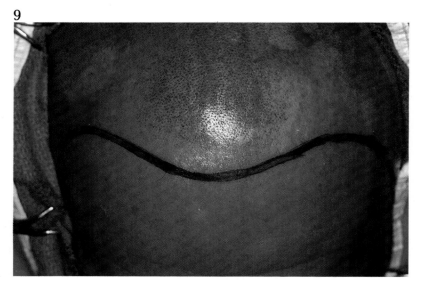

10

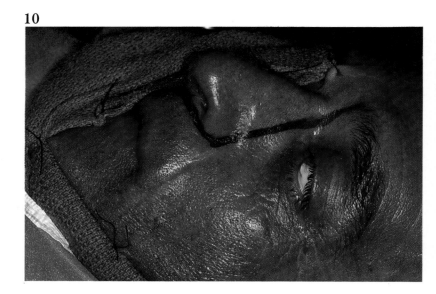

11

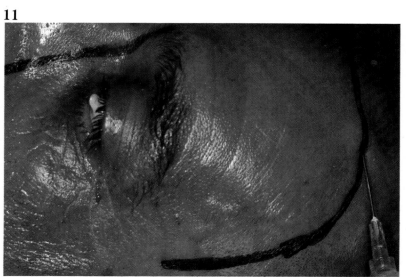

12

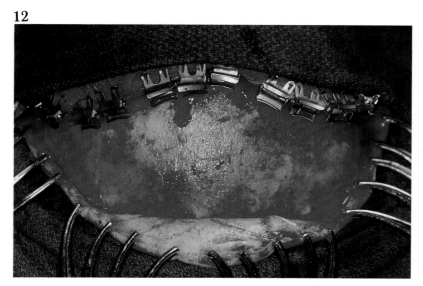

13

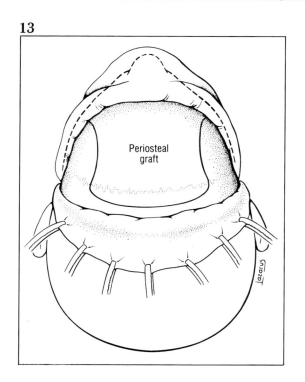

Periosteal
graft

14

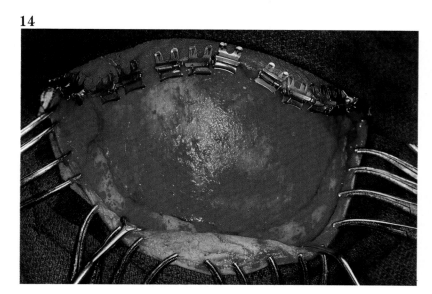

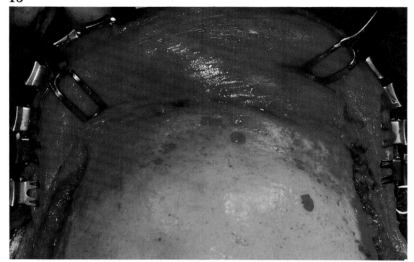

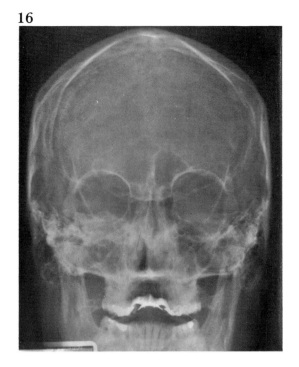

The skin of the entire scalp and face is prepared with Betadine solution. Appropriate drapes are applied to keep the area of craniotomy exposed as is shown in **(9)**. The left side of the face is exposed and isolated with the use of the drapes **(10)**. The patient is under general anesthesia with an endotracheal tube, which is brought out through the commissure of the oral cavity on the right side and isolated by sterile drapes. The left eye will remain in the surgical field and is therefore protected with a ceramic corneal shield. Cloth drape towels are sutured to the skin with silk sutures to maintain strict asepsis and isolation of the field.

Bifrontal craniotomy is begun first. The entire length of the proposed incision of the scalp is infiltrated with 1/100 000 epinephrine in saline solution to reduce bleeding during incision **(11)**.

The scalp is incised through its full thickness but up to a plane between the galea aponeurotica and the pericranium **(12)**. The plane of loose areolar tissue between the galea and the pericranium permits easy mobilization of the posterior aspect of the scalp flap. The posterior scalp flap is mobilized several centimeters remaining superficial to the pericranium. Hemostasis on the cut edges of the scalp can be obtained by using several hemostats or, alternatively, children's hospital clips may be used as is shown on the anterior edge of the scalp incision in **(12)**.

The proposed line of incision (U-shaped) in the pericranium for the elevation of a pedicled periosteal flap for subsequent use during repair of the skull base defect is shown in **(13)**.

Incision in the pericranium has been made as described above. Note that the posterior scalp flap is retracted significantly to obtain a generous portion of the pericranium for the pedicled flap **(14)**. Using a periosteal elevator, the pericranium is then elevated very carefully over the calvarium all the way up to the supraorbital ridges; any injury to the pericranium causing buttonholes must be avoided.

The exposed calvarium is shown here **(15)** demonstrating full elevation of the pericranium up to the supraorbital ridges on both the sides. Note that the pericranial flap is not separated from the anterior scalp flap so as to maintain its blood supply which is derived from the supraorbital and supratrochlear vessels. The scalp with the attached pericranial flap is retracted with loop retractors showing here the supraorbital ridges on both sides.

A plain posteroanterior X-ray of the skull clearly demonstrates the extent of the frontal sinus **(16)**. A template of paper is made to estimate the shape of the frontal sinus, sterilized and placed over the frontal bone to outline the proposed area of removal of the anterior wall of the frontal sinus. This is made in preference to a central burr hole for gaining access to the frontal sinus.

17

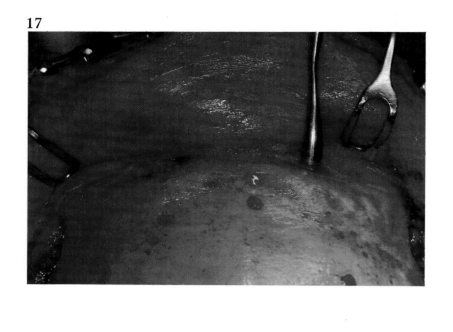

18

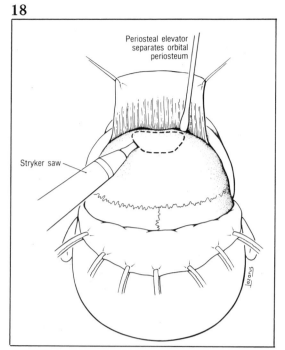

Periosteal elevator
separates orbital
periosteum

Stryker saw

19

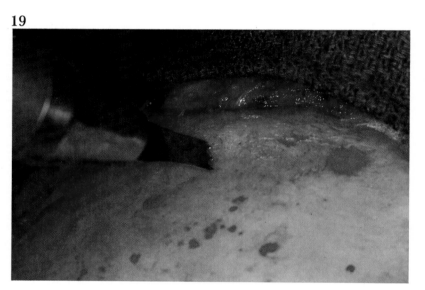

20

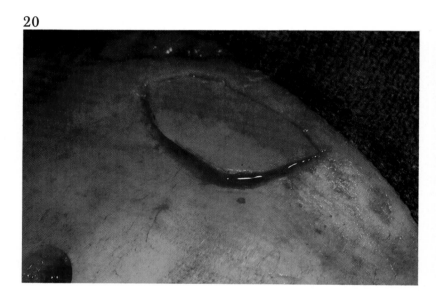

21

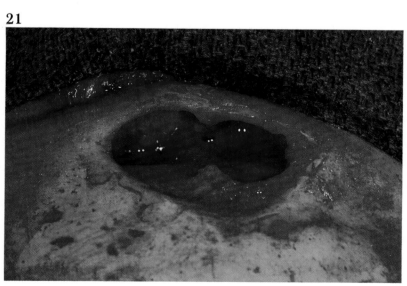

22

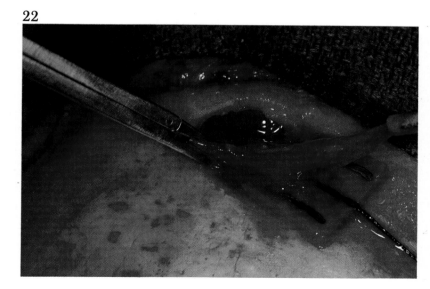

23

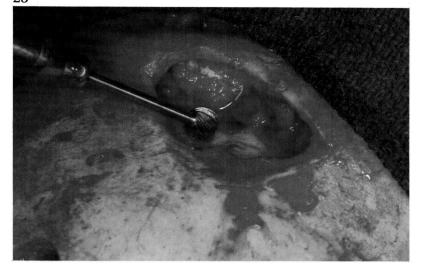

24

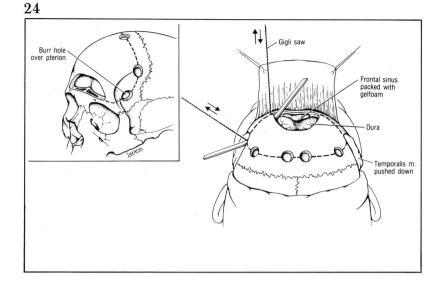

25

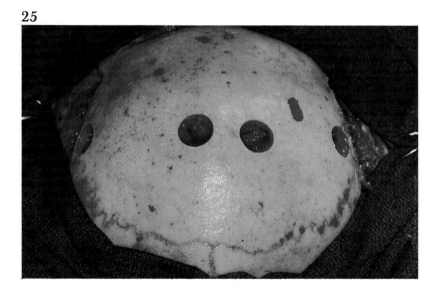

26

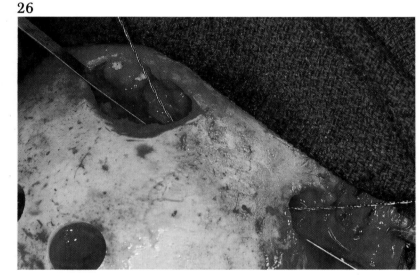

The periosteum of the roof of the orbit is separated on its medial aspect to provide *en bloc* removal of the lamina papyracea with the surgical specimen **(17)**.

The proposed line of bone cut to be made in the frontal bone along the confines of the frontal sinus is shown in **(18)**. The template of the frontal sinus is used to mark out the line of bone division and the bone cuts are made obliquely with a high-speed saw, preferably a sagittal saw with a flat blade **(19)**. Then a circumferential bone cut is made remaining within the confines of the frontal sinus for removal of the anterior wall of the frontal sinus **(20)**, and to gain entry into it **(21)**. If no tumor is seen in the frontal sinus, then its mucosa is curetted out. On the other hand, if there is a tumor then the entire frontal sinus including the floor of the frontal sinus and posterior wall would be removed *en bloc* with the tumor. In this patient no tumor could be seen in the

frontal sinus which is relatively clean and has normal glistening mucosa.

The bony septa in the frontal sinus are removed with a rongeur and Kerrison forceps **(22)**. All the sharp, bony spicules are smoothed out with a high speed burr **(23)**. The mucosa of the sinus is curetted out, and the openings of the nasofrontal ducts are plugged with gel foam.

Multiple burr holes (which can be made very rapidly with a craniotome) are now made in the frontal bone to permit elevation of the frontal bone flap; in **(24)** the relative positions of the burr holes to allow removal of the bone flap are shown. All the burr holes are completed, as shown in **(25)**. A gigli saw is then used to connect the burr holes. A close-up view of the area of two adjacent burr holes **(26)** shows the gigli saw in position for division of the bone. A guide strip is passed underneath the saw to prevent injury to the underlying dura during division of the bone.

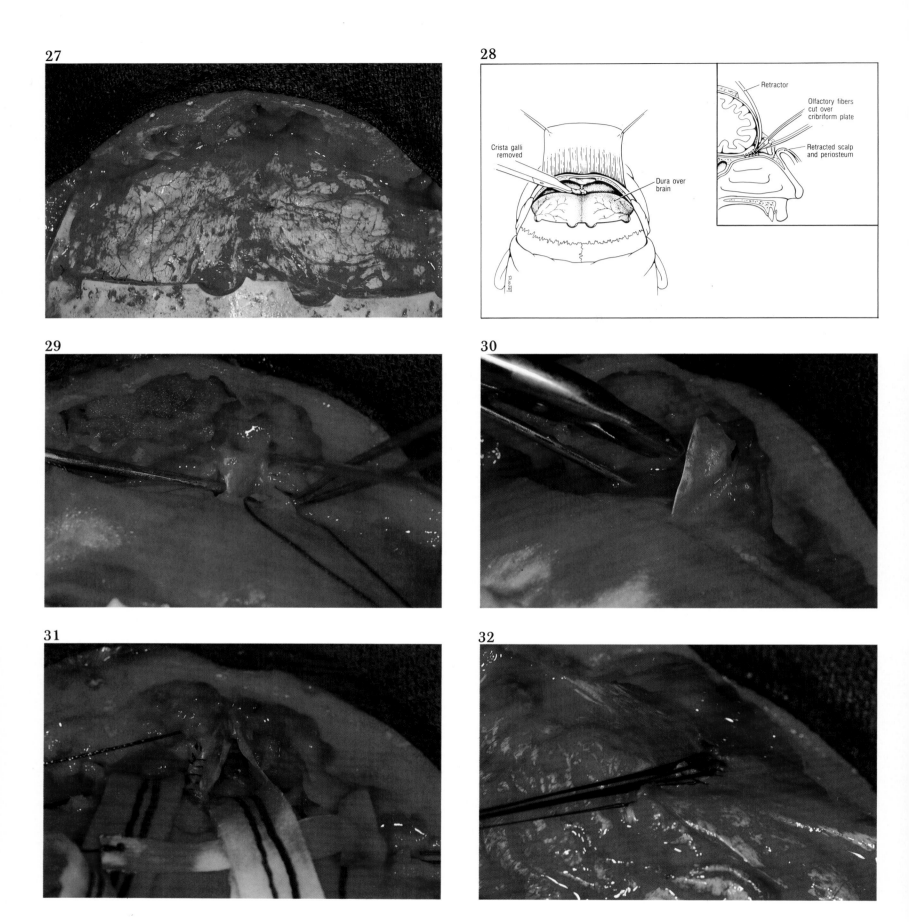

27

28

Crista galli
removed

Dura over
brain

Retractor

Olfactory fibers
cut over
cribriform plate

Retracted scalp
and periosteum

29

30

31

32

146

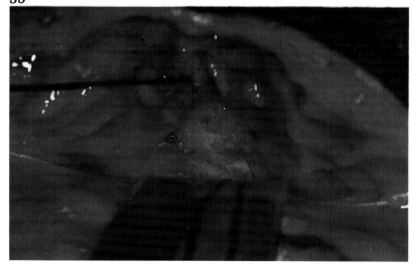

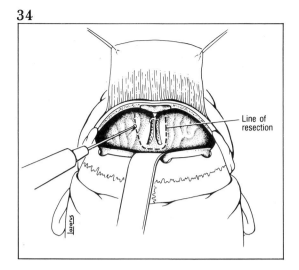

Line of resection

All the burr holes have been connected and the frontal bone flap is removed and saved for replacement during closure of the craniotomy **(27)**. During elevation of the bone flap, meticulous attention should be paid to the underlying dura which may be adherent to the undersurface of the frontal bone, in which case it should be carefully separated with appropriate dural elevators to prevent any inadvertent tears in the dura.

Attention is now focussed, as shown in **(28)**, on elevation of the dura from the floor of the anterior cranial fossa. Attachments of the dura to the crista galii require sharp division, and the dural sleeves along the olfactory nerves are individually divided and ligated.

Elevation of the dura is shown in **(29)**; the crista galii is exposed and, using a rongeur, removed giving access to the cribriform plate region **(30)**. Meticulous attention should be paid to avoid any inadvertent tear in the dura during removal of the crista galii.

As the dura is separated from the crista galii, any tears in it are immediately repaired using 4-0 neurolon sutures **(31)**. Attention is now focussed on the fibers of the olfactory nerve with its dural sleeves traversing the cribriform plate. Each of these sleeves is individually identified, dissected, divided and ligated. Immediate ligation of the dural sleeves is desirable to avoid contamination of the brain during subsequent phase of the operation.

All the dural sleeves have been divided and ligated **(32)**, with the sutures left long for demonstration. The long sutures over the dural sleeves are now cut. Approximately 10–12 mls of cerebrospinal fluid is removed at this time to allow slackening of the brain. A malleable retractor is used along the midline over the sagittal sinus to expose the posterior part of the cribriform plate and planum sphenoidale **(33)**.

As is shown in **(34)**, a high-speed drill is now used to cut the bone on the floor of the anterior cranial fossa to mobilize the proposed specimen. Since this patient's tumor involves the ethmoid air cells on the left side, the bone cut will go through the medial aspect of the orbit, allowing removal of the lamina papyracea on the left side with the specimen. On the right side, however, the bone cut will go through the ethmoid air cells since the right ethmoid air cells are completely clear as seen preoperatively on the CT scan.

35

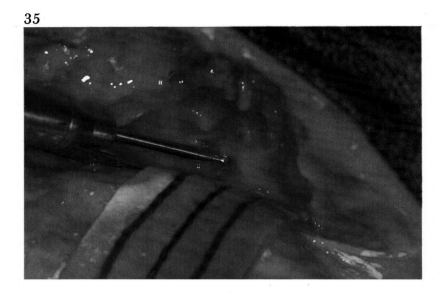

36

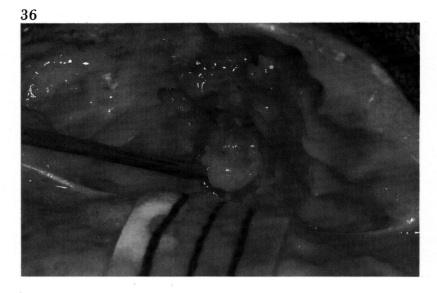

37

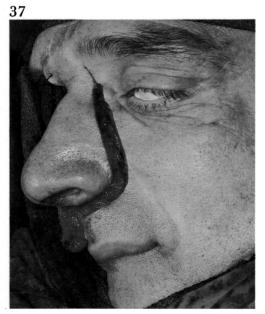

38

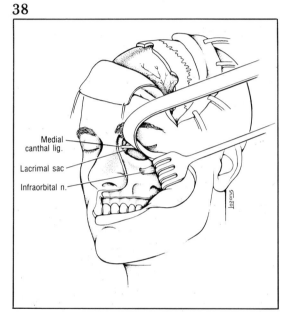

Medial
canthal lig.

Lacrimal sac

Infraorbital n.

39

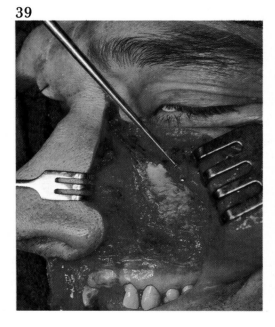

40

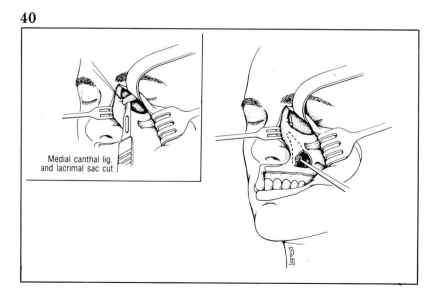

Medial canthal lig.
and lacrimal sac cut

41

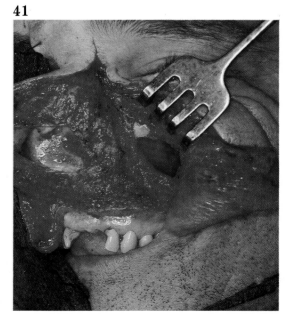

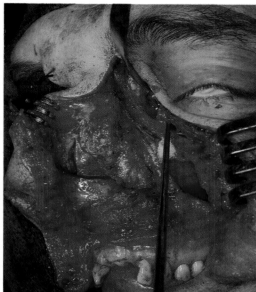

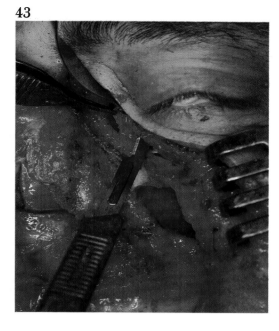

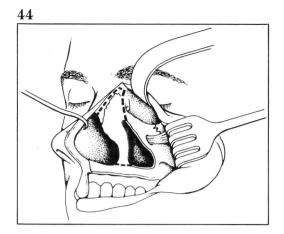

The high-speed drill is now used to make the bone cuts through the floor of the anterior cranial fossa **(35)**. The circumferential bone cut around the cribriform plate is completed **(36)**. Note that the bone cut has completely mobilized the superior aspect of the surgical specimen. At this point, the first phase of the operative procedure by mobilization of the specimen through craniotomy is complete.

The facial approach begins with the Weber–Ferguson incision **(37)**, which is taken up to the medial aspect of the eyebrow through full thickness of the soft tissues and musculature of the face.

The cheek flap is elevated directly over the anterior bony wall of the maxilla, but carefully preserving the infraorbital nerve as it exits from the infraorbital foramen **(38)**. Periosteum of the orbit is also elevated to keep the contents of the orbit within its periosteum, but this would need detachment of the medial canthal ligament as well as division of the nasolacrimal duct.

The cheek flap is retracted laterally showing the infraorbital nerve coming out of the infraorbital foramen and going to the cheek **(39)**. The nerve is carefully preserved to maintain sensation of the cheek skin.

The nasolacrimal duct and the lacrimal sac are delivered from the lacrimal fossa using fine periosteal eleva-

tors, and are divided flush with the rim of the orbit. The medial canthal ligament is divided and tagged with a suture **(40)**. The nasolacrimal duct is grasped with a fine-toothed forceps and divided with a scalpel, as shown here **(41)**.

The anterior wall of the maxillary antrum is opened with the use of a high speed drill **(42)**, large enough to permit easy insertion of an index finger. Careful inspection of the interior of the antrum is made to see whether there is any tumor present—no tumor could be seen in this patient. The soft tissues of the nose are elevated over the nasal bone and the nasal septum.

A periosteal elevator is used to raise the lacrimal duct from the lacrimal fossa. Similarly, the orbital periosteum is elevated from the bony orbit in its medial half. A malleable retractor is introduced into the orbit, retracting the globe laterally and putting the nasolacrimal duct on tension. The latter is grasped with a fine-toothed forceps and the duct divided with a scalpel **(43)**.

Bone cuts are now made through the nasal process of maxilla as well as the nasal bone and the medial wall of the maxillary antrum **(44)**, to allow complete mobilization of the lateral wall of the nasal cavity, including lamina papyracea of the left side.

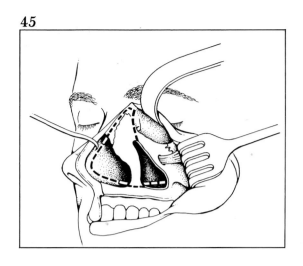

45

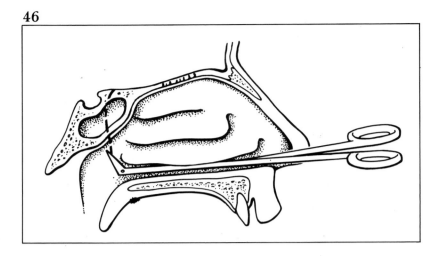

46

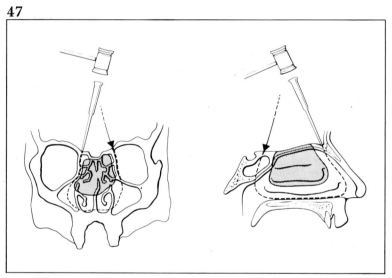

47

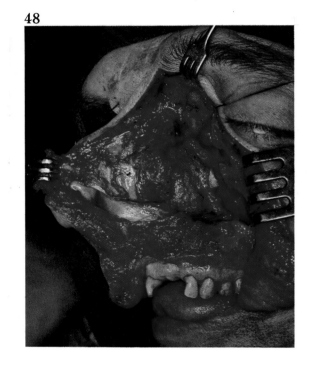

48

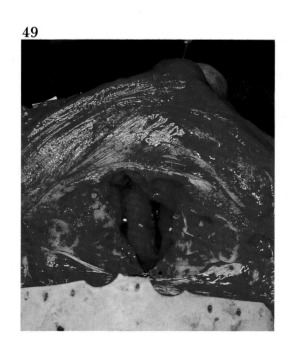

49

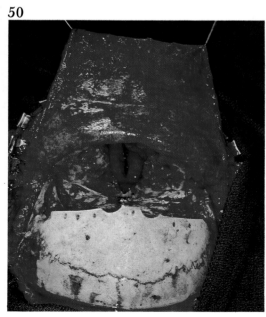

50

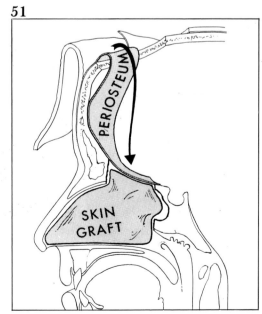

51

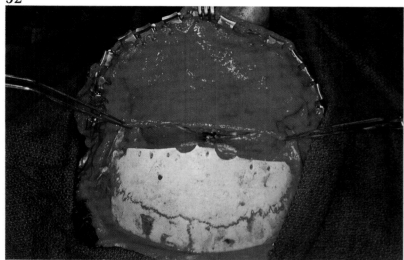

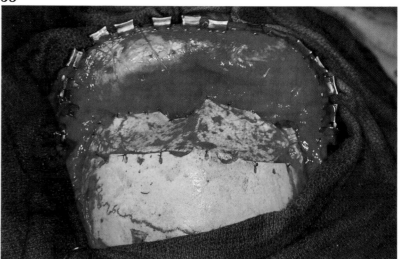

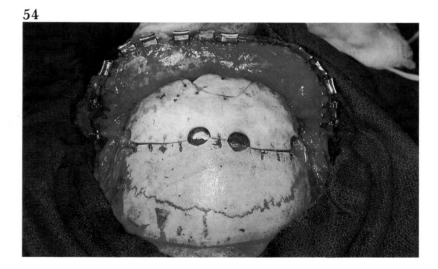

An incision is also made in the nasal septum, as shown in (45) to complete medial mobilization of the surgical specimen and totally remove the tumor in the ethmoid air cells.

Angled scissors are now used to cut through the posterior aspect of the lateral wall of the nasal cavity (46), being introduced through the nostril and guided with a finger from the antrum to cut cephalad.

The cranial aspect of the surgical field is now exposed, and with digital and visual guidance provided by the head and neck surgeon from the facial aspect, the specimen is finally removed (47). Straight osteotomes are used from the cranial cavity, mobilizing the specimen laterally through the medial aspect of the left orbit and through the ethmoid air cells on the right side as well as through the sphenoid sinus posteriorly, as shown in (47). Gentle strokes with a mallet on the osteotome are necessary to complete the fracture of remaining bony attachments and allow delivery of the specimen.

The surgical defect is seen from the facial aspect showing complete exenteration of the nasal cavity and removal of the lateral wall of the nasal cavity (48). Note the silk suture overlying the upper eyelid that identifies the medial canthal ligament to be resutured to the remaining nasal bone for repositioning of the medial canthus in its normal position.

The surgical defect seen from the cranial cavity (49) shows a through-and-through resection of the bony floor of the anterior cranial fossa in the region of the cribriform plate.

The previously elevated pericranial flap is now brought in the field (50) to cover the bony defect in the anterior skull base. For this, several drill holes are made in the cut edges of the bony floor of the anterior cranial fossa. This will involve making drill holes through the roof of the orbit on the left side, through the shelf of the bone along the right ethmoid air cells, and through the planum sphenoidale posteriorly.

A diagrammatic representation of how the periosteal pedicled flap is swung down to cover the bony defect in the skull base is shown in (51).

The pericranial flap is now sutured to the bony skull base, providing complete closure of the bony defect in the skull (52). Several interrupted sutures are taken between the pericranium and the drill holes through the floor of the anterior cranial fossa.

The previously withdrawn cerebrospinal fluid is now reintroduced, and the brain is allowed to expand. Meticulous hemostasis is confirmed at this stage of the operation prior to closure of the craniotomy, and the wound is irrigated with Bacitracin solution. Several drill holes are made obliquely, so as to go only through the outer table of the cut edges of the frontal bone to reapproximate the bone flap to the rest of the calvarium (53). Several neurolon sutures are taken between the dura and the drill holes through the outer table in the frontal bone to cause tenting of the dura, a maneuver that prevents a dissecting extradural hematoma.

The bone flap is now returned and secured in position with several neurolon sutures (54), and the bony tem-

55

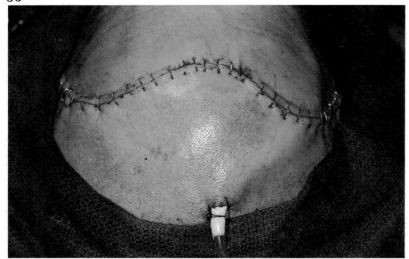

56

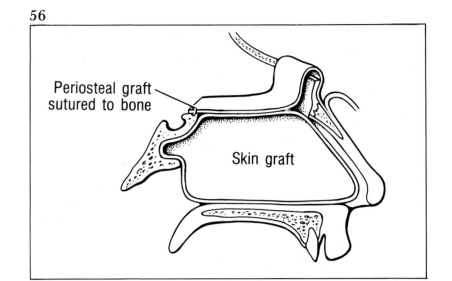

Periosteal graft sutured to bone

Skin graft

57

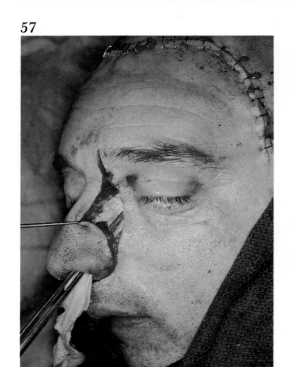

58

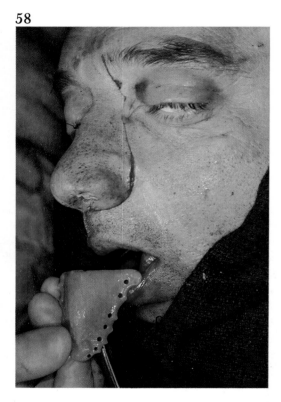

59

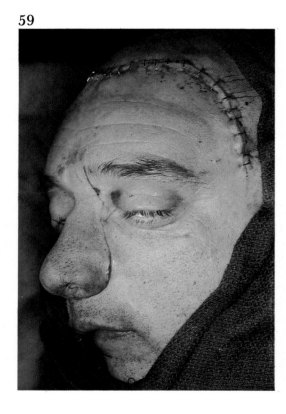

60

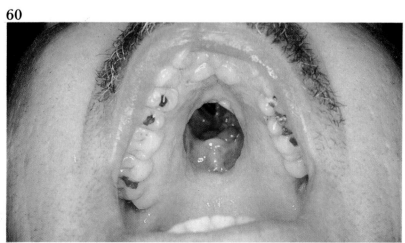

61

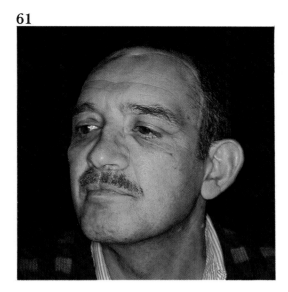

62

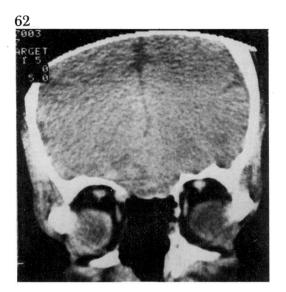

63

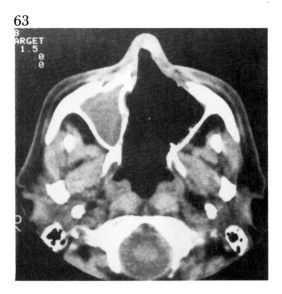

plate of the anterior wall of the frontal sinus is replaced similarly. A suction drain is placed under the scalp and the scalp wound is closed in two layers (**55**).

From the facial aspect, the previously harvested split-thickness skin graft is applied to the raw areas in the nasal cavity (**56**), directly approximating the nasal aspect of the pericranial flap at the skull base. The skin graft is retained in position by xeroform gauze packing introduced through the nasal cavity to support the graft which will line the raw areas in the nasal cavity and appose the pericranium at the roof of the nasal cavity (**57**). The bony defect at the skull base will thus be repaired with two layers consisting of the pedicled pericranial flap and split-thickness skin graft. The medial canthal ligament is sutured through a drill hole to the left nasal bone with non-absorbable suture. The two medial canthi are positioned at exactly the same level.

The facial incision is then closed in layers (**58**). A central palatal fenestration is made providing access through the oral cavity into the surgical defect in the nose. The packing in the nose is retained and the pala-

tal fenestration plugged with a surgical dental obturator wired to the remaining teeth. This obturator remains for 1 week and is then removed, as is the packing, through the oral cavity. Following insertion of the dental obturator, the facial incision is closed (**59**).

The postoperative appearance of the patient at approximately 3 months after surgery (**60**) shows the palatal fenestration in the oral cavity—the surgical defect can be visualized. This fenestration gives access to the nasal cavity for irrigation and debridement of crusts and excess shreads of skin graft to maintain adequate hygiene.

The postoperative appearance of the patient at approximately 3 months (**61**) shows well-healed incisions. The external facial deformity is minimal, the patient has binocular vision, and the disposition of the globe on the left side is essentially normal.

Postoperative CT scans in transverse and coronal cuts show total exenteration of the nasal cavity and contents of the left maxillary antrum demonstrating complete removal of the tumor of the nasal cavity (**62, 63**).

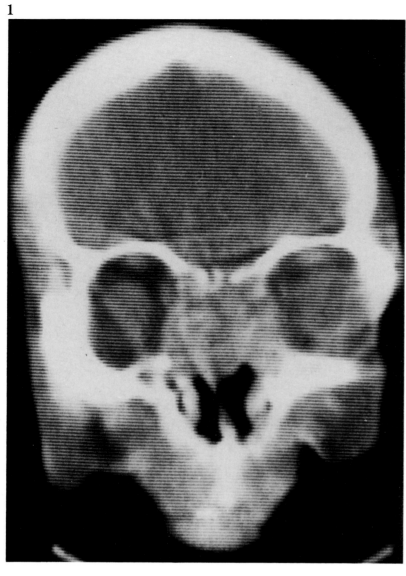

1

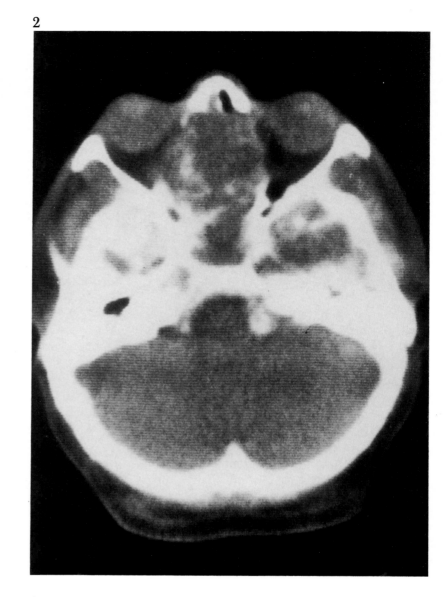

2

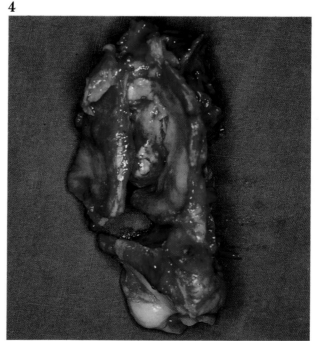

3

Crista
galli

Nasal
septum

Medial
wall
of orbit

Tumor

Inferior
turbinate

Hard
palate

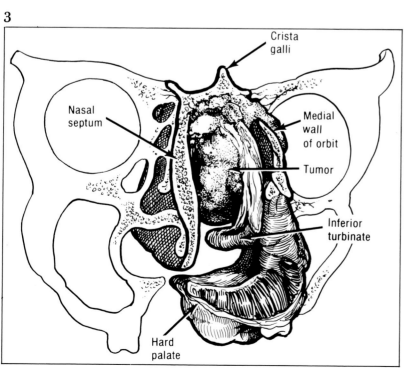

4

A two-team simultaneous craniofacial resection for tumors involving the bony anterior skull base is an extremely satisfactory operative procedure which permits monobloc resection of tumors that are otherwise not amenable to satisfactory surgical resection. If the orbit is involved by the tumor, it may have to be exenterated, but if the primary tumor is confined strictly to the nasal cavity and ethmoid complex then contents of both orbits can be safely preserved. An additional example of craniofacial resection for carcinoma of the ethmoid complex with exenteration of the nasal cavity but preservation of both orbits is demonstrated in this patient who presented with epistaxis and nasal obstruction. A biopsy of the nasal tumor confirmed the diagnosis of Schneiderian carcinoma of the ethmoid.

A radiographic assessment of the patient's tumor as seen here (1) in a coronal cut of CT scan shows the primary tumor completely replacing the ethmoid complex with extension of tumor up to the cribriform plate on both sides, although it does not involve the orbit or maxilla on either side. Inferiorly, the tumor is clear of the hard palate.

A transverse cut of the CT scan taken through the midplane of the orbit shows an extensive tumor extending from the anterior aspect of the nasal cavity to fill up the entire ethmoid complex with secondary obstructive changes in the sphenoid sinus (2). The lamina papyracea on the left side appears to be destroyed, although at the time of surgery there was no gross extension of tumor into the orbital socket.

The artist's rendering of the extent of surgical resection (3) demonstrates the proposed surgical specimen as shown by the shaded area. The entire nasal cavity on the left side will be exenterated including the medial wall of the orbit, the medial wall of the maxilla, the left half of the hard palate, nasal septum, as well as the crista galii and cribriform plate.

The surgical specimen as shown in (4) demonstrates the nasal septum, the tumor in the ethmoid complex, and the lateral wall of the nasal cavity on the left side along with the floor of the nasal cavity and a portion of the hard palate on the left side. At the upper end of the surgical specimen, one can clearly see the crista galii and cribriform plate on both sides giving a satisfactory monobloc resection of the tumor.

The postoperative CT scan of the patient (5) demonstrates the surgical defect following resection of the tumor. Note that the displaced orbit on the left side has now returned to its normal position with removal of the lamina papyracea on the left side. The entire nasal cavity from the nasal bones through the posterior wall of the sphenoid sinus is totally exenterated as seen here.

5

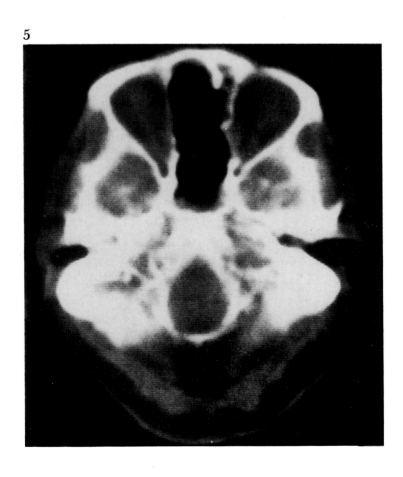

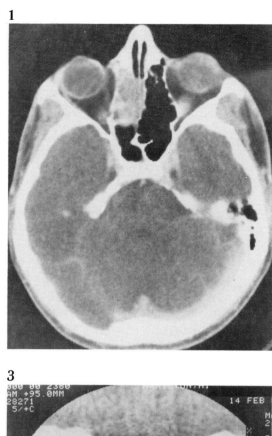

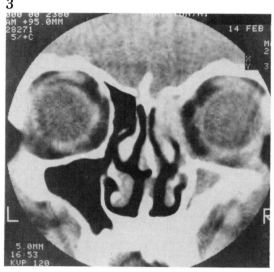

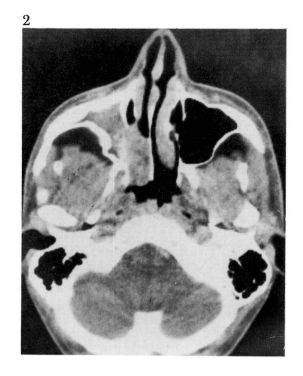

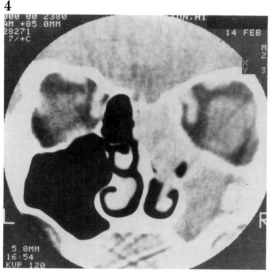

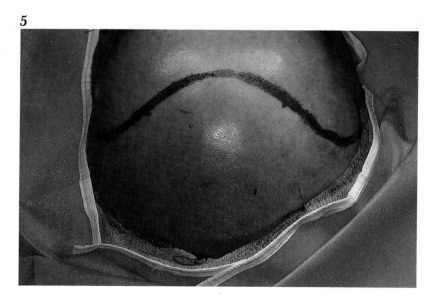

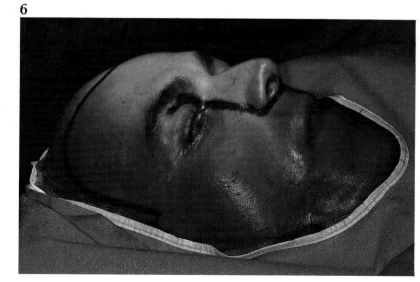

156

Craniofacial resection for carcinoma of the ethmoid with extension to maxilla

This surgical procedure requires the expertise of two surgical teams working simultaneously to facilitate *en bloc* resection of the tumor. The patient presented here had an adenoidcystic carcinoma arising in the ethmoid air cells on the right side with extension to involve the cribriform plate cephalad, and the nasal cavity and maxillary antrum caudad, but not the contents of the orbit. The surgical procedure contemplated here will resect the entire primary tumor in continuity with the crista galii, cribriform plate, ethmoid complex, contents of the nasal cavity and right maxilla by partial maxillectomy.

A review of the CT scans shows the tumor arising in right ethmoid air cells but not extending into the orbit (1). A lower section of CT scan clearly shows tumor extension in the right maxillary antrum (2).

The coronal cut of a CT scan through the region of the crista galii shows the tumor extending up to the cribriform plate (3), and a posterior section shows extension from the cribriform plate down to the maxillary antrum, but the orbit is not involved (4).

After induction of general endotracheal anesthesia, a split-thickness skin graft (1/18 000″) is obtained from the anterolateral aspect of the thigh for subsequent use during the course of the operation; a single sheet of split graft measuring approximately 7.5 × 20 cm is sufficient to cover the surgical defect. The donor site on the thigh is covered with xeroform gauze and appropriate dressings are applied.

The patient is now turned over on his side and a lumbar puncture performed with the insertion of a flexible indwelling spinal drainage catheter introduced into the lumbar subarachnoid space and connected to a closed drainage system for removal of cerebrospinal fluid as needed.

The entire scalp is shaved. The head is placed in a straight supine position with appropriate neurosurgical tongs and vice, or alternatively kept rested on a U-shaped head rest. General anesthesia is maintained through an orotracheal anesthetic tube which is kept outside the surgical field with appropriate drapes (5). The entire face and scalp are now prepared with Betadine solution, and a bicoronal scalp incision and Weber–Ferguson incision with Lynch extension is marked out (6). A ceramic corneal shield is introduced in the right eye.

After appropriate draping and isolation of the face and head, the face is covered with a sterile drape, and the neurosurgical team begins the operative procedure. A bifrontal craniotomy is performed through a coronal incision on the scalp extending from the region of the tragus of one ear and following the hairline up to the tragus of the opposite ear. The scalp is incised through the galea but remaining superficial to the pericranium.

Brisk hemorrhage is encountered from the cut edges of the scalp on both sides (7). This can be easily controlled with a series of hemostats or by using children's hospital clips tacked to the cut edge of the scalp, and a cloth towel. Both anterior and posterior flaps are elevated superficial to the pericranium.

The posterior portion of the incised scalp is, however, elevated further back significantly to allow for exposure of a large area of the pericranium (8). An incision is now made in the pericranium as far back as possible to permit elevation of a pedicled periosteal flap. The incision is made transversely first and then extended on each side anteriorly up to the anterior aspect of the scalp.

7

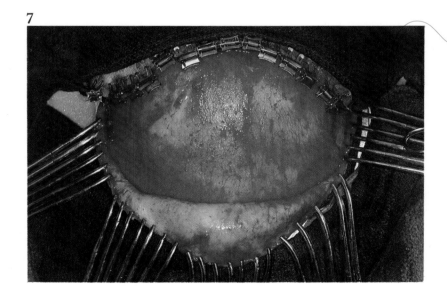

8

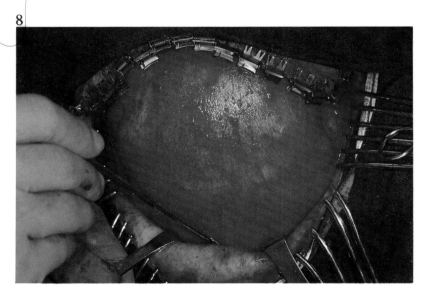

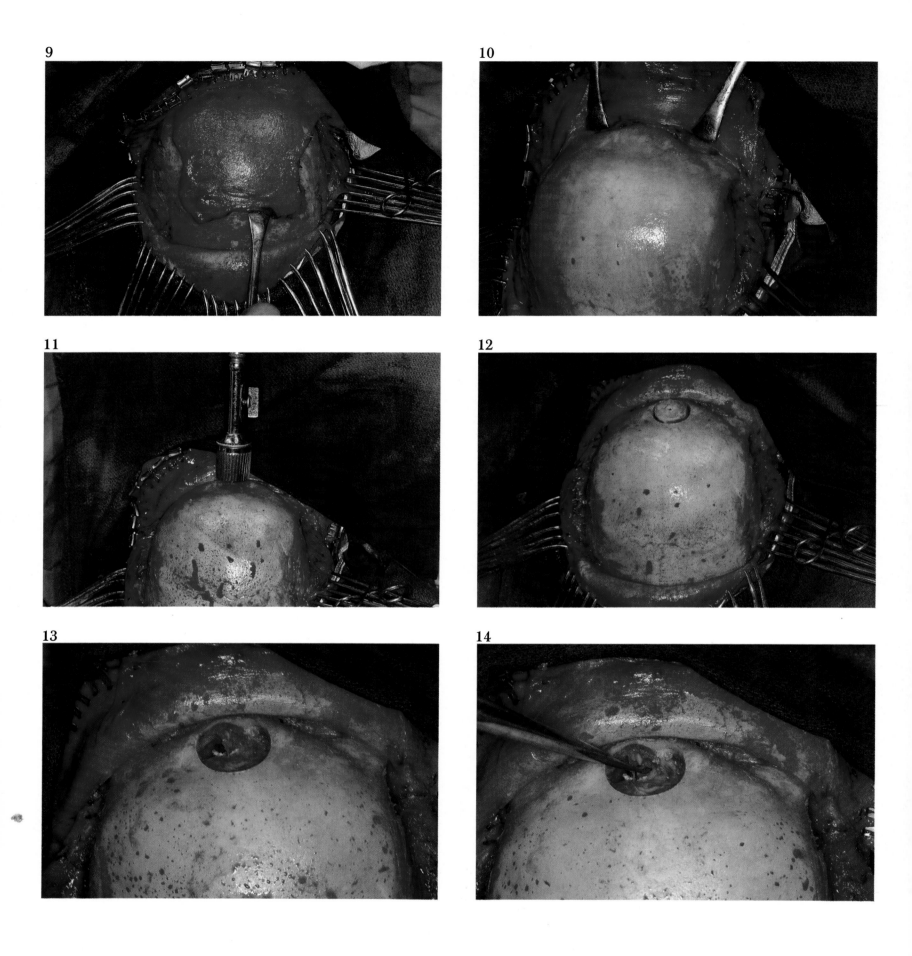

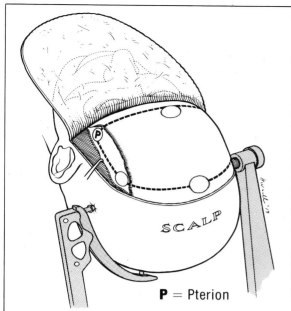

P = Pterion

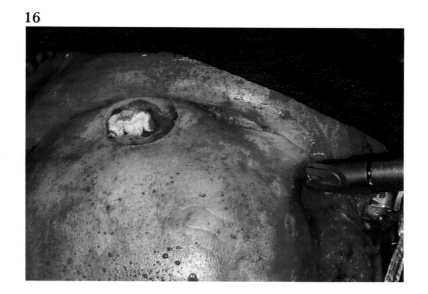

Using a periosteal elevator, the pericranium is elevated over the calvarium (9), very carefully to avoid any buttonholes in the pericranium. The entire elevated pericranium should be raised as a single sheet of periosteum subsequently to be used for repair of the skull base.

Elevation of the pericranium over the calvarium extends anteriorly all the way up to the supraorbital region (10). In the frontal region, the pericranium is separated from the calvarium but remains attached to the frontalis muscle and scalp. Blood supply to this pericranial flap is derived from the supratrochlear and supraorbital vessels.

A burr is now used to create a large central burr hole in the midline of the forehead in the frontal bone overlying the frontal sinus (11). Alternatively, a template of the frontal sinus can be made from the plain X-ray picture of the frontal bone and a high speed drill used to remove the anterior wall of the frontal sinus along the template which can subsequently be replaced at the time of closure. Using a template rather than a large

burr hole in this fashion does away with the midline deformity of depression created by the large burr hole.

Once the hole is made, the disk of bone (the anterior wall of the frontal sinus) is removed and saved for subsequent replacement (12). Alternatively, if the anterior wall of the frontal sinus is excised along the line of the template, then it is saved for subsequent use during closure of the craniotomy. The frontal sinus is exposed through the large burr hole as seen here (13), and mucosa of the sinus and its septa are clearly visible.

Using appropriate curettes and a rongeur, the mucosa of the frontal sinus is curetted out and all septa are divided to completely clean out the frontal sinus (14), which is packed with gel foam to plug its openings into the nasal cavity, as seen in (16).

Lateral burr holes are now made through the pterion (15), several are then placed thorough the coronal suture as shown in (16). Brisk bleeding from the bone is encountered at the site of the burr holes, but this can be easily controlled with bone wax.

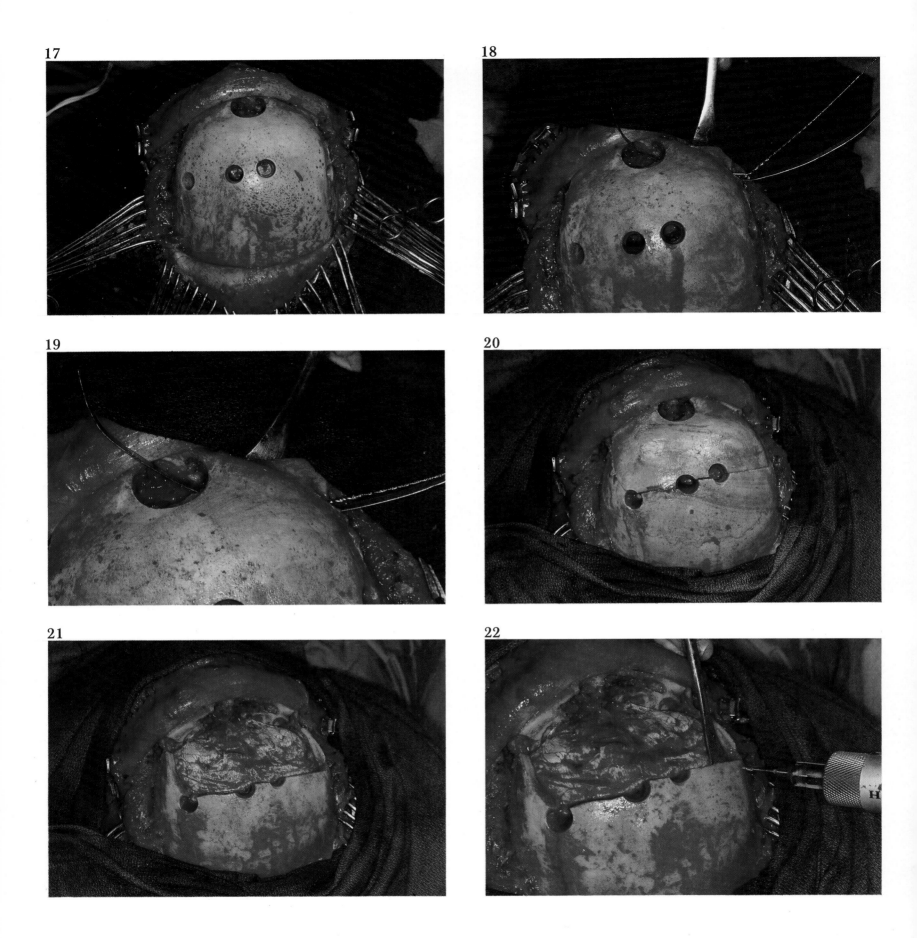

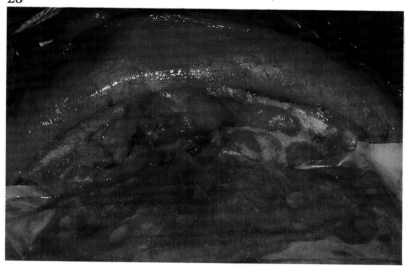

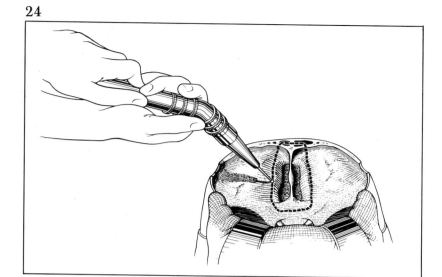

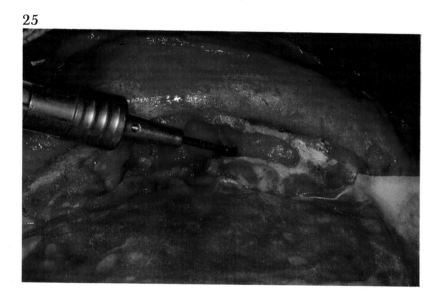

After completion of the burr holes, dural elevators are used to separate the dura from the undersurface of the calvarium and a guide strip is passed for use of a gigli saw (**17**). The guide strip protects the underlying dura and allows an easy sweep of the gigli saw for division of the bone flap as shown in (**18**).

The close-up view of the gigli saw in action is shown in (**19**), dividing the bone flap between the midline burr hole and that through the pterion. The entire bone flap is now divided connecting all the burr holes with the gigli saw (**20**).

The bone flap is now carefully lifted off making sure that no tears are created in the dura (**21**), which is carefully and meticulously stripped away from the undersurface of the bone flap allowing easy removal. The bone flap is now rapped in a moist saline towel and saved for subsequent replacement. The exposure obtained by removal of the frontal bone flap demonstrates the dura of the anterior cranial fossa which is still intact and *in situ.* Bleeding from the cut edges of the calvarium is easily controlled with the use of bone wax, and bleeding from the surface of the dura with bipolar cautery.

Using a high speed drill and a very fine drill bit, several holes are now made obliquely through the outer table of the transected edges of the calvarium, and through all the edges of the craniotomy (**22**). These drill holes will allow subsequent placement of sutures to retain the bone flap in its proper position during closure of the craniotomy.

Meticulous and careful dissection of elevation of the dura now takes place with fine dural elevators (**23**). Extreme care should be exercised to avoid any tears or rents in the dura during this step. The dura is carefully elevated from the floor of the anterior cranial fossa. The dural sleeves of the olfactory nerves will be traversing through the cribriform plate, in the central part of the

anterior cranial fossa over the region of the cribriform plate. Each dural sleeve is carefully identified, transected and oversewn to prevent leakage of cerebrospinal fluid, so the entire group of dural sleeves traversing from the olfactory bulbs along the olfactory fibers through the cribriform plate is totally transected and closed before any further mobilization is undertaken. Careful division of the dura in this fashion allows complete exposure of the central part of the floor of the anterior cranial fossa. Dense dural attachments over the crista galii may have to be transected and/or the latter may have to be removed with a rongeur. A rubber dam is now placed over the mobilized dura to keep it moist and protected.

A high speed drill is used to demarcate the line of transection of the bony floor of the anterior cranial fossa as shown in (**24**). The drill is used to burr off the posterior wall of the frontal sinus as shown in (**25**). Once that

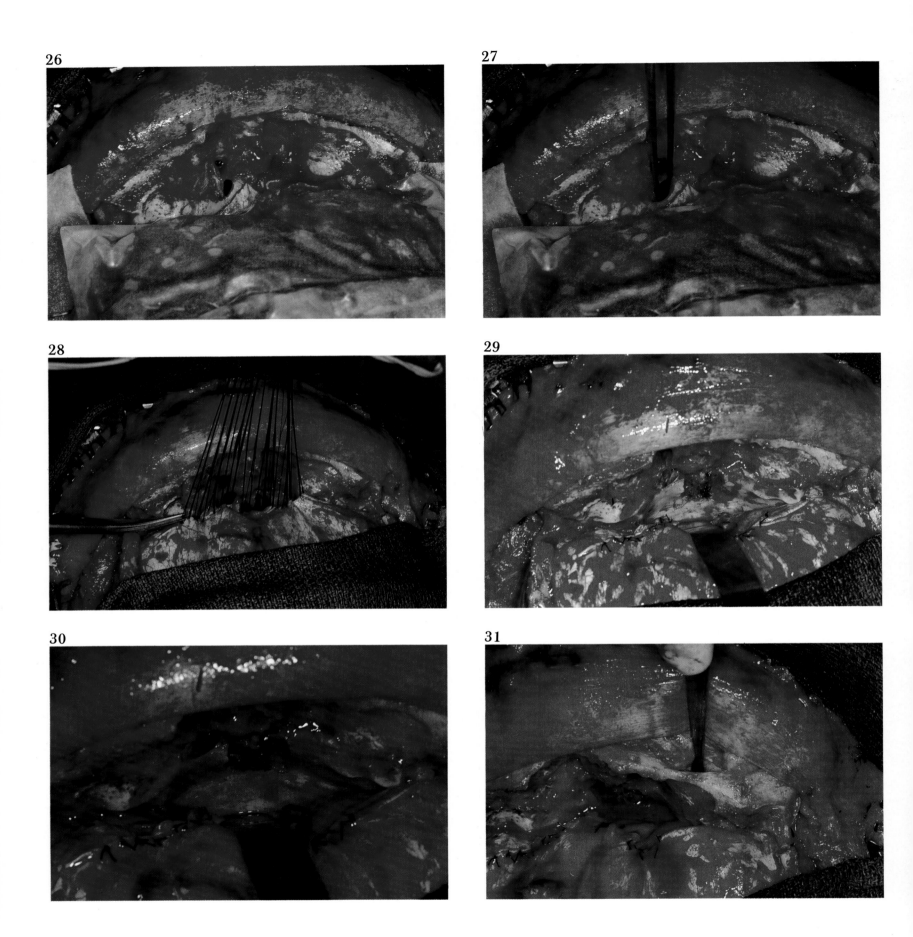

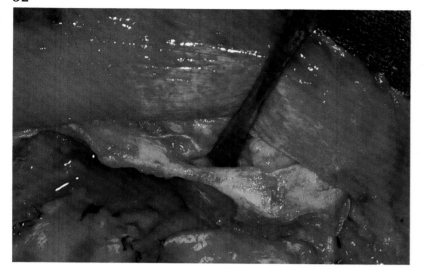

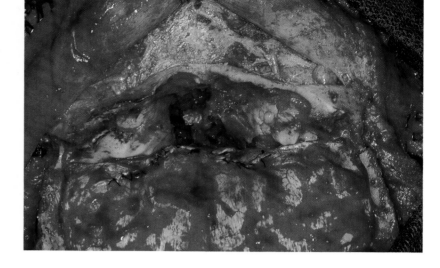

is completed, the exposed floor of the anterior cranial fossa will show the entire cribriform plate up to the region of the planum sphenoidale for adequate assessment of the intracranial component of the tumor or its extensions (26). Minor bleeding from the surface of the dura or the transected margins of the dural sleeves is easily controlled using bipolar cautery (27).

The ligated dural sleeves are demonstrated here (28) with sutures over each of them, carefully closed to maintain watertight closure of the dura and minimize contamination of the brain during the rest of the surgical procedure. Each of the sutures are now divided to allow the rest of the brain to retract posteriorly and provide exposure of the anterior fossa. At this point, approximately 10 mls of cerebrospinal fluid is removed from the spinal canal to allow slackening of brain and its contraction, and letting it drop posteriorly without any manual retraction. Up to 30–40 mls of cerebrospinal fluid may have to be removed, and this is done in aliquots of 10 mls each at half-hour intervals.

Exposure of the floor of the anterior cranial fossa is now complete, and the cribriform plate and crista galii can be seen in (29).

A close-up view of the floor of the anterior cranial fossa in its central compartment (30) shows the planum sphenoidale, the cribriform plate and the medial part of the roof of the orbit on both sides. At this point, the high speed drill, mentioned above, is used again to outline and divide the bony skull base through the proposed line of resection.

Since this patient's tumor extends up to the lamina papyracea of the orbit on the right side, it will be sacrificed but keeping the orbital periosteum intact. A periosteal elevator is now introduced inferior to the supraorbital ridge in the upper part of the right orbit, to allow separation of the periosteum of the orbit from the roof, and the lamina papyracea medially (31).

Further exposure of the bony roof and medial wall of the orbit is obtained with a malleable retractor introduced in the superior medial quadrant of the orbit to retract the globe inferiorly and laterally (32).

Intracranial mobilization of the tumor, at this point, is complete (33), and the neurosurgical team can take a break.

34

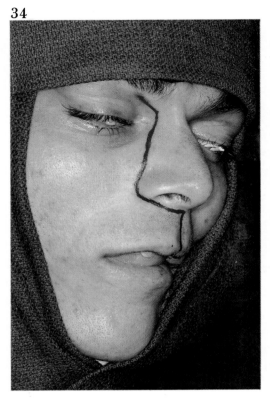

35

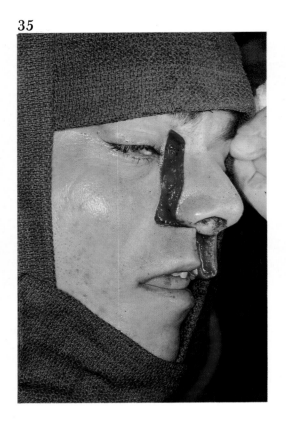

36

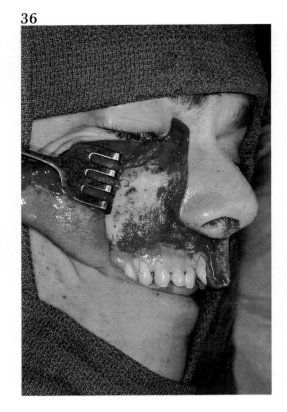

37

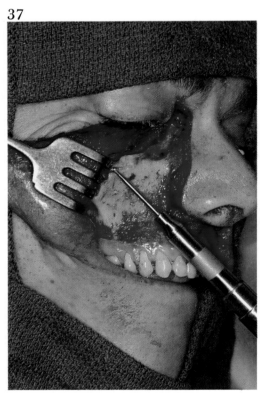

38

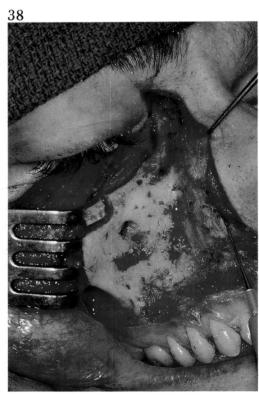

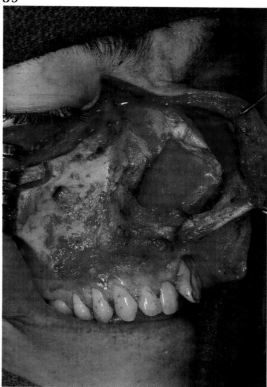

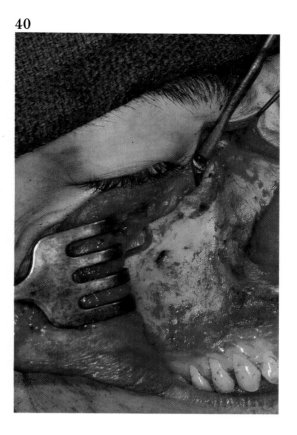

The head and neck surgical team now proceeds with the facial aspect of the operative procedure (34). A Weber–Ferguson incision is taken with a Lynch extension going up to the medial end of the right eyebrow. The skin incision is deepened through the soft tissues along the nasolabial fold up to the bony anterior wall of the maxillary antrum (35). Superiorly, the incision is deepened through all the soft tissues over the nasal bone and the medial bony rim of the orbit.

Using electrocautery, the upper cheek flap is elevated directly over the anterior bony wall of the maxilla (36), identifying the infraorbital nerve as it exits from the infraorbital foramen. To obtain adequate lateral exposure, the nerve will have to be divided, and blood vessels accompanying it will require ligation on its distal stump in the soft tissues of the cheek. Proximally, however, electrocoagulation in the infraorbital canal with a cautery will control bleeding. Generous exposure of the anterior aspect of the maxilla should be obtained by significant retraction on the cheek flap with rake retractors to facilitate a satisfactory resection. The orbicularis oculi muscle is, however, carefully preserved since the contents of the right orbit are to be retained. Thus, during elevation of the cheek flap it must be noted that all the soft tissues, including the orbicularis oculi muscle, are elevated with the skin, keeping the plane of dissection directly over the bone.

Using a high speed drill with a very fine drill bit, an incision is made along the anterior wall of the maxillary antrum to outline the proposed line of transection for removal of the surgical specimen (37). In this patient, the medial third of the orbital floor is resected to remove the lamina papyracea, the ethmoid complex and the entire right maxilla *en bloc*.

The close-up view of the transected floor of the orbit and the line of bone division along the anterior wall of the maxilla and the zygomatic process of maxilla is shown in (38). Using electrocautery entry is made into the nasal cavity by dividing all the soft tissues along the nasal process of maxilla and retracting the soft tissues and the ala of the nose medially.

Retraction of the nostril gives satisfactory exposure of the nasal septum, the nasal bone, nasal process of maxilla, and the contents of the nasal cavity on the involved side (39). Note that the mobilization of the orbital periosteum from its medial aspect has already given satisfactory mobilization of the surgical specimen isolating the contents of the orbit. At this point, the medial canthal ligament must be detached to further free the bony attachment of the orbital periosteum allowing lateral retraction of the globe and exposing the medial wall of the orbit. A small periosteal elevator is now used to isolate and dissect the lacrimal duct from the lacrimal fossa (40). The nasolacrimal duct is transected at this point permitting further lateral retraction of the globe.

41 **42**

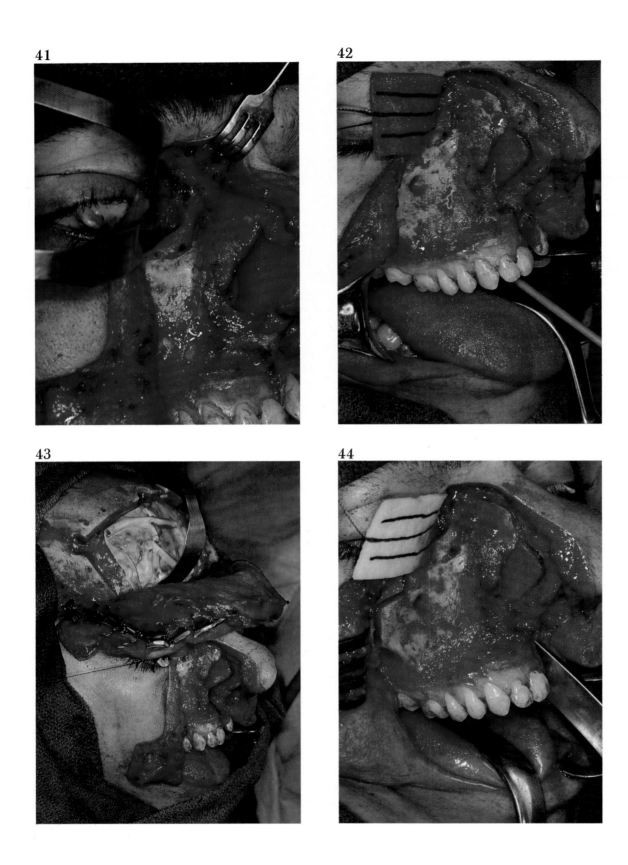

43 **44**

45

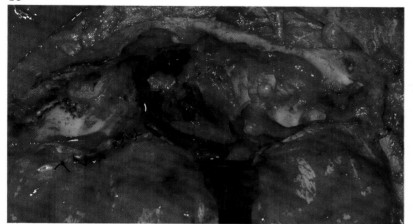

46

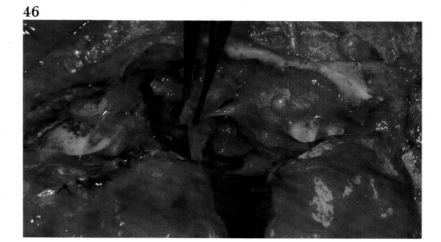

Malleable retractors are now introduced into the orbit retracting the globe laterally and exposing the medial wall of the orbit to demonstrate the lamina papyracea as shown in (**41**). The silk suture seen overlying the upper eyelid between two malleable retractors is anchored to the medial canthal ligament and will be used subsequently during closure for repositioning of the medial canthus. Superomedial retraction of the glabellar region exposes the root of the nose in the frontal sinus area. A cotton pattie is now introduced between the globe and the orbit medially to protect the globe. Using a high speed drill, the right nasal bone is transected from the upper part of the orbital rim up to its free edge inferiorly as shown here. Thus, the nasal process of maxilla and attached portion of the nasal bone would be removed *en bloc* with the surgical specimen.

Using electrocautery, the nasal septum is divided through-and-through as shown in (**42**). Care must be taken to preserve the columella and the tip of the nasal septum leaving a rim on its dorsal aspect to maintain the shape of the nose. Again using a high speed drill, the anterior lower part of maxilla is divided from the floor of the nasal cavity through the premaxilla between the two central incisor teeth. Using electrocautery an incision is made in the mucosa and mucoperiosteum of the hard palate extending from the central incisor teeth in the midline up to the junction of the hard and soft palate, at which point the mucosal incision is turned laterally to reach the maxillary tubercle. A sagittal saw is used to transect the hard palate partly through the line of the mucosal incision.

The neurosurgical team rejoins the operation at this point (**43**).

Using a straight osteotome, as shown in (**44**), the hard palate is fractured through its midline along the previous line of partial division achieved by the sagittal saw. At this point, the specimen is practically mobilized from all its aspects. Both the intracranial and facial aspects of the surgical specimen are also now exposed. From the facial aspect, fine attachments of soft tissue and mucosa are divided under direct vision through the cranial cavity to provide complete mobilization and freeing of the upper aspect of the surgical specimen.

As shown in (**45**), the entire surgical specimen is fully mobilized and freed from the cranial aspect. It contains the crista galii, cribriform plate, medial aspect of the roof of the orbit and part of the posterior wall and floor of the frontal sinus, all of which are totally mobilized.

The specimen at this point should be free enough to be rocked with the use of a plain forceps grasping the crista galii, as is shown in (**46**). Minor attachments of soft tissues are divided such that the specimen does not fracture and come out piecemeal. The specimen is rocked from the facial aspect, and soft tissues in the region of the pterygomaxillary fossa are divided to complete the maxillectomy. Muscular attachments of the soft palate and pterygoid region are also divided under direct vision to allow *en bloc* removal of the specimen.

The surgical defect is seen here (**47**) from the cranial aspect showing a through-and-through resection achieved by removing the bony floor of the anterior cranial fossa. Note that the contents of the orbit on the right side are prolapsing into the nasal cavity due to resection of the lamina papyracea. The orbital periosteum, which is still maintained intact, is seen prolapsing in the space from which the ethmoid complex is removed.

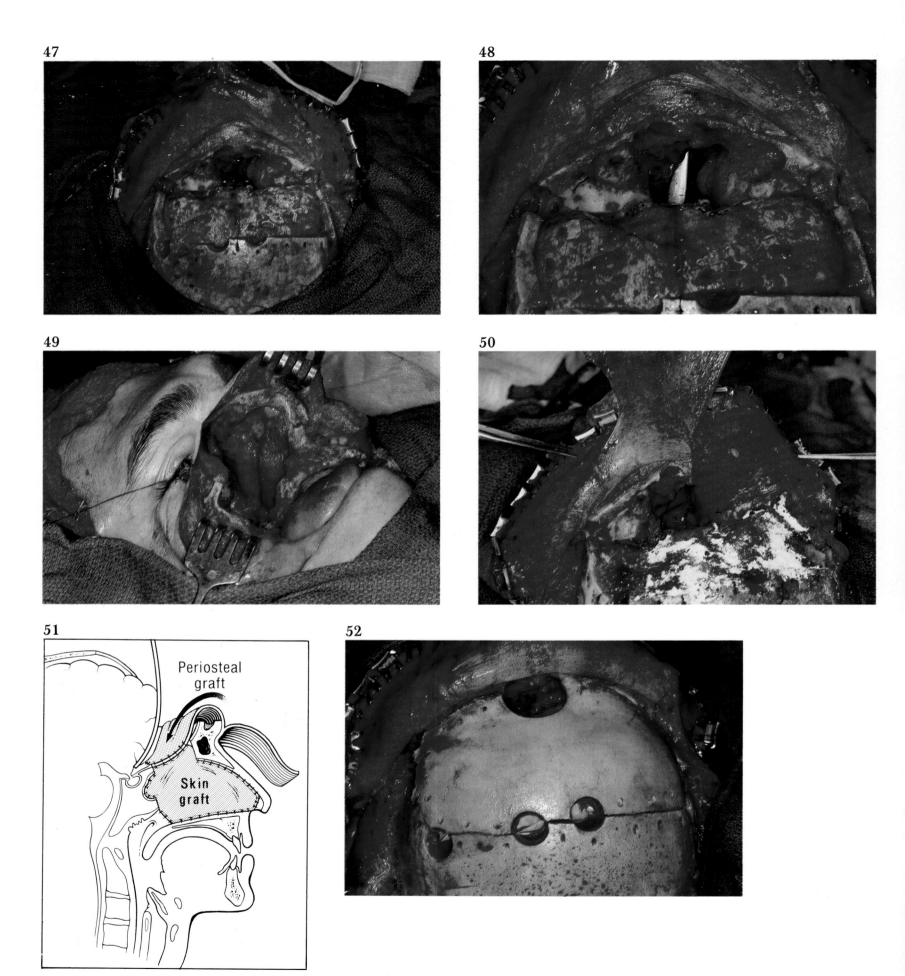

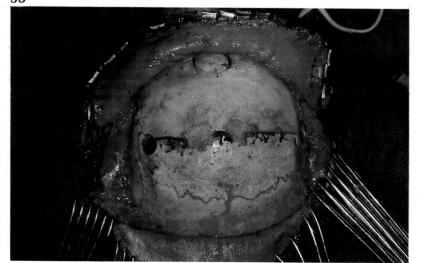

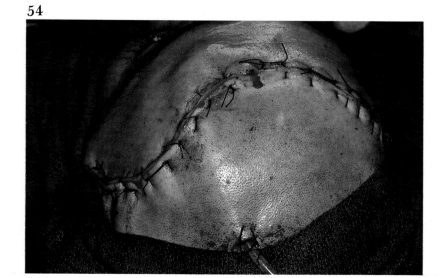

A close-up view of the surgical defect in the floor of the anterior cranial fossa is shown in (48). A metallic instrument introduced in the nasal cavity from the facial aspect is seen here in the center of the surgical defect demonstrating a through-and-through resection of the ethmoid complex. Note also the prolapse of the orbital contents on the right side due to removal of the lamina papyracea.

The surgical defect, as seen from the facial aspect, demonstrates complete removal of the right maxilla and right ethmoid complex and nasal septum (49). Note that the bony support of the medial wall of the orbit and the medial third of the floor of the orbit is resected causing prolapse of the orbital contents medially and inferiorly in the nasal cavity. The medial and inferior turbinates of the left nasal cavity are visualized secondary to resection of the nasal septum. Note, however, that the columella, tip and hump of the nose are preserved as a result of leaving a rim of the nasal septum to maintain the contour and the shape of the nose.

Repair of the surgical defect in the bony floor of the anterior cranial fossa begins now (50). Complete hemostasis in the cranial cavity is absolutely essential prior to closure of the craniotomy, and can be achieved using ligation of major bleeders, and bipolar cautery for small bleeding points over the dura; microfibrillar collagen in powder form can also be sprinkled on the dura.

The previously elevated, pedicled periosteum is now brought into the surgical field and reflected down to drape over the bony defect in the anterior cranial fossa (51). Its free edge is sutured to the cut edge of the planum sphenoidale and the roof of the orbit on both sides through several tiny drill holes. No bony replacement is necessary to fill the defect in the floor of the anterior cranial fossa. Previously withdrawn cerebrospinal fluid is now reintroduced and the brain is allowed to expand.

The bone flap is replaced and sutured in position with several interrupted neurolon sutures taken through the previously drilled holes in the outer table of the calvarium at both ends (52). The discs of bone removed from the site of previous burr holes are replaced and also sutured in position (53). The entire craniotomy wound is completely evacuated of all blood clots and is irrigated out with saline.

A suction drain is introduced below the scalp through a separate stab wound, and the scalp incision closed with non-absorbable suture material (54).

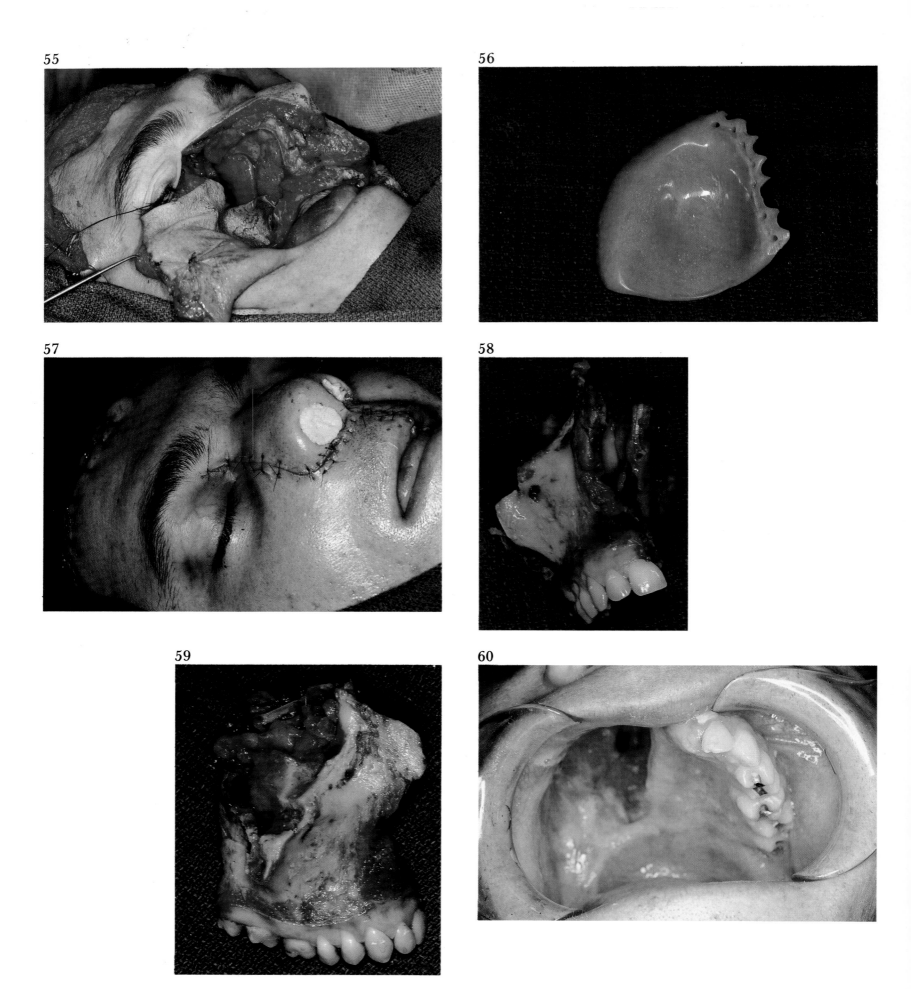

61 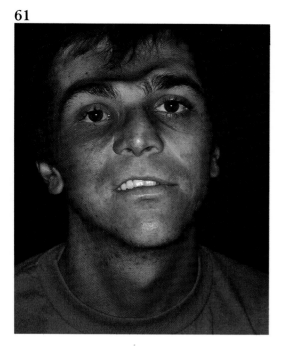 **62** 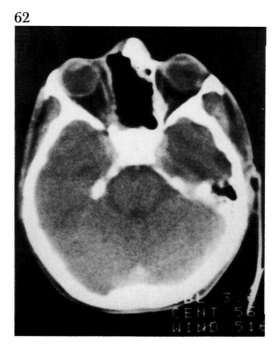 **63**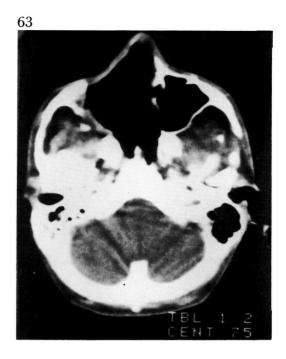

On the facial aspect, the previously obtained skin graft is used to line the raw areas in the surgical defect created by the maxillectomy (**55**). The skin graft is sutured to the cut edges of the cheek mucosa using interrupted chromic catgut sutures; it is then draped over the maxillectomy defect, extended over superomedially to provide lining over the orbital periosteum and then draped over the roof of the nasal cavity. At this point, it is applied directly against the pedicled periosteal flap used to repair the bony skull base; it is snugly applied to all the raw areas and kept in position with xeroform gauze packing, which is retained in the defect using a previously fabricated surgical dental obturator wired to the remaining teeth of the opposite upper alveolus in the oral cavity (**56**). The medial canthal ligament is reapproximated through a drill hole in the stump of the nasal bone, keeping the alignment of the medial canthus of the right eye at the same level as that of the opposite eye. The cheek flap is returned in its normal position and is closed in two layers using chromic catgut interrupted sutures for subcutaneous tissue and 5-0 nylon for skin (**57**). Meticulous attention is necessary in accurate reapproximation of the skin edges to provide an esthetically acceptable scar. The vermilion border and philtrum should be accurately realigned. Additional packing is introduced through the nasal cavity to minimize postoperative bleeding from the nasal cavity and also retain the skin graft in position.

The surgical specimen is seen from the anterior aspect and shows the right maxilla, contents of the right nasal cavity, nasal septum, ethmoid complex, lamina papyracea and crista galii with cribriform plate (**58**).

Note that the entire specimen is removed *en bloc* keeping the contents of the right nasal cavity intact and undisturbed to allow a satisfactory monobloc surgical resection of the tumor.

The surgical specimen is seen here from the lateral aspect showing the right maxilla, floor of the medial aspect of the orbit, tumor in the upper ethmoid air cells with the crista galii and cribriform plate removed intact in a monobloc fashion (**59**).

The postoperative appearance of the intraoral surgical defect is shown in (**60**). Note that the right half of the hard palate is missing and the surgical defect is lined with a healed skin graft. In the posterior aspect of the surgical defect, the sphenoid sinus is visible. The patient at this point uses the permanent dental obturator which obliterates the defect in the hard palate and allows normal mastication and swallowing as well as speech.

The postoperative appearance of the patient shows well-healed external incisions (**61**), but note the obvious deformity in the frontal region. In this patient the frontal bone flap had to be removed due to infection in the suture line of the scalp. If sepsis in the suture line of the scalp is evident, then the frontal bone flap must be removed promptly to prevent the risk of meningitis. The bony defect, in this instance, will require secondary reconstruction either using the same bone flap, which may be cryopreserved, or metallic bone plate or bone cement.

Postoperative CT scans of the patient (**62, 63**) show complete removal of the tumor.

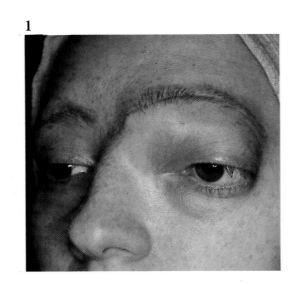

1

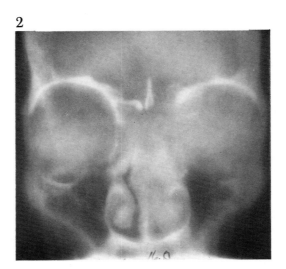

2

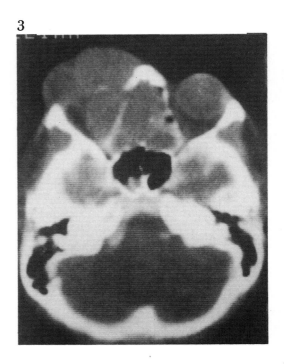

3

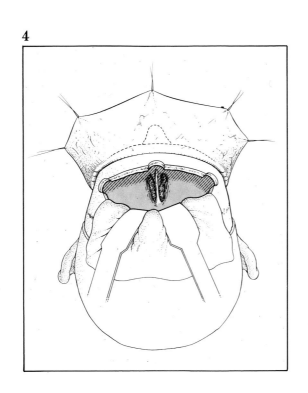

4

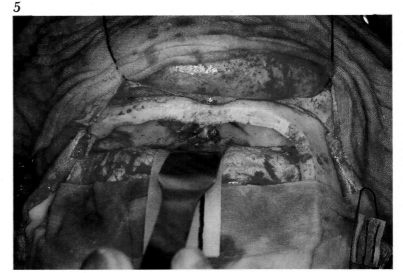

5

Craniofacial resection for tumor of the orbit and anterior fossa

When primary tumors of the nasal cavity and paranasal sinuses extend to the orbit, then consideration should be given to orbital exenteration for satisfactory removal of the tumor. On the other hand, if a primary tumor begins in the orbit, arising from the lacrimal apparatus, ocular adenexa or the globe itself, orbital exenteration becomes mandatory. The patient presented here (1) has recurrent chondrosarcoma arising in the orbit. This patient had previously undergone an attempt at supraorbital surgical resection. The primary tumor arose in the soft tissues of the orbit and frontal bone with displacement of the globe laterally and inferiorly. The patient had diplopia, and intractable pain secondary to tumor invasion.

Coronal tomogram of the facial skeleton taken through the anterior ethmoid air cells (2) shows extension of tumor to destroy the cribriform plate on the left side with destruction of the medial wall of the orbit and adjacent frontal bone. The tumor had clearly extended into the frontal sinus and the ethmoid air cells. The transverse cut of CT scan through the midplane of the orbits shows a massive tumor in the medial aspect of the left orbit with extension to fill the nasal cavity (3). The tumor, however, did not involve the sphenoid sinus or the apex of the orbit into the middle cranial fossa.

Surgical exposure for resection of this tumor is through a standard bifrontal craniotomy as described above (4). The usual precautions are taken for elevation of the pedicled periosteal flap. A frontal bone flap is also elevated as usual to provide satisfactory exposure of the bony floor of the anterior cranial fossa.

As shown in (5), the frontal bone flap has been elevated and the dura of the anterior cranial fossa is separated giving exposure of the roof of the orbit and the region of the cribriform plate.

The close-up view of the floor of the anterior cranial fossa (6) shows the tumor bulging through the frontal sinus and cribriform plate on the left side. At this point it became apparent that the tumor had indeed involved the dura and the decision was made to resect the attached portion of the dura with the primary tumor. The dura was opened and there was no extension of tumor in the subdural space. A cuff of dura adherent and involved by the tumor was resected to remain in continuity with the main tumor mass.

The bony cuts around the tumor from the cranial aspect are completed as shown in (7). Note that the entire frontal sinus is resected with the crista galii, cribriform plate and roof of the orbit on the left side. The bony cut on the left side passes through the lateral aspect of the roof of the orbit. Posteriorly, the bony cut through the floor of the anterior cranial fossa passes through the roof of the sphenoid sinus and the planum sphenoidale, and on the right side the bone cut goes through the ethmoid air cells.

6

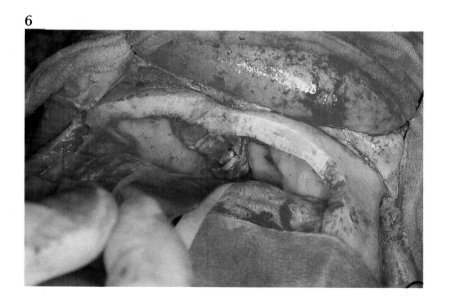

7

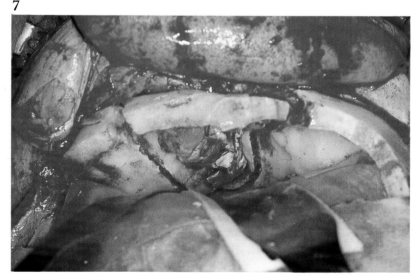

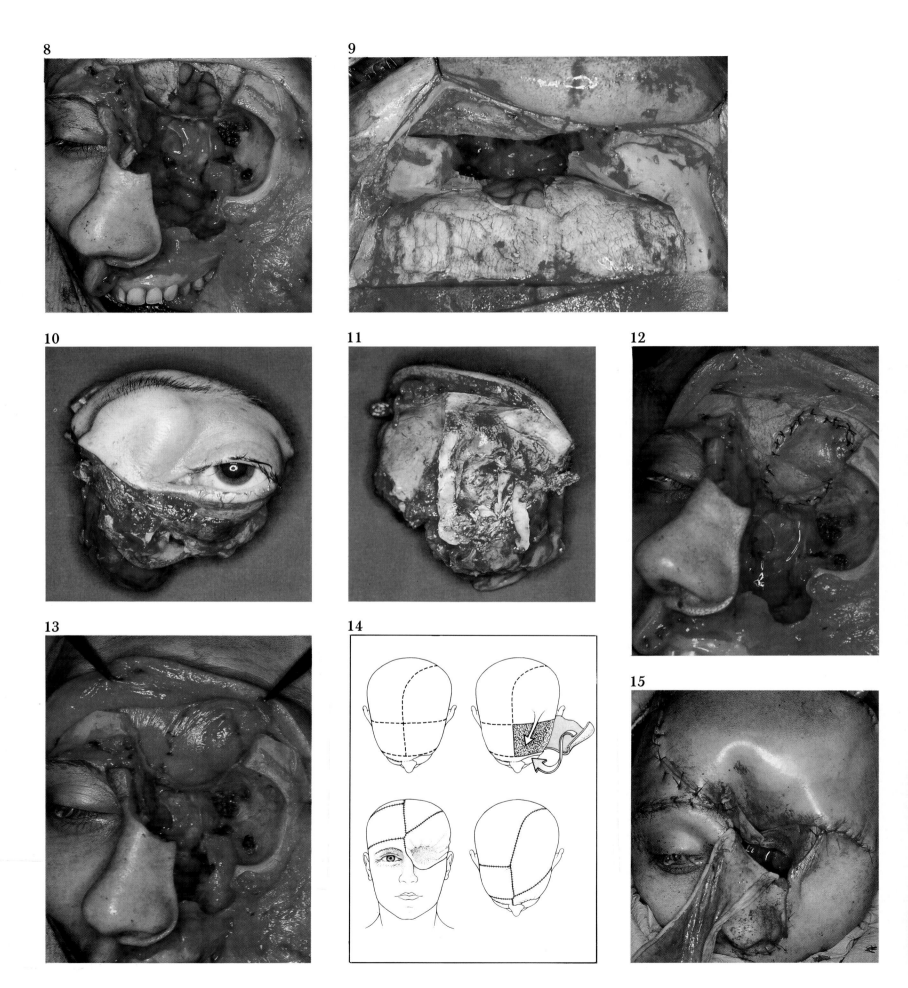

16 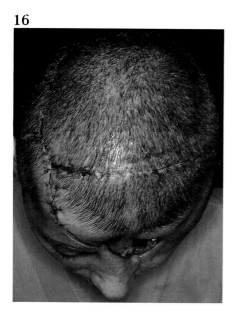 **17**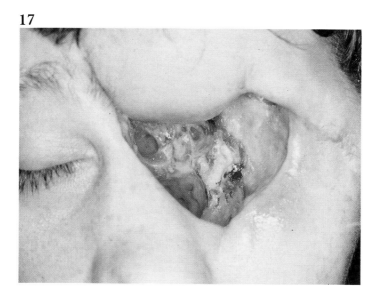

The facial exposure is obtained through a routine Weber–Ferguson incision with generous sacrifice of the skin and soft tissues around the left orbit. Both the upper and lower eyelids as well as the eyebrow and the skin of the cheek and the glabellar region of the nose are resected *en bloc* with the primary tumor.

The surgical defect is seen from the facial aspect showing total excision of the tumor with orbital exenteration **(8)**. Note the dural defect exposing the brain with remaining lateral half of the bony wall of the orbit. The entire medial half of the bony orbit with the contents of the nasal cavity and the roof of the antrum are resected in conjunction with the frontal bone in a monobloc fashion.

The surgical defect is seen from the craniotomy aspect following removal of the specimen **(9)**. Note that a segment of the dura is resected exposing the brain with a through-and-through resection including the floor of the anterior cranial fossa with full-thickness resection of the frontal bone to encompass the entire tumor.

The surgical specimen is viewed from the frontal aspect showing the left orbit, glabellar region and the contents of the nasal cavity and roof of the antrum removed in one piece **(10)**. The surgical specimen in **(11)** is seen from the cranial aspect showing the skin of the forehead, frontal bone, crista galii, cribriform plate and roof and contents of the orbit.

The defect in the dura is repaired first using a free fascial graft obtained from the temporalis fascia **(12)**. Alternatively, a piece of the pericranium can be used to repair the dural defect. Several interrupted 4-0 neurolon sutures are used to apply the patch to repair the dura, and a watertight closure is obtained. Previously withdrawn cerebrospinal fluid is now reintroduced and the

brain is allowed to expand to check for any minor leakage of cerebrospinal fluid.

The previously elevated, pedicled periosteal flap is now reflected downwards and sutured to the bony edges of the surgical defect in the floor of the anterior cranial fossa **(13)**. The periosteal flap will thus be supporting the repaired dura and brain in the surgical defect; it is anchored to the edges of the bony defect with several neurolon sutures taken through tiny drill holes made in the edges of the bony defect.

Because of the large size of the bony resection of the floor of the anterior cranial fossa, herniation of the brain in this patient is a good possibility. Therefore, instead of applying a split-thickness skin graft, a rotated scalp flap is used to support the brain in the orbital defect to prevent herniation. As shown in **(14)**, the scalp over the calvarium is divided in four flaps, and the anterior left scalp flap is rotated inferomedially to cover the defect created by the resected skull base. The left posterior scalp is moved anteriorly and a split-thickness skin graft is applied in the occipital region.

The scalp flap is shown here **(15)** rotated in the orbital defect to support the brain. A split-thickness skin graft is used to line the rest of the surgical defect and the nasal cavity. Craniotomy and facial incisions are thereafter closed in the usual fashion.

The postoperative appearance of the patient approximately 3 weeks after surgery **(16)** shows primary healing of the incisions in the scalp and the scalp flap.

The close-up view of the orbital defect **(17)** shows a well-healed scalp flap supporting the brain at the site of resected skull base with the rest of the defect of orbital exenteration lined by a skin graft. Note the exposed sphenoid sinus in the depth of the orbit.

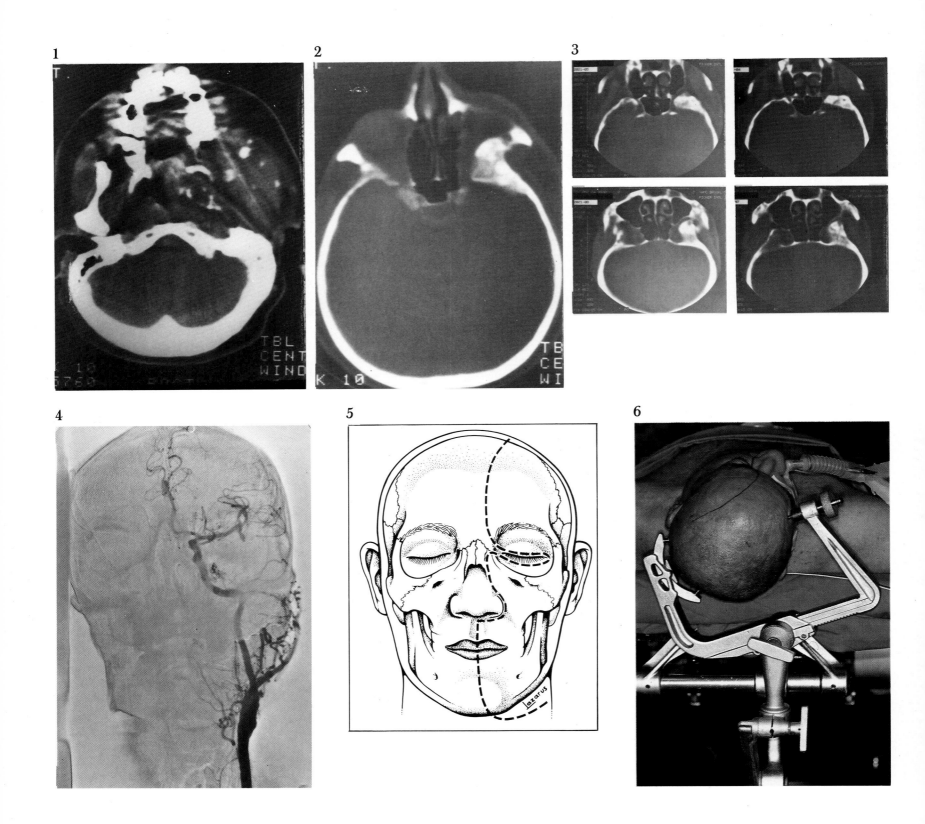

Resection of tumor involving pterygoid fossa and base of the middle cranial fossa

Surgical resection of tumors presenting in the pterygoid fossa with secondary extension to the infratemporal fossa and base of the middle cranial fossa require extensive exposure for protection of vital structures and adequate *en bloc* resection of the tumor. Surgical access to this area is extremely difficult unless a very generous exposure is provided by appropriate incisions.

The patient presented in this procedure had recurrent ameloblastoma involving the bed of the ascending ramus of the mandible with extension to the infratemporal fossa, secondary invasion of the floor of the middle cranial fossa, and extension into the orbit through its posterolateral wall. He had previously undergone segmental mandibulectomy for ameloblastoma.

The CT scan at the level of the upper alveolar process (1) demonstrates an extensive tumor involving the pterygomaxillary fissure with medial extension into the parapharyngeal space. Posteriorly, the tumor extends up to the prevertebral plane and laterally it displaces the parotid gland.

A higher cut through the midplane of the orbit shows bone invasion by tumor involving the lateral wall of the orbit and the inferolateral wall of the middle cranial fossa (2). The tumor, however, does not extend medially to involve the optic foramen.

Coronal cuts through the skull base clearly show that tumor extension involves the floor of the middle cranial fossa as well as the lateral wall of the orbit (3), but no intracranial extension is seen, nor is the cavernous sinus involved.

Carotid angiography (4) shows displacement of the terminal branches of the external carotid artery which are the main feeding vessels for this tumor. The internal carotid artery, however, is in its normal disposition with only slight medial displacement. The carotid canal is undisturbed and the intracranial portion of the carotid artery is uninvolved.

The plan of surgical excision includes a midfacial incision extending from the occipitoparietal region, up to the medial end of the eyebrow on the left side (5). At that point the incision is continued along the tarsal plate of the upper eyelid up to the lateral canthus, then turning medially along the tarsal plate of the lower eyelid up to the medial canthus and then carried on as a Weber–Ferguson incision dividing the upper lip in the midline. The incision is then continued for elevation of the lower cheek flap dividing the lower lip and chin in the midline and extending in the upper part of the neck on the left side along the scar of the patient's previous surgical procedure. The incision will thus provide elevation of all the soft tissues of the face along with the skin flap. The flap will be taken full thickness directly up to the bone, elevating all the facial musculature, including orbicularis oculi, on the flap, thus preserving the nerve supply to facial muscles through terminal branches of the facial nerve. Laterally, the flap will contain the parotid gland and will be elevated in a plane deep to the parotid gland, carefully identifying and preserving the main trunk of the facial nerve to remain in continuity with the rest of the flap.

After induction of general anesthesia, with an endotracheal tube passed through the oral cavity (6), an indwelling spinal catheter is placed for drainage of cerebrospinal fluid during the course of the operation. The patient's head is properly positioned and held with pins. The endotracheal tube is fixed to the oral commissure on the right side and would be isolated from the surgical field.

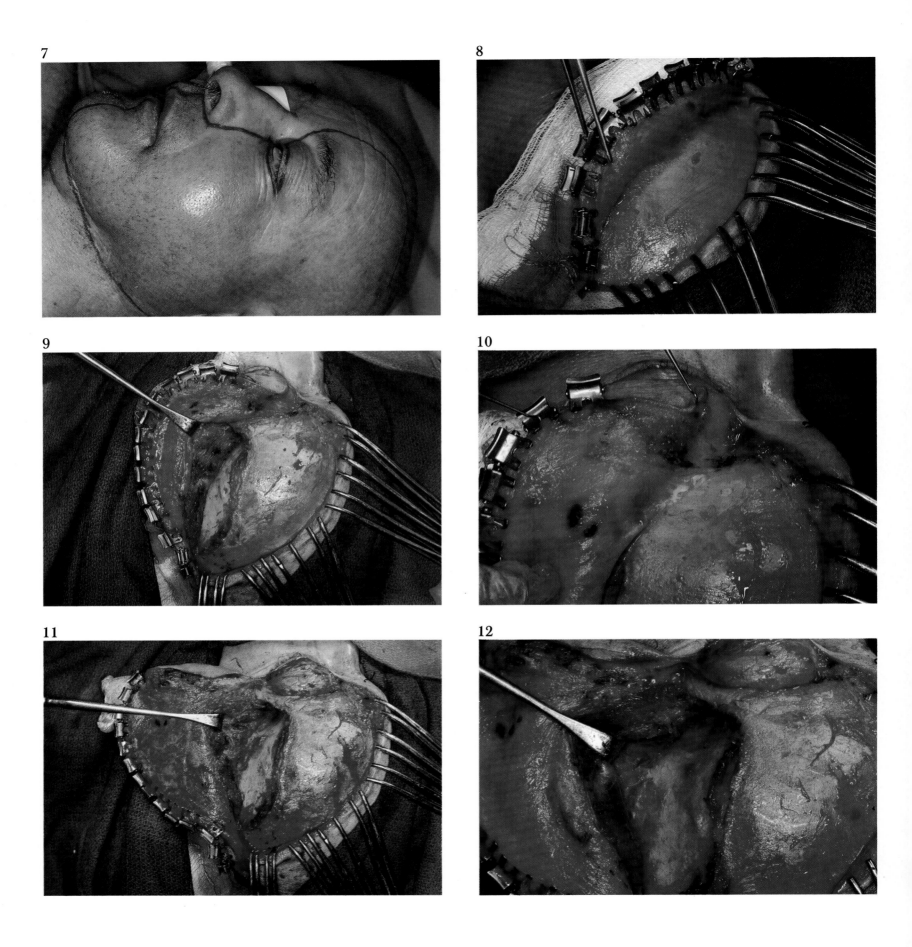

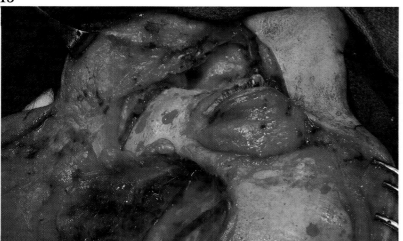

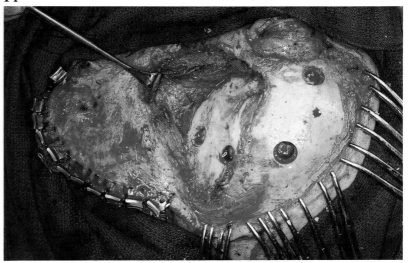

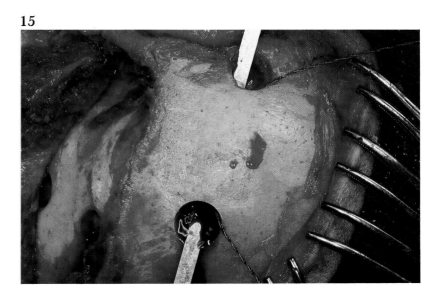

The incision is marked out as shown here (7), extending from the parieto-occipital region on the left side, up to the midline, and then turning slightly to the left up to the medial canthus. The left eye is protected with a corneal shield.

The craniotomy aspect of the operation begins first with the parieto-occipital incision taken through the scalp up to and including the pericranium (8). Hemostasis is obtained with appropriate use of hemostats and children's hospital clips.

The temporalis muscle is detached from its insertion over the temporal bone, and elevated in a subperiosteal plane as far down as possible from this exposure (9). Elevation of the temporalis muscle brings into view the zygomatic arch and the lateral rim of the orbit providing access to and exposure of the infratemporal fossa. The plane of dissection remains directly over the bony base of the skull of the middle cranial fossa. At this juncture, no tumor is visualized. Anteriorly, the skin of the upper eyelid is also elevated with the rest of the flap remaining in a plane deep to the orbicularis oculi muscle directly over the periosteum of the globe and superficial to the bulbar conjunctiva (10).

Further elevation of the lower flap continues to provide exposure of the infratemporal fossa with elevation of the soft tissues from the lateral orbital rim and zygomatic arch (11). In the depth of the field, bone invasion by tumor becomes apparent as the region of the medial aspect of the floor of the middle cranial fossa comes into view. The close-up view of the infratemporal fossa is shown in (12). The temporalis muscle is retracted laterally exposing the area of bone involved by tumor.

In order to gain further exposure in this area, the facial incision is now continued from the lateral canthus along the tarsal plate of the lower eyelid up to the medial canthus, and then carried on to complete the Weber–Ferguson incision (13). The entire cheek flap is then elevated remaining superficial to the anterior surface of maxilla and zygoma. Extreme care is taken to preserve the orbicularis oculi muscle on the cheek flap to maintain its nerve supply and integrity. The plane between the orbicularis oculi muscle and the periorbita is very delicate and should be handled with extreme care. Musculature of the face is completely reflected in the cheek flap, keeping intact both the muscular interdigitations and the nerve supply. The zygoma as well as the anterior wall of the maxilla are seen exposed here with the temporalis muscle freed but remaining deep to the zygomatic arch.

Four burr holes are now made through the frontal and temporal bones to proceed with the craniotomy (14), and are connected with the use of a gigli saw passed with a guide strip giving safe division of the bone plate, which is removed and preserved for subsequent replacement during closure of the craniotomy (15).

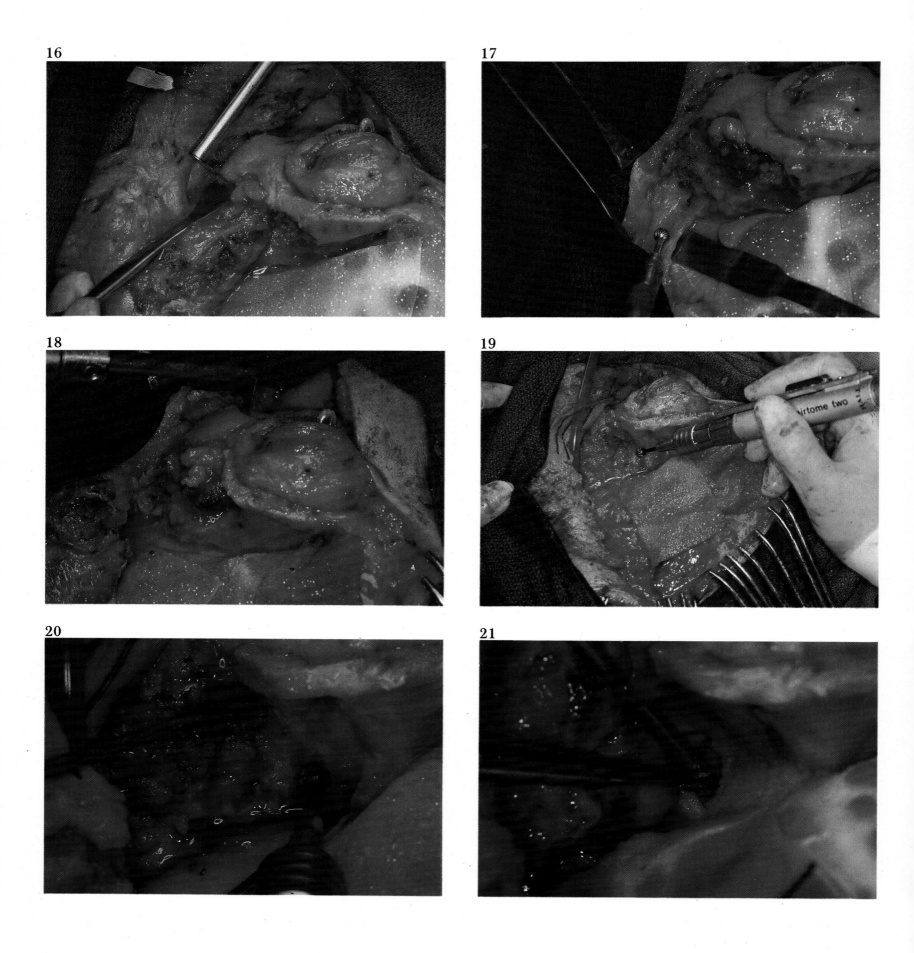

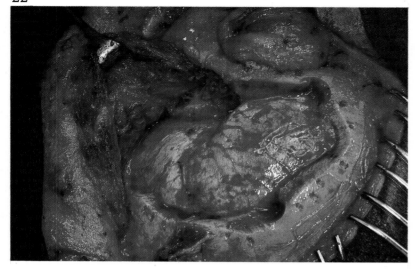

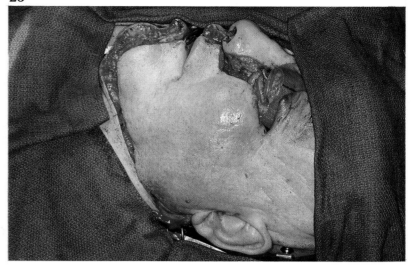

In order to gain direct access to the infratemporai fossa, the zygomatic arch as well as the zygoma will have to be removed. The lateral aspect of the zygoma is divided first with a Strycker saw to allow removal of the zygomatic arch **(16)**; the posterior end of the zygomatic arch is divided with a high speed drill **(17)**.

To gain further access to the infratemporal fossa, it would be necessary to excise the zygoma itself **(18)**. Using the Strycker saw, the zygoma is divided in order to preserve the continuity of the rim of the orbit, but remove the body of the zygoma.

The bony floor of the middle cranial fossa is removed with a high speed drill **(19)**. Remaining lateral to the area of gross involvement by tumor, the bony skull base is drilled out, carefully protecting the underlying dura with malleable retractors. The bone cut is made lateral to the area of tumor involvement as seen grossly and radiographically.

The close-up view of the high speed drill used to divide the bony skull base is shown in **(20)**. As the bone division proceeds medially, the region of the foramen ovale comes into view. The fifth cranial nerve as it exits

from the foramen ovale is divided under direct vision **(21)**. Brisk hemorrhage from accompanying dural veins is likely to result in this area, and should be carefully controlled with bipolar cautery or suture ligature, or occasionally a packing of gel foam in the bleeding area, as is shown in **(21)**.

The craniotomy aspect of the surgical procedure is nearly complete at this point **(22)**. Note that the bony skull base has been removed completely to free the area of tumor involvement medially. Wide access to the infratemporal fossa gained by the frontotemporal craniotomy and removal of the zygoma will facilitate *en bloc* removal of tumor. The entire surgical procedure so far has been extradural, and since there was no intracranial extension of tumor, no portion of dura had to be sacrificed.

The facial procedure begins now with completion of the lower cheek flap which would be elevated at this point **(23)**. The division of lower lip and chin goes through its full thickness, carefully preserving the musculature of the lip and chin to allow it and the cheek flap to maintain its blood and nerve supply.

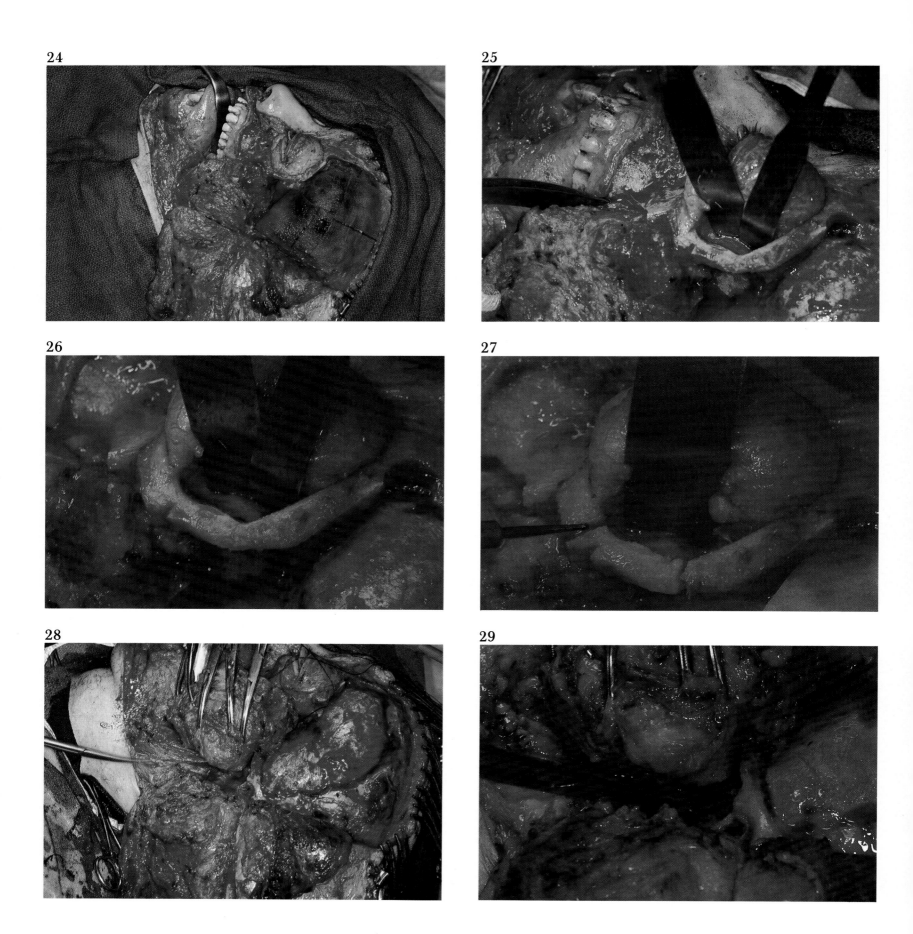

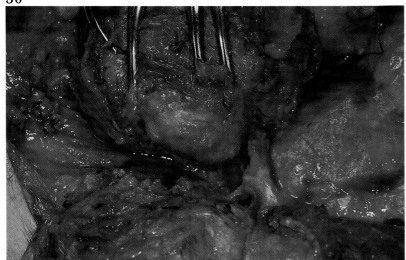

The entire cheek flap is now reflected laterally giving wide exposure of the lateral aspect of maxilla and the pterygomaxillary and infratemporal regions (24). Meticulous attention should be paid to keep the plane of dissection deep to the parotid gland to preserve the integrity of the facial nerve. If the ascending ramus of the mandible is intact, then the plane of dissection should be deep to the masseter muscle giving safe elevation of the facial nerve.

The orbital periosteum is now elevated in its lateral half and the globe retracted medially with malleable retractors (25) to provide access to the posterolateral aspect of the orbit. As seen here, a curved osteotome is used to fracture the tuberosity of the maxilla which would be the anterior margin of the surgical specimen. The close-up view of the orbit (26) shows the extension of tumor in the orbital socket through its lateral wall.

To obtain a monobloc resection of the lateral bony wall of the orbit, a small segment of the latter will also be sacrificed (27). Bone cuts are made with a high-speed drill in the anterior rim of the orbit. Using a small, curved osteotome, the rest of the lateral wall of the orbit will be fractured to mobilize the specimen in this area.

The surgical specimen now has to be further dissected from the cervical exposure upwards (28). The internal jugular vein and common carotid artery as well as the bifurcation of the carotid artery are identified. The plane of dissection now remains anterolateral to the carotid sheath. The internal carotid artery is found to be free and clear of the tumor; the vagus nerve was also uninvolved by tumor, but the hypoglossal nerve was directly involved and had to be sacrificed. The dissection proceeds slowly and carefully cephalad towards the jugular foramen. The posterior belly of the digastric muscle is excised to remain in continuity with the specimen. Dissection continues up to the cartilagenous portion of the auditory canal. At this point, the main trunk of the facial nerve is identified and carefully retracted laterally with the cheek flap.

The close-up view of the plane of surgical dissection near the jugular foramen (29) shows the heavy Mayo scissors separating the specimen from the anterior aspect of the jugular foramen remaining just inferomedial to the auditory canal.

The posterior attachments of the surgical specimen have been separated, and the only attachments that remain to be divided are those in the pterygoid fossa requiring fracture of the pterygoid plates from the sphenoid bone and detachment of the medial aspect of the specimen from the parapharyngeal space (30). The plane of dissection, medially, is along the parapharyngeal space. Having divided the maxillary tubercle, the plane of dissection remains just lateral to the soft palate and the lateral wall of the nasopharynx. With gentle rocking movements, remaining soft tissue attachments of the specimen are divided with heavy Mayo scissors and the specimen is delivered.

The surgical field following removal of the specimen (31) shows the resected lateral bony wall of the orbit, the floor of the middle cranial fossa and the tumor from the infratemporal fossa and pterygopalatine region.

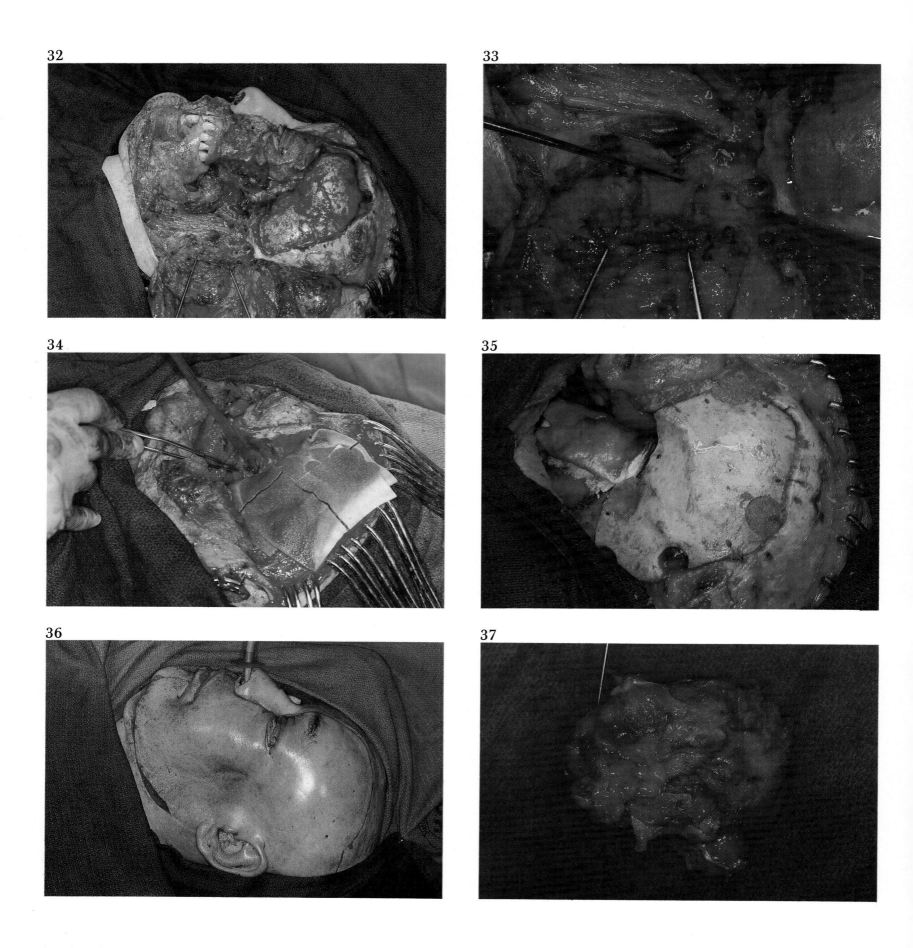

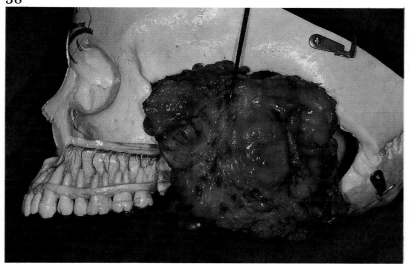

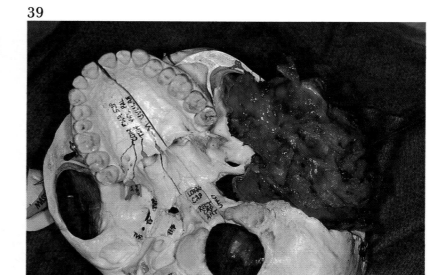

The parotid gland is retracted laterally showing the jugular foramen with exiting internal jugular vein and vagus nerve. The bony auditory canal is also seen here with the main trunk of the facial nerve protruding from the stylomastoid foramen (32).

The close-up view of the skull base near the region of the jugular foramen (33) shows the internal jugular vein and vagus nerve as well as the internal carotid artery entering the carotid canal. A nerve hook shows the main trunk of the facial nerve lifted up with the rest of the parotid gland and retracted laterally with hooks.

The foramen ovale is demonstrated here with fine-tipped forceps (34). As mentioned earlier, venous oozing from the region of the foramen ovale is not uncommon and can be sometimes tedious to control, but gel foam packing with pressure is occasionally sufficient to control this. The wound is now irrigated, previously withdrawn cerebrospinal fluid is reintroduced, and the brain is allowed to expand. The dura is inspected for any cerebrospinal fluid leakage. Following this, closure of the craniotomy begins first. The bone plate is returned and sutured in position with neurolon sutures (35). The temporalis muscle is used to fill the surgical defect created by removal of the tumor. A watertight mucosal closure in the oral cavity is completed by suturing the mucosa of the cheek to that of the floor of the mouth and the upper gum.

The orbicularis oculi muscle is sutured back to the upper and lower eyelids with absorbable sutures. The rest of the skin incision is closed in two layers with a suction drain brought out through a separate stab incision in the neck. A suction drain is also placed under the scalp (36).

The surgical specimen in (37) shows monobloc resection of the tumor. The surgical specimen superimposed on a skull (38) shows from where it was removed. Note that the specimen was removed from the area of tumor involvement which extended into the infratemporal fossa, the posterior wall of the maxilla, the pterygopalatine fossa and the upper part of the neck.

The basal view of the skull (39) shows the location of the tumor from where the surgical specimen was removed. Note the extension of tumor medially into the skull base in the region of the jugular foramen as well as in the infratemporal fossa.

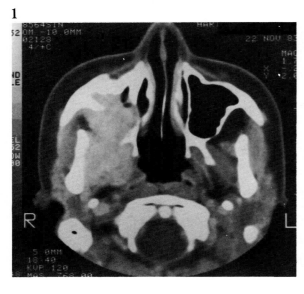

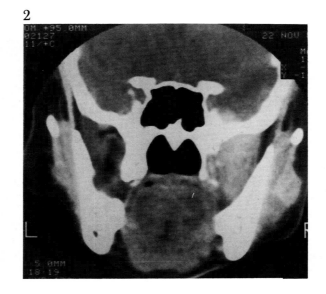

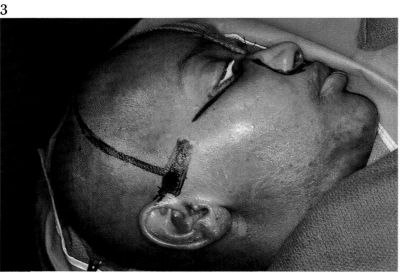

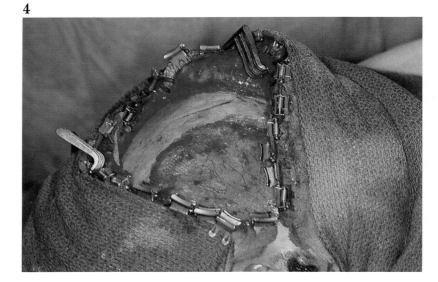

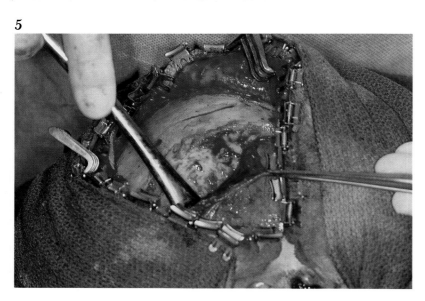

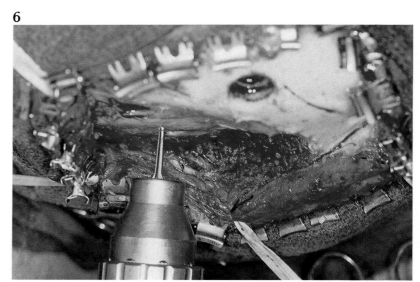

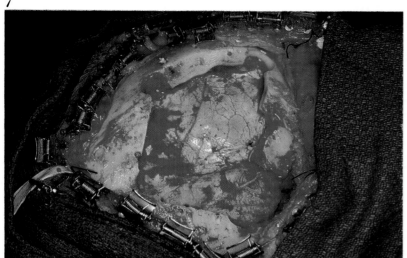

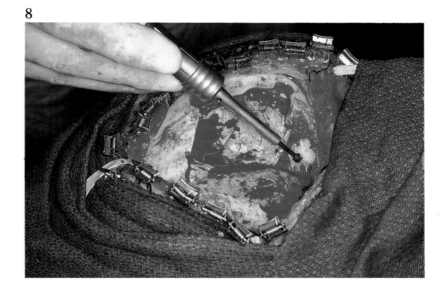

Resection of tumor of the maxilla extending into the pterygoid and infratemporal fossae

Excision of tumors of the maxilla extending into the pterygoid fossa and infratemporal fossa with secondary extension in the middle cranial fossa require a two-team simultaneous craniofacial approach.

The patient presented here has an aggressive fibromatosis for which she had undergone multiple surgical procedures in the past. The patient presented with total trismus and severe pain on the side of the face.

A review of the CT scan (1) showed the presence of a contrast-enhancing lesion extending from the posterolateral aspect of the maxillary antrum into the pterygoid space and infratemporal fossa. The tumor had involved both medial and lateral pterygoid muscles which were replaced by tumor infiltration extending up to the medial wall of the ascending ramus of the mandible.

The coronal cut of the CT scan (2) shows extension of tumor from the pterygoid fossa through the greater wing of sphenoid into the middle cranial fossa. Note that the lateral pterygoid plate is completely destroyed by the tumor.

Surgical exposure of the middle cranial fossa in this patient required a temporal craniotomy via a vertical incision in the temporoparietal scalp (3). The incision begins approximately 1.5 cm anterior to the attachment of the helix and extending towards the vertex, and curved anteriorly towards the hairline. A Weber–Ferguson incision is also outlined with a Diffenbach extension up to the lateral canthus, as shown here. A ceramic corneal shield is placed in the conjunctival sac to protect the cornea.

A split-thickness skin graft is obtained and an in-dwelling spinal catheter is introduced through lumbar puncture.

The scalp incision has been taken and both posterior and anterior scalp flaps are elevated (4). The parietal and squamous part of the temporal bone is exposed along with the attached temporalis muscle. The anterior flap is elevated as low as the zygomatic arch to provide sufficient exposure necessary for proceeding with temporal craniotomy.

The temporalis muscle is elevated from its insertion over the calvarium (5). The lower part of the parietal bone as well as the squamous part of the temporal bone is completely exposed. The temporalis muscle is excised after its tendinous insertion is detached from the coronoid process of the mandible.

To proceed with the craniotomy five burr holes are now made, and connected by a craniotome (6). Alternately, one can use a gigli saw to remove the bone flap. In this case the bone flap removed is approximately 4 × 6 cm; it is preserved for subsequent replacement during closure of the operation.

The dura of the temporal lobe is now carefully elevated over the floor of the middle cranial fossa (7).

Using a high speed drill, a subtemporal craniectomy is performed from the lower edge of the bone flap, curving medially towards the floor of the middle cranial fossa (8). Appropriate malleable retractors provide adequate protection to the brain. The entire length of the floor of the middle cranial fossa along the length of the craniectomy is drilled out.

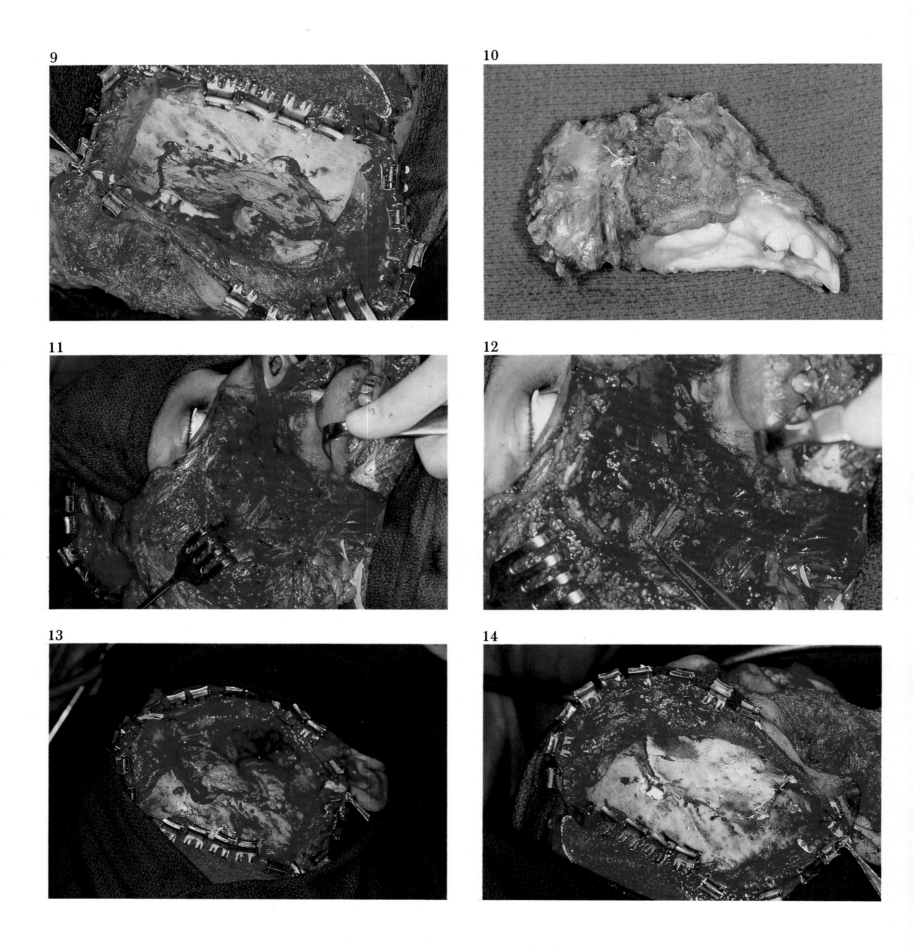

As the craniectomy proceeds medially and the dura is elevated, the foramina ovale, rotundum and spinosum come into view (9). At this point, the intracranial exposure is sufficiently wide to proceed with facial exposure for removal of the tumor. Superior mobilization of the surgical specimen from the bony floor of the middle cranial fossa is complete.

The facial exposure begins with a Weber–Ferguson incision with the Diffenbach extension almost up to the anterior aspect of the zygomatic arch. The skin flap is elevated by making an incision in the mucosa of the oral cavity through the gingivobuccal sulcus. Mucosal incision from the region of the maxillary tubercle is continued along the retromolar gingiva into the gingivobuccal sulcus of the lower alveolus up to the midline of the inner aspect of the lower lip. The latter is divided in the midline, and the lower cheek flap elevated. The skin incision is in the midline, dividing the chin, and curving to the right in the upper part of the neck. The masseter muscle is detached from the ascending ramus of the mandible and retracted laterally to protect the parotid gland containing the main trunk and peripheral branches of the facial nerve. The ascending ramus of the mandible is then excised by dividing the mandible through its body between the second and third molar teeth on the right side. The condyloid process is dislocated and the ascending ramus is removed after detaching the attachments of the pterygoid muscles. This then provides direct access to the infratemporal fossa.

A cut is then made, with a Strycker saw, about 2 mm below the floor of the orbit anteriorly which extends into the nasal bone medially; the cut is then carried from the nasal process of maxilla through the midline of the hard palate, again using a Strycker saw. A straight osteotome is then used to fracture the hard palate in the midline. Soft tissue attachments of both hard and soft palate are divided using electrocautery.

With the exposure available so far, and with guidance from the craniotomy side, superior mobilization of the specimen is continued. Medially, mobilization of the specimen requires working through the submucosal plane in the lateral wall of the nasopharynx. The pterygoid musculature and both pterygoid plates remain attached to the specimen. Since the latter was freed from the intracranial aspect, its posterior attachments with soft tissues around the internal carotid artery are gently divided. At this point, the third division of the trigeminal nerve appears to be the only attachment to the patient. The third division of the fifth nerve is divided intracranially and its stump is suture-ligated.

With a gentle rocking motion, the specimen containing the right maxilla with both pterygoid plates, all pterygoid muscles and extensive tumor of the infratemporal fossa was removed en bloc, including the lateral wall of the nasal cavity on the right side (10). The surgical defect as seen from the facial aspect is shown in (11). Complete removal of the tumor is effected. A close-up view of the surgical defect (12) shows the resected floor of the middle cranial fossa. The forceps in the center of the field shows the lateral wall of cavernous sinus.

The surgical defect as seen from the craniotomy aspect (13) shows a through-and-through defect in the bony floor of the middle cranial fossa extending into the infratemporal fossa and the upper part of the neck. After complete hemostasis is obtained, the craniotomy wound is closed.

Previously withdrawn cerebrospinal fluid is reintroduced and the brain is allowed to expand. The bone plate is returned to its place (14).

15

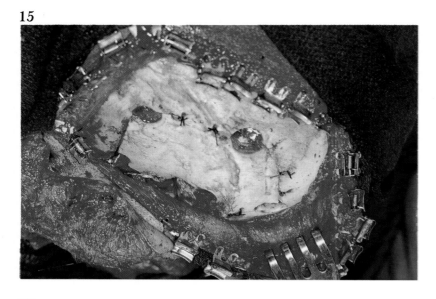

16

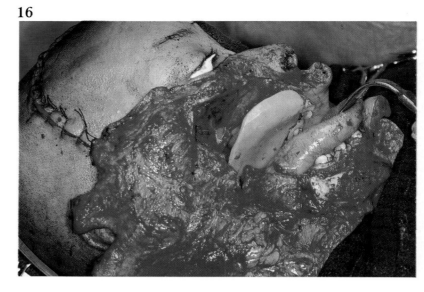

17

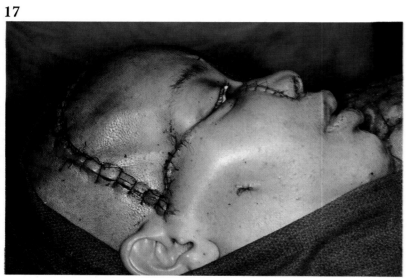

18

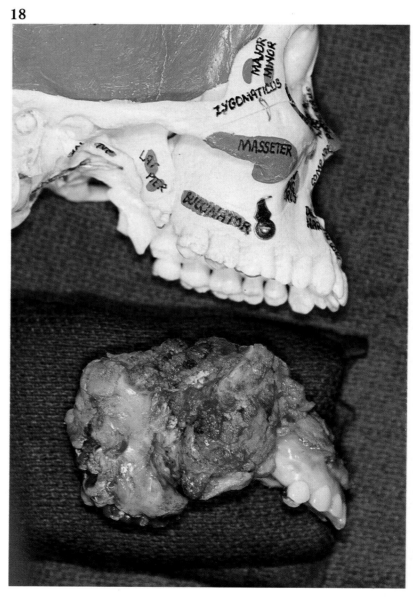

Several neurolon sutures are taken to retain the bone plate in its place (15), and the craniotomy wound is then closed in layers with a suction drain under the scalp.

On the facial aspect, an immediate palatal obturator is wired to the remaining upper teeth on the left side (16). Then the previously obtained skin graft is applied to the raw areas on the inner surface of the cheek flap, and the facial incision is closed in layers. The skin graft is retained in position with snug packing using xerofoam gauze.

Meticulous attention should be paid to closure of the skin incision on the face. The lateral extension of the Weber–Ferguson incision is closed with fine sutures, paying specific attention to accurate reapproximation of the skin edges (17). A subcuticular absorbable suture with 4-0 Dexon provides a superior esthetic result.

The surgical specimen of the massive tumor of infra-temporal fossa removed *en bloc* with maxillectomy is shown next to the skull for comparison (18). Note that the bulk of the tumor is posterior to the last molar tooth in the infratemporal fossa. *En bloc* resection of tumors presenting in the infratemporal fossa can thus be safely achieved via a temporal craniotomy and maxillectomy approach with either mandibulectomy or mandibulotomy.

The postoperative appearance of the patient 6 weeks after surgery (19) shows a clean, well-healed surgical defect of right-sided maxillectomy with removal of the tumor from the infratemporal fossa. Note that the patient is now able to open her mouth completely without any pain or discomfort.

A permanent dental obturator is now in place providing obliteration of the maxillectomy defect and restoration of the functions of speech, mastication and swallowing (20).

19

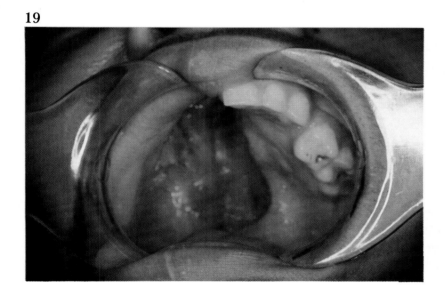

20

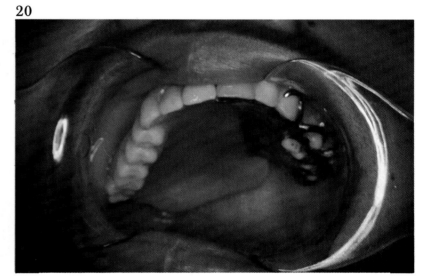

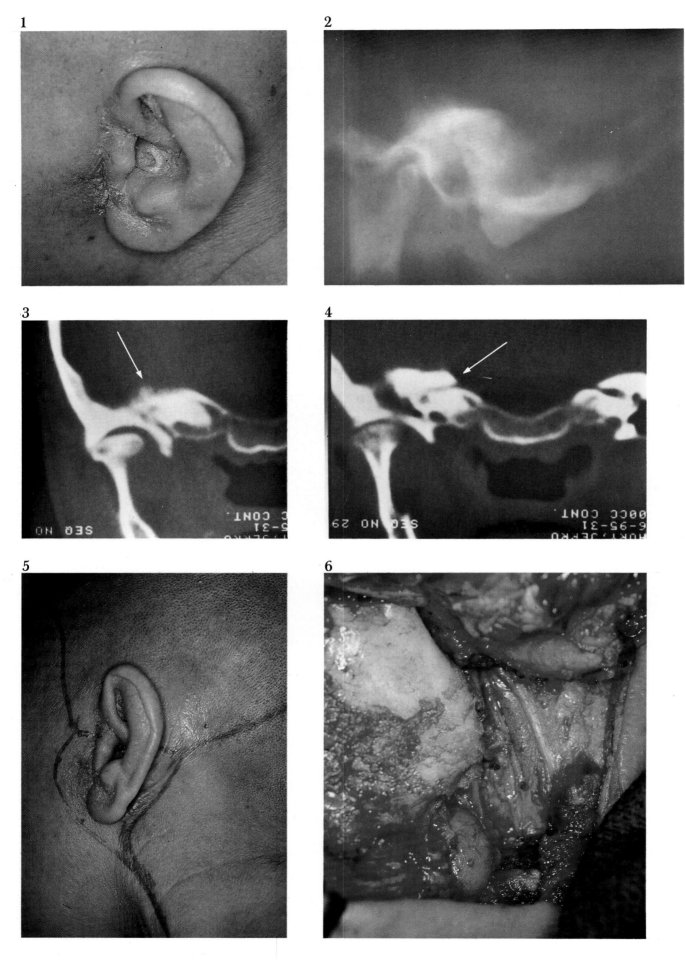

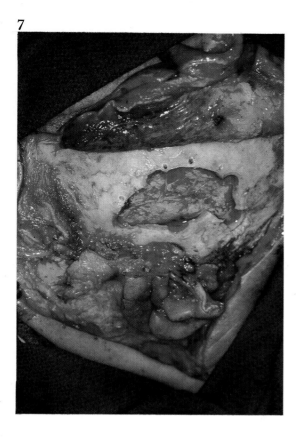

7

Temporal bone resection

Excision of tumors arising in the auditory canal either in its cartilagenous or bony part call for temporal bone resection. In the past malignant tumors arising in the auditory canal were treated by external irradiation with poor results. *En bloc* resection of the tumors presenting in the cartilagenous portion of the auditory canal or the lateral portion of the bony canal are amenable to satisfactory surgical resection with significant improvement in locoregional control rate and survival.

The patient presented here (1) has carcinoma of the auditory canal fungating through the external ear. She had previously been treated with external irradiation which failed to control the cancer. There is significant induration in the parotid region with fibrosis and scarring, but the facial nerve function is intact.

Sagittal tomograms through the bony auditory canal show involvement of the upper half of the ear canal in the petrous part of the temporal bone (2). The CT scan in a coronal plane taken through the anterior aspect of the petrous portion of the temporal bone shows erosion of the superior surface of the temporal bone, raising the possibility of involvement of the petrous temporal bone intracranially (3). However, at the time of surgery, no tumor was seen in the cranial cavity. The CT scan in a coronal plane further posterior (4) shows that the internal acoustic meatus is clear of tumor, and the patient is therefore a suitable candidate for temporal bone resection.

The plan of surgical incisions is outlined here (5). The lower half of the external ear will be sacrificed along with the skin of both preauricular and postauricular regions to encompass the fungating tumor. The pinna will remain attached to the auditory canal with which it will be removed *en bloc* in continuity with the temporal bone. The scalp is elevated from the outlined incisions with a wide base as outlined here on the skin. An indwelling spinal catheter is introduced through a lumbar puncture.

The anterior skin incision is taken first. A radical total parotidectomy is performed to remain in continuity with the specimen of the temporal bone. After the skin flap is elevated, the plane of dissection is directly over the lateral aspect of the ascending ramus of the mandible, remaining deep to the masseter muscle which is detached from both the mandible and the zygomatic arch. As shown here, the mandible is exposed, and the condyloid process of the mandible is divided to aid removal of the temporal bone *en bloc* (6). The posterior skin incision is taken next, and the scalp flap is elevated. Incision on the scalp is taken straight down to the cranium through the temporalis muscle which remains attached over the scalp flap (7). Thus, the lower part of the temporalis muscle is transected as the incision goes through it to the squamous part of the temporal bone, which is exposed using a periosteal elevator. Five burr holes are made and a temporal craniotomy performed using a craniotome or gigli saw to connect the burr holes. The bone plate is preserved for subsequent closure of the wound. Dura of the middle cranial fossa is carefully elevated to avoid any injury to it. Following temporal craniotomy, approximately 15 mls of cerebrospinal fluid is removed from the lumbar spinal drainage catheter. The dura is then gently stripped away from the floor of the middle cranial fossa and from the mastoid process, and posteriorly from the posterior fossa. A high speed drill is now used to proceed with mastoidectomy.

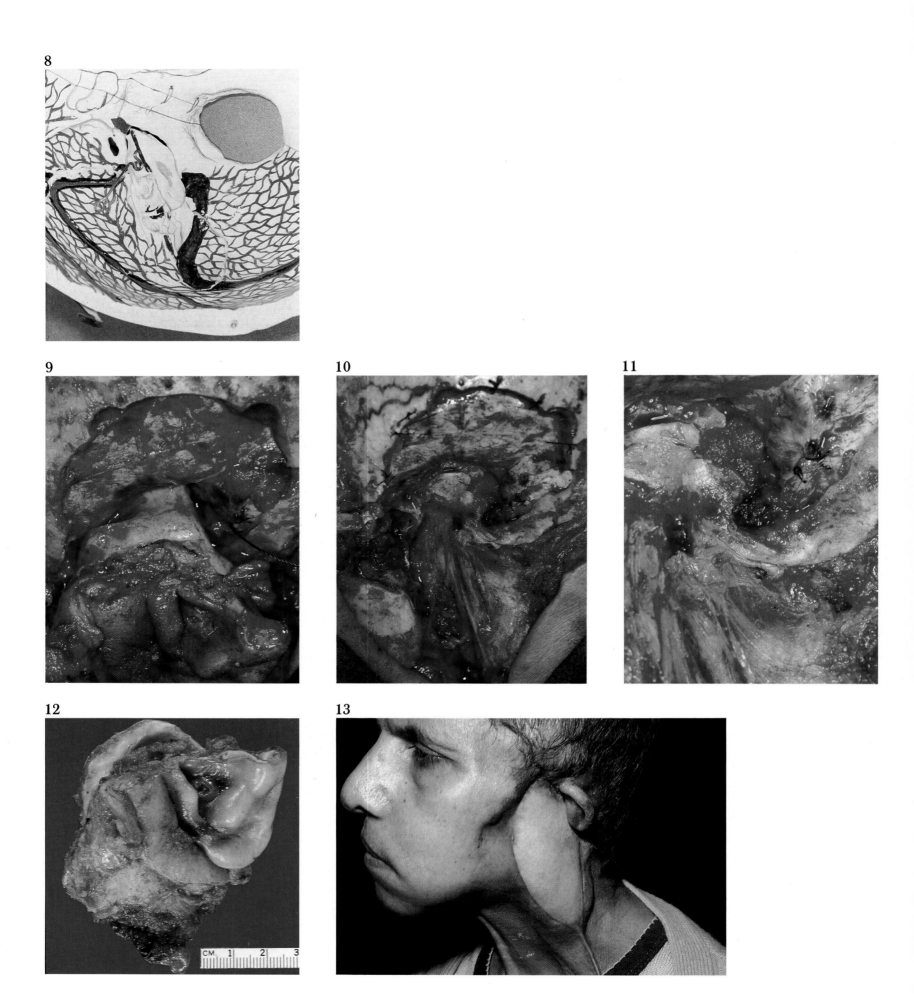

The plan of surgical procedure at this point is to expose the superior aspect of the sigmoid sinus skirting the temporal bone posteriorly, as demonstrated on the skull (8). Meticulous attention should be paid to leaving a thin shell of bone over the sigmoid sinus to prevent any unnecessary hemorrhage. This is a tedious, slow dissection, but it can be expedited using a high speed drill and suction irrigator. As the sigmoid sinus is approached, a thin shell of bone is left over it beneath which one can see the bluish sinus. Elevation of the dura over the petrous part of the temporal bone continues. Very careful and meticulous dissection is now undertaken with fine dural elevators to elevate the sigmoid sinus from its bed, exposing the posterior part of the petrous temporal bone. Bleeding, at this point, is usually encountered from the superior petrosal sinus, and can be controlled by gel foam or bone wax.

The zygomatic process is now divided using a Strycker saw. The sternomastoid muscle is detached from the mastoid process, and the posterior belly of the digastric muscle is also detached from the digastric groove over the temporal bone. Using a high speed drill and fine drill bit, the line of transection on the petrous part of the temporal bone, remaining just lateral to the internal acoustic meatus, is demarcated. Similarly, using the high speed drill, a bone cut is made over the floor of the middle cranial fossa through the squamous part of the temporal bone just anterior to the auditory canal and the petrous temporal bone up to the temporal craniotomy. Now all the vascular connections of the temporal bone are carefully dissected off, including the sigmoid sinus from its posterior aspect. The bone cut through the medial part of the petrous temporal bone is deepened using a fine drill bit. The specimen is completely mobilized from all its attachments except medially, as shown here (9).

Using a medium curved osteotome, the petrous temporal bone is fractured through the previously demarcated cut made by the drill bit. Similarly, using the osteotome, the anterior part of the petrous temporal bone is fractured through the line of previously demarcated bone cut made with the drill. Once this fracture is made the specimen can be mobilized laterally and anteriorly to detach the lateral pterygoid muscle attached to the condyloid process of the mandible. Remaining soft tissue attachments are divided and the specimen is delivered.

Once the specimen is removed, the upper part of the jugular vein and the jugular foramen come into view (10). The soft tissue attachments must be divided meticulously and carefully in order to preserve the contents of the jugular foramen, that is, the neurovascular structures that exit from the skull. The internal jugular vein, hypoglossal and vagus nerves are carefully identified and preserved. The internal carotid artery remains medial as it enters the carotid canal, and is also carefully isolated and preserved. The lateral wall of the jugular foramen may have to be excised with the surgical specimen, depending upon the extent of the tumor.

A close-up view of the surgical field following removal of the specimen (11) shows the stump of the apex of the petrous temporal bone medially, with the internal jugular vein entering the jugular foramen and the jugular bulb forming the sigmoid sinus through the base of the skull. This completes the monobloc resection of the temporal bone, extending from the lateral lip of the internal acoustic meatus and including the lateral wall of the jugular foramen all the way up to the skin.

The surgical specimen (12) shows the lower half of the external ear with the auditory canal, periauricular skin, parotid gland, masseter muscle and temporal bone all removed en bloc. In this patient, a total temporal bone resection has been performed remaining medial to the cochlea; she will therefore have a transient disturbance of balance as well as complete facial paralysis.

The resection of external ear and periauricular skin resulted in loss of a large portion of skin requiring appropriate skin coverage, using a pectoralis major myocutaneous flap (13). A lateral tarsorrhaphy is performed to prevent corneal damage.

The procedure is generally well tolerated by most patients, although both complete loss of hearing and facial paralysis are to be expected on the side of surgery. Loss of balance, however, is transient and lasts from 2 to 3 weeks. If there is any cerebrospinal fluid leakage at the time of surgery, it should be meticulously repaired to prevent leakage of fluid and subsequent meningitis. Most patients are ambulatory by the third postoperative day, although the vertigo resulting from the surgery will take approximately 2–3 weeks to resolve.

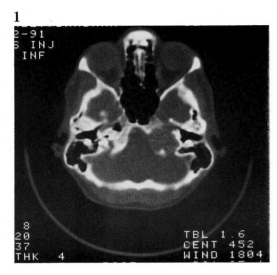

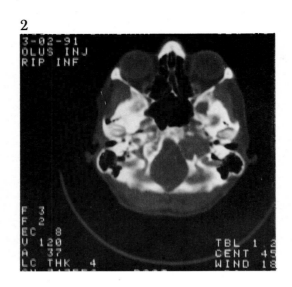

1

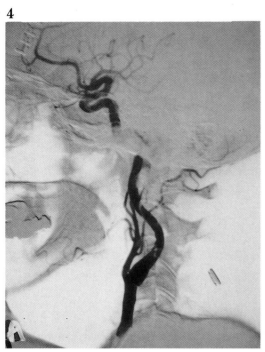

2

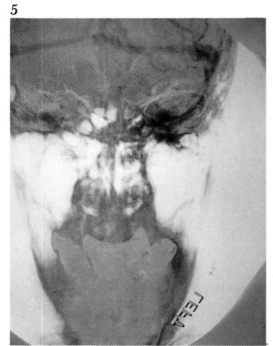

3

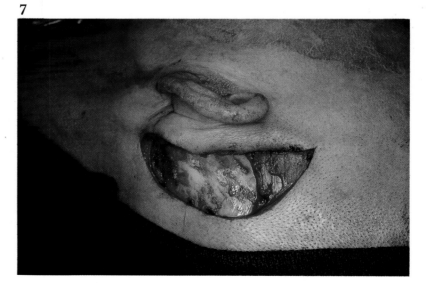

4

5

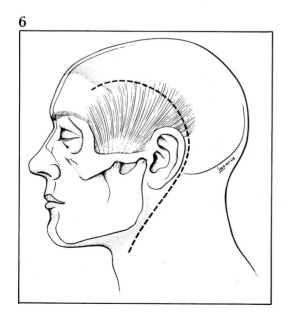

6

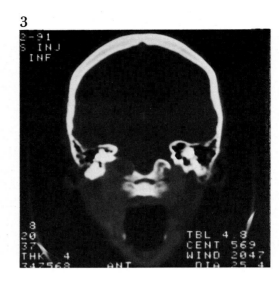

7

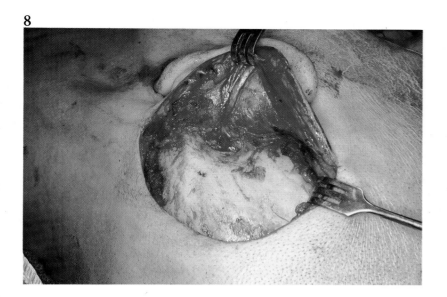

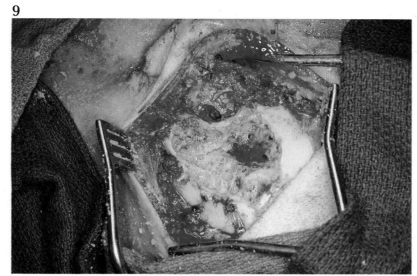

Infratemporal fossa approach for removal of glomus jugulare tumor

The infratemporal fossa approach is an excellent surgical procedure for tumors in the vicinity of the petrous portion of the temporal bone. It also provides a very good approach for extensive tumors of the jugular foramen extending to the clivus and parasellar region. The operative procedure demands permanent anterior transposition of the facial nerve, obliteration of the pneumatic spaces of the temporal bone via a mastoidectomy, and permanent occlusion of the eustachian tube. The external auditory canal is closed like a blind sac which prevents postoperative infection and permits primary wound healing, but the function of the inner ear is preserved by this approach.

The patient presented in this surgical procedure had a previous history of breast carcinoma from which she had been cured for several years. At this time, she presented with tinnitus and dizziness and on work up was found to have a glomus tumor on the left side.

A review of CT scans show the presence of a tumor in the region of the apex of the petrous temporal bone presenting posteriorly adjacent to the clivus (1), a large lesion that had partially destroyed the bone. The CT scan lower down (2) showed the tumor extending up to the lateral lip of foramen magnum, although the margin of the latter was intact. The CT scan in a coronal plane show significant enlargement of the jugular foramen compared to the opposite side (3).

Carotid angiography showed this to be a vascular lesion. During the arterial phase of the angiographic study, minimal visualization of the tumor could be seen (4). During the venous phase, however, a large lesion is seen involving the region of the jugular bulb and medial aspect of the sigmoid sinus (5).

The patient is positioned on the operating table with an indwelling spinal catheter for drainage of cerebrospinal fluid. The head is turned to the right side and a postauricular incision is planned (6), extending into the upper part of the neck inferiorly and over the temporoparietal scalp anteriorly.

The incision on the postauricular skin has been taken and deepened through the soft tissue attachments to expose the mastoid process (7). The cartilagenous portion of the auditory canal is retracted with the external ear, anteriorly (8). Elevation of the skin incision on the scalp is taken posteriorly up to the mastoid emissary vein.

Self-retaining retractors are now placed in and mastoidectomy is started (9), performed with a high speed drill, a fine drill bit and a suction irrigator equipment. Cortex of the temporal bone, in this area, is first drilled as far back as approximately 1 cm posterior to the sigmoid sinus, inferiorly up to the tip of the mastoid process, and anteriorly as far as the root of the zygoma. Medially, the drilling is first directed towards the antrum which is identified as is the horizontal semicircular canal.

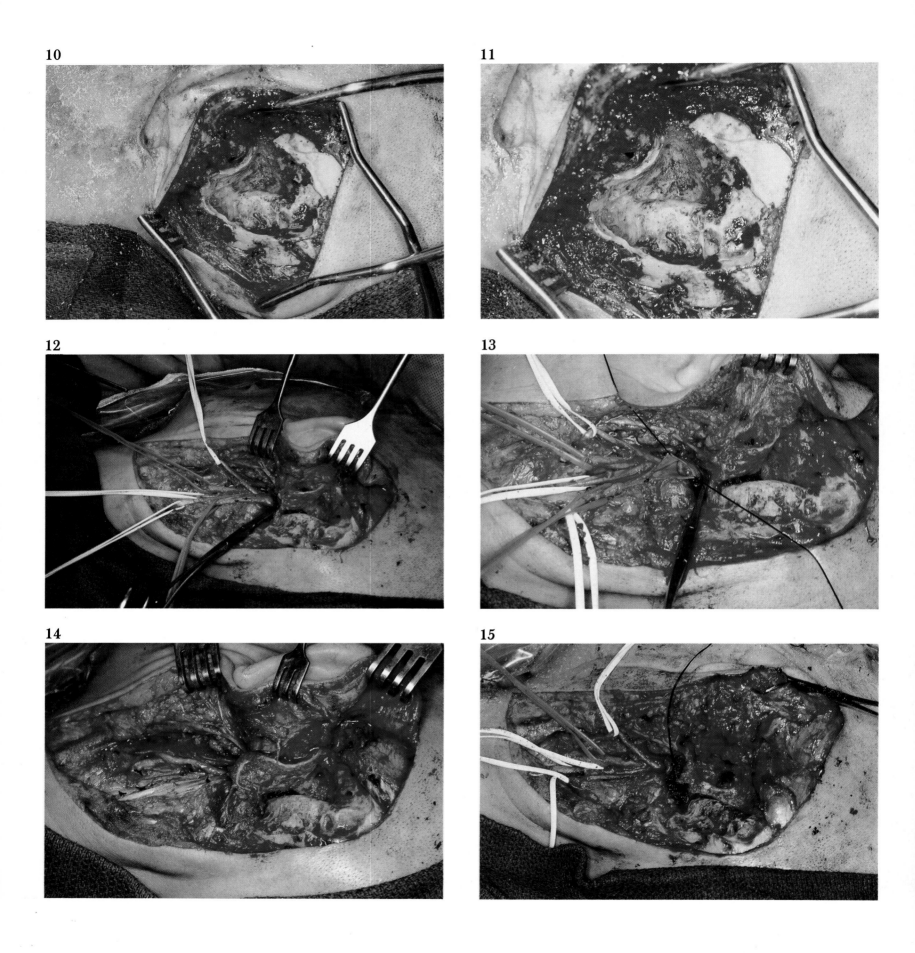

At this point, the edges of the mastoidectomy cavity are saucerized with the high speed drill, and the mastoidectomy is carried further to expose the sigmoid sinus along its entire length down to the level of the jugular bulb (10). The facial nerve is still protected in its canal and is not visualized. The landmarks identified at this point are the short process of incus as well as the digastric ridge, inferiorly. The posterior fossa is also exposed along the sigmoid sinus up to the level of the posterior semicircular canal. A thin shell of bone, however, is left over the semicircular canal as well as the entire length of the sigmoid sinus. The area of the jugular bulb is now identified and no tumor can be seen as yet at that level (11).

At this stage, the intracranial portion of the operative procedure is held, and the C-shaped incision extended into the upper part of the neck (12). The anterior and posterior skin flaps are elevated as usual. The anterior border of the sternomastoid muscle is identified, and is retracted posteriorly so as to expose the carotid bulb, the internal jugular vein, the hypoglossal, vagus, the superior laryngeal, and glossopharyngeal nerves. Rubber tapes are placed around each of these structures, particular attention being paid to achieving control of the left internal jugular vein. Note, in (12), that the white rubber tapes are round the hypoglossal, vagus and accessory nerves, the blue tape is round the internal jugular vein, and the red tape round the internal carotid artery. On palpation of the jugular vein near the jugular foramen, firm tumor could be felt in its lumen. In this case, because of the previous history of breast cancer in this patient, it was mandatory to establish a tissue diagnosis before proceeding with the surgical procedure for removal of the glomus tumor. A vascular clamp is, therefore, applied on the jugular vein at the jugular foramen and a vessel loop placed lower down in the neck around the vein.

Then the vein is opened next and an open biopsy of the tumor presenting in its lumen performed. The tumor is clearly seen here as it presents itself in the lumen of the jugular vein (13). A small wedge from the tumor is removed and sent for frozen section examination, this confirming the diagnosis of paraganglioma. The vein is, therefore, ligated below the presenting tumor and divided, and the vascular clamp removed. Following this, a superficial parotidectomy is performed as usual, and the main trunk and peripheral branches of the facial nerve identified and dissected to expose the entry of the main trunk into the stylomastoid foramen (14).

Attention is now directed back to the intracranial portion of the operative procedure. The cartilagenous ear canal is transected and reflected anteriorly, and the posterior canal wall is removed. The tympanic membrane is dissected off the malleus. The incusostapedial joint is dislocated and the incus also freed from its junction with the malleus, and removed. Following this, using a cup forceps, the malleus is also removed. All of this is done to prevent transmission of vibrations through the ossicles to the inner ear. The facial nerve is then identified along its entire course after drilling the bone around the facial canal to identify it from the geniculate ganglion superiorly, and down to its exit through the stylomastoid foramen inferiorly. Using a diamond burr all around the facial canal, the bone is removed from nearly 270° around the canal, leaving a very thin covering which is removed using curettes and hooks. The nerve is then identified in its full length, and the deep branch of the *chorda tympanii* as well as the stapedius branches cut. The nerve is carefully elevated from its exit through the stylomastoid foramen and from the surrounding structures using sharp dissection so as to minimize traction, and carefully delivered from its fallopian canal using blunt and sharp dissection where necessary. The entire dissection of the facial nerve requires the use of the operating microscope, high speed drill with a diamond drill bit and suction irrigator. Dissection and delivery of the nerve continues up to the geniculate ganglion.

Following this maneuver, the nerve is rerouted both anteriorly and superiorly leaving no nerve structure in the bone between the mastoid, the hypotympanum and the jugular foramen (15). Following identification of the posterior semicircular canal, the bone is drilled out from that level to the area of the jugular foramen, and the mastoid tip taken out using rongeurs. The lateral lip of the carotid canal is also removed using Kerrison forceps. At this point, distal but not proximal control of the jugular vein is secured. Therefore, the thin shell of bone over the sigmoid sinus is drilled out and peeled off the sigmoid sinus. Incisions in the dura are made on each side of the sigmoid sinus and a blunt needle passed along the medial surface of the sinus, and through the dural holes a large vascular clip is applied, the dural openings being sutured with 4-0 neurolon sutures. The lateral wall of the sigmoid sinus is then opened and followed to the area of the jugular bulb. Some bleeding is encountered at this time, but the sinus is distally packed with gel foam.

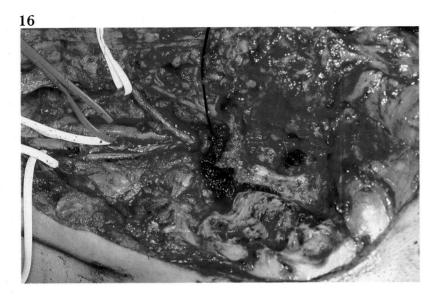

16

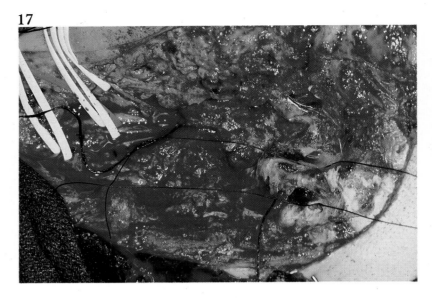

17

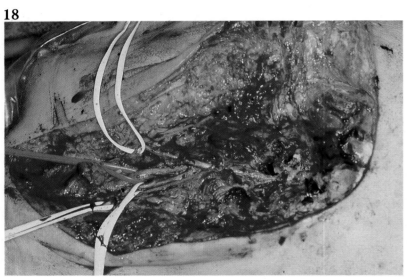

18

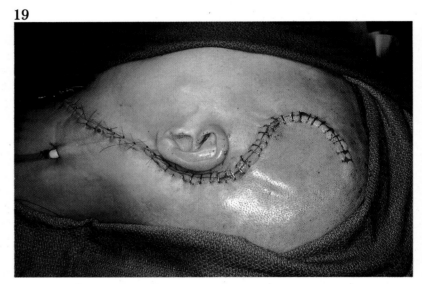

19

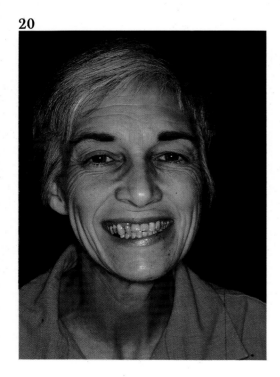

20

Dissection of the stump of the jugular vein along with the contents of the sigmoid sinus including intravascular tumor is then undertaken (**16**). When the sigmoid sinus is opened, some bleeding is to be expected from the inferior petrosal sinus which is packed with muscle. In this patient, additional tumor extension was found to extend beyond the vein in the area anterior and medial to the jugular bulb. The tumor is then dissected off from the carotid artery, and also from all the nerves that leave the skull through the jugular foramen (**17**). Following this dissection, if the tumor extends further medially towards the foramen magnum, it is removed using an ultrasonic suction aspirator.

Gross total removal of the tumor is accomplished. The surgical field shows the open area of the excised sigmoid sinus and the jugular foramen with its lateral lip missing. Cranial nerves exiting from the jugular foramen are shown here (**18**). The proximal part of the sigmoid sinus, which has been clipped, is seen. The wound is reinspected for bleeding and then irrigated.

The rerouted facial nerve is placed over the zygomatic bone and the incision is closed. The posterior aspect of the auditory canal is closed with suture of soft tissues to create a blind sac of the auditory canal. All the vessel loops around the identified nerves and vessels are removed. A suction drain is placed through a separate stab incision and the skin incision is closed in layers (**19**).

The postoperative appearance of the patient approximately 5 months after surgery (**20**) shows complete recovery of the facial nerve function which was transiently paretic.

Excision of glomus jugulare tumors is a complex surgical procedure demanding a high degree of technical expertise and great familiarity with the anatomy of this area. Radiographic findings on CT scan should be correlated with the skull prior to the surgical procedure, and a skull should also be available in the operating room. The intracranial part of the operative procedure should be undertaken by a neurosurgeon or a neurotologist.

9: Cysts and Tumors of the Mandible

Introduction

The mandible, a membranous bone which supports the lower dentition, is the most important supporting bony structure for the function of mastication. The blood supply, nerve supply and muscular attachments to the mandible are bilaterally symmetrical, and are such that the dynamic forces supporting the movements of the mandible are balanced. The principal blood supply is derived from the terminal branches of the external carotid artery via the internal maxillary artery. The nerve supply to the teeth is derived from the mandibular division of the trigeminal nerve. The latter leaves the skull through the foramen ovale and traverses medially to the mandible where it gives off its lingual branch and then enters the mandibular canal through the medial aspect of the ascending ramus of the mandible. Within the mandibular canal it is called the inferior alveolar nerve. It provides nerve supply to the roots of the teeth and gives off its terminal mental branch which exits through the mental foramen to provide nerve supply to the skin of the lower lip and chin.

The mandibular canal is well below the sockets of the teeth in the mandible; however, in the edentulous mandible, as the alveolar process recedes the mandibular canal comes closer to the alveolar surface of the mandible. The principal muscular attachments to the mandible consists of the temporalis muscle attached to the coronoid process and the medial and lateral pterygoid muscles attached to the ascending ramus and condyloid process of the mandible respectively. The masseter muscle is attached to the mandible on the lateral surface of the ascending ramus, and the myelohyoid muscle is attached to the myelohyoid groove on the inner aspect of the body of the mandible. The genioglossus and geniohyoid muscles are attached in the midline on the lingual aspect over the genial tubercle.

Radiographic evaluation

Plain films of the mandible often provide satisfactory radiographic evaluation of its bony architecture and pathology, but oblique views must be obtained. The entire mandible is, however, screened by a panoramic view (panorex), which provides good visualization of the ascending ramus and the body of the mandible on both sides, though not of the symphysis region since the panoramic view is often not clear in the midline. More adequate and finer details of the bony architecture around the roots of the teeth and any early pathological changes are best seen through dental films and occlusal views of the mandible. Computerized tomography of the mandible is also a satisfactory screening device for bone pathology, but this is of limited value since the fine details of bony architecture do not show up well on a computerized tomogram.

Technetium bone scans are often of value since they may detect early neoplastic invasion before radiographic demonstration of bone invasion. In that respect, bone scans will be positive earlier than radiographic demonstration of bone invasion by a tumor. It must be borne in mind, however, that the bone scans can be positive with inflammatory processes and in situations of benign tumors with increased vascularity.

Preoperative preparation

Any patient in whom surgery on the mandible is anticipated must be seen by a dental surgeon for appropriate preoperative dental evaluation and management as indicated. This may include obtaining impressions and dental cast models for subsequent fabrication of dental splints and/or obturators. If septic teeth are present they should be attended to prior to contemplated surgery, but septic and/or loose teeth within the tumor-bearing area of the bone are best not disturbed until surgical resection. If a mandibulotomy is contemplated, the patient may require archbars for intermaxillary fixation and they should be applied, if possible, prior to the contemplated surgical resection. A dental surgeon should be available in the operating room if intraoperative dental assistance is necessary.

Excision and curettage of cysts of the mandible

The most common cysts encountered in the mandible are dental root and dentigerous cysts (1). Dental root cysts are secondary to a septic focus at the root of the involved tooth which goes on to form a destructive, mostly unilocular, cystic lesion. Dentigerous cysts form around an unerupted tooth, either unilocular or multilocular, and generally present with a tooth within the cystic area.

After appropriate radiographic evaluation, surgical treatment is undertaken via a peroral approach. Mucosa over the mandible is incised through the gingivolabial sulcus and the underlying bone is exposed. Using a periosteal elevator, a generous surface of the lateral aspect of the bone is exposed in the patient with teeth, or the alveolar process itself is exposed in the edentulous patient. Using an osteotome and a mallet, entry is made into the mandibular cyst. The cyst wall is usually eggshell thin and breaks very easily. The fluid encountered in the cystic space is evacuated, the unerupted tooth is removed, and the lining mucosa is totally curetted out. Meticulous attention should be paid to breaking the septa within the cystic lesion and in curetting out as much or all of the lining mucosa as possible.

Several other methods are available to destroy the lining of the mucosa, such as cryosurgery which involves pouring liquid nitrogen into the cystic cavity to destroy the lining mucosa. After complete curettage and irrigation of the cystic space, hemostasis is achieved by the use of electrocautery. Extreme care and delicacy should be used in curetting mandible since the thin wall of the cystic cavity may occasionally lead to mandible fracture.

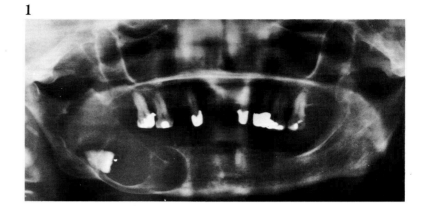

1

Following complete curettage, the cavity is left open and packed with xeroform gauze packing, both for hemostasis and to prevent closure of the cystic space from its roof causing the cyst to recur.

The initial packing placed in the operating room is changed within 48 hours and is replaced by a repeat packing. This is changed daily, and after several days the patient is taught to pack the cavity himself or herself until the space fills in from the bottom and heals without a cyst recurring. The cystic space will initially be filled with granulation tissue which will eventually calcify. Within 6 months to 1 year the cystic space will be completely obliterated and radiographic documentation will show new bone formation. With adequate curettage and proper postoperative care, cystic lesions of the mandible are unlikely to recur.

Mandible resection for fibrous dysplasia

Fibrous dysplasia is a benign disorder usually seen in the growing child. The lesion may present as a painful or painless bony swelling which, on radiographic evaluation, may either show osteoblastic or osteolytic areas, or occasionally a mixed picture. The indications for surgical excision are increasing pain and/or increasing mass causing deformity. The patient presented here (1) is an 11-year-old male with history of a progressive, enlarging mass in the region of the angle of the left-sided mandible of 3 years' duration. He had continuous and progressive pain with increasing mass demonstrated on serial radiographs over the previous few years, so surgical intervention was indicated.

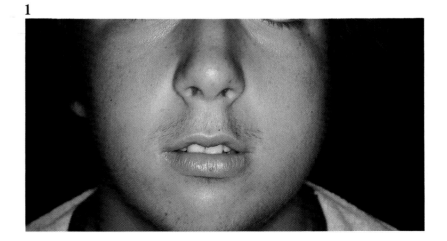

1

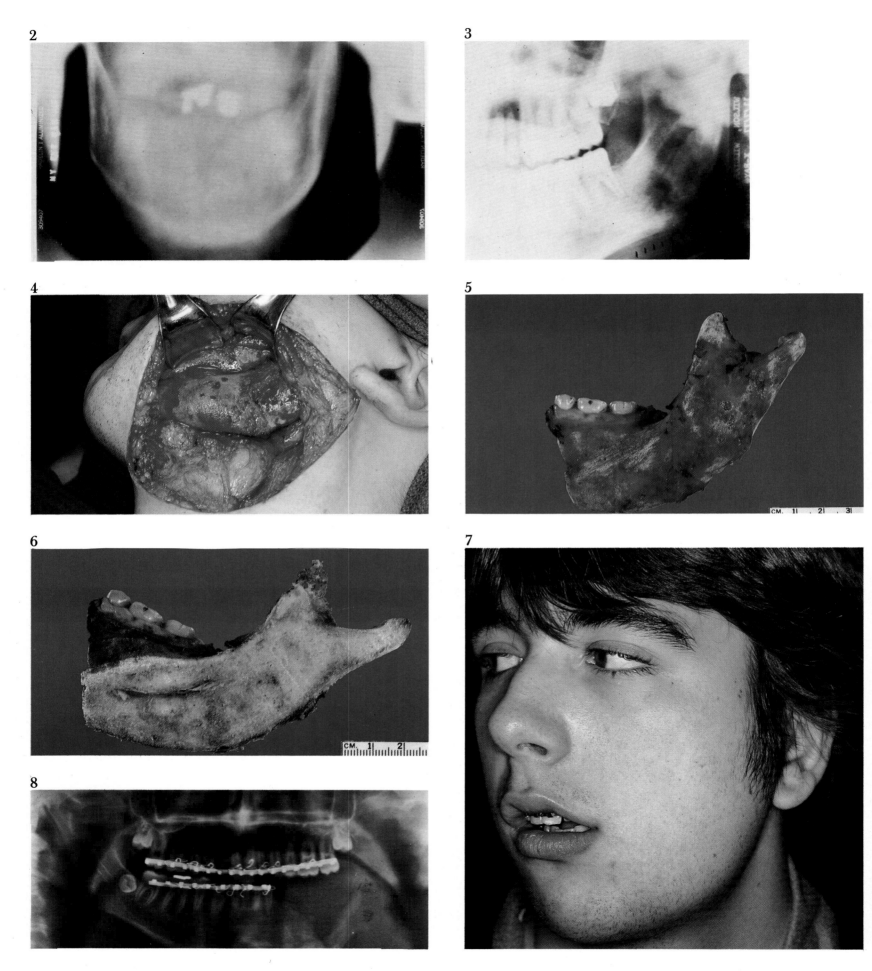

Radiographs of the mandible show a partly ossified and partly destructive bone lesion with periosteal reaction (2). The mandible also gives a ground-glass appearance at the site of involvement (3). The disease extends from the region of the notch of the mandible all the way up to the canine tooth.

Surgical exposure of the area intended for resection is easily achieved through a upper neck transverse incision extending from the mastoid process, following the upper neck skin crease up to the region of the hyoid bone (4). After skin incision, the platysma is incised along the line of the incision and meticulous dissection is undertaken while raising the upper skin flap. The mandibular branch of the facial nerve is carefully identified and preserved. Both anterior and posterior facial veins will be encountered during elevation of the skin flap, and these are divided, ligated and retracted cephalad with the cheek flap. Similarly, the facial artery will have to be divided, ligated and retracted with the cheek flap, cephalad, exposing the mandible in the region of the angle as well as the body. The entire dissection is kept in a plane just superficial to the mandible.

In (4) the area of bone involvement is exposed showing a pinkish-brown lesion on the outer cortex of the body of the mandible near the angle. The masseter muscle is detached from the mandible and is allowed to retract cephalad, and by further retraction and progressive detachment of the masseter, the notch of the mandible is reached. At this point, the tendon of the temporalis muscle attached to the coronoid process becomes evident and, using electrocautery, is completely detached. The oral cavity is now entered through the gingivolabial sulcus. The canine tooth is extracted and, through the socket of the canine tooth, the body of the mandible is divided using a Strycker saw, and an attempt is made to retract it laterally; this is prevented by muscular attachments of the myelohyoid muscle as well as the mucosa of the floor of the mouth.

An incision is made into the mucosa of the floor of the mouth where the mandible is divided along the lingual gingiva, and this is taken up to the retromolar trigone, meeting the incision in the gingivolabial sulcus, so the alveolar process is completely detached all round its mucosal attachments. The mandible is now retracted laterally and, as the myelohyoid muscle is divided, the surgical specimen can be retracted and rotated externally. The medial pterygoid muscle now comes into view, and under direct vision is divided from the mandible. Brisk hemorrhage from several branches of the internal maxillary artery is to be expected during this maneuver. The branches of the internal maxillary artery are clamped and tied or suture-ligated. Finally, the lateral pterygoid muscle is detached by dividing its tendinous attachment to the condyloid process on its medial

surface. The mandible now remains attached only through the capsule of the temporomandibular joint. The capsule is incised and the condyloid process dislocated from the mandibular socket, leaving the intra-articular disc behind.

The surgical specimen (5) shows the body and the ascending ramus of the mandible with both the coronoid and the condyloid processes completely removed in one piece with the dentition posterior to the canine tooth in the specimen. The specimen is bisected to show complete loss of normal architecture of bone and replacement with fibrous dysplasia (6). The wound is irrigated with Bacitracin solution, and a suction drain is placed. The mucosa of the floor of the mouth is closed by approximation to the cheek mucosa with interrupted chromic catgut sutures. The skin incision is closed in two layers using 3-0 chromic catgut interrupted sutures for platysma and 5-0 nylon sutures for skin. The patient is placed in intermaxillary fixation, postoperatively, to retain the right side of the mandible in occlusion with the upper dentition.

The postoperative appearance of the patient is shown approximately 3 years after surgery (7). Note minimal esthetic deformity after resection of the posterior part of the body and the ascending ramus of the mandible. Since the patient is wearing archbars and is in intermaxillary fixation, the drift of the remaining mandible is not evident. The archbars are initially maintained in full intermaxillary fixation for a period of 3 weeks, at which point the intermaxillary wires are removed leaving the archbars in place with ivy loops and rubber bands. This allows minimal motion of the mandible, but still maintains the upper and lower teeth on the right side in adequate occlusion. The patient is asked to keep the rubber bands for a period of up to 6 months, during which time the remaining musculature of the mandible on the right side is trained enough to close the lower jaw in proper occlusion during mastication.

The postoperative panoramic view of the mandible at 3 years (8) shows new bone formation through the retained periosteum of the mandible on the left side. Since this patient is still growing, the periosteum is active and has already regenerated new bone along its bed to replace the resected mandible. This patient's spontaneous regeneration of mandible through the retained periosteum provided satisfactory replacement for the resected bone, and mandibular reconstruction was not needed. Thus if mandible resection is necessary for a benign disease process in the growing child, then every attempt should be made to retain the periosteum to promote new born formation and regenerate a 'new mandible' at the site of the resected bone. If, however, there is no new bone formation, or the patient is an adult, secondary mandible reconstruction may be considered.

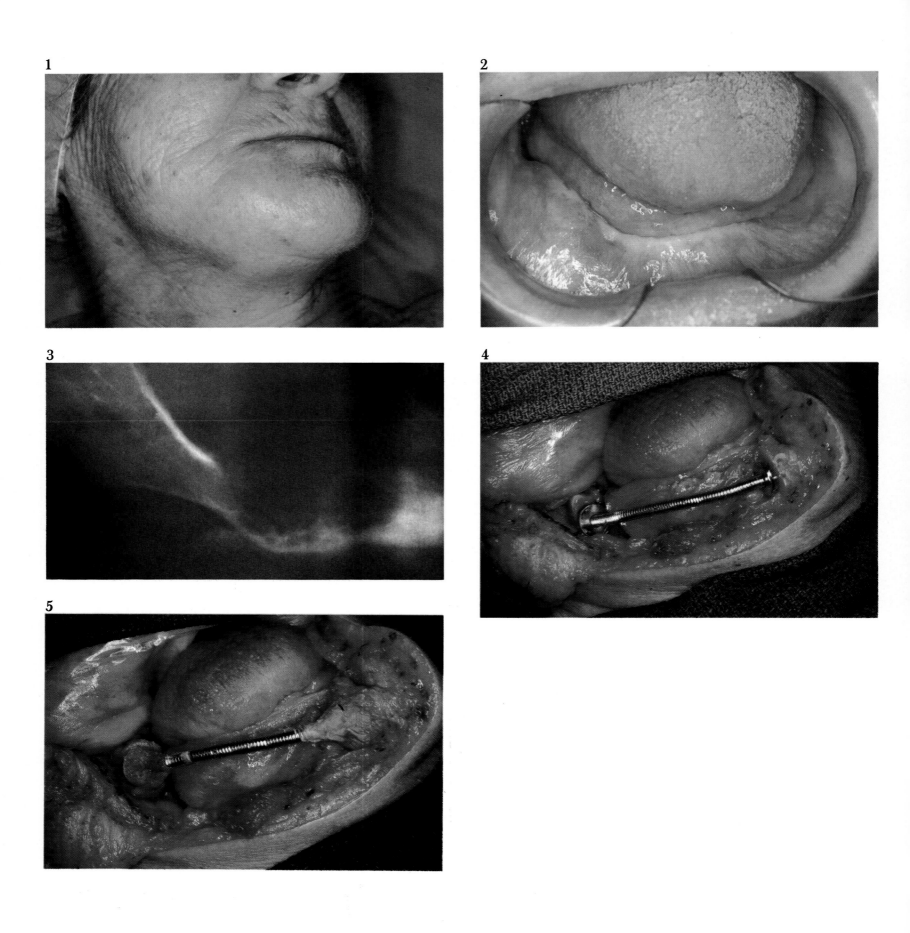

Limited resection of mandible and stabilization with a Steinmann pin

A variety of methods of mandible reconstruction are available to the operating surgeon. However, every method has its pros and cons and these should be weighed carefully before a particular method of reconstruction, replacement or stabilization of the mandible prior to surgical resection is selected. When the mandible is resected for palliation of a metastatic lesion, and the patient's life expectancy is very short, an elaborate reconstructive effort is unnecessary. If the patient is a poor surgical risk for a long operative procedure, or when primary mandible reconstruction is contraindicated, then stabilization of the bony stumps of the mandible with internal fixation using a Steinmann pin and bone cement are indicated. This is a very simple and easy method of restoration of continuity of the mandible arch which preserves the function of speech and swallowing. The patient presented here (1) is an 86-year-old woman with metastatic renal cell carcinoma in the mandible which had caused a painful, pathological fracture, the lesion presenting as a mass along the body of the mandible.

The intraoral view of the lesion (2) shows an expansile, soft lesion involving the outer cortex and alveolar process of the mandible, and a small part of the lingual plate of the mandible.

The radiograph of the mandible (3) shows a large, lytic lesion causing bone destruction with pathological fracture through the site of the tumor. There is complete dissolution of the bony architecture in the area of the metastatic lesion, but the adjacent bone in the ascending ramus of the mandible, and the body of the mandible beyond the midline, were completely within normal limits. The surgical procedure contemplated here would require a segmental mandibulectomy for total excision of the lesion with immediate stabilization using a Steinmann pin and bone cement.

A lower lip-splitting incision is taken, extended downwards dividing the chin in the midline and turning to the right side through the upper neck skin crease. the right lower cheek flap is elevated in the usual way carefully preserving the mandibular branch of the facial nerve. The facial vessels are divided and retracted with the cheek flap. The lateral aspect of the mandible is exposed from the midline up to the angle of the mandible. A portion of the masseter muscle is detached from the anterior aspect of the ascending ramus of the mandible near the junction of the body and the ascending ramus, giving adequate exposure of the site of resection. A mucosal incision is now made in the floor of the mouth near the lingual gingiva, and this is extended to divide the mucosa over the alveolar process both anteriorly

and posteriorly to the proposed site of excision of the mandible. Following this, the mandible is divided with a Strycker saw, giving satisfactory anterior and posterior margins around the tumor.

The remaining muscular attachment on the surgical specimen is that of the myelohyoid muscle which is detached next delivering the tumor-containing specimen of the mandible, and thus completing the segmental mandibulectomy. The length of the body of the mandible excised is now measured; this is vitally important since the Steinmann pin (available in a standard length of 15 cm) used for replacement of the resected segment of the mandible should be no longer than the resected segment. The Steinmann pin is now brought into the operating field. In this patient, the extent of the resected mandible was 5 cm, so 8 cm is cut from the full length of the pin, two nuts are threaded, one at each end of the segment of the pin to be used, in such a way that the length between the two nuts remains at 5 cm. Using a spanner and pliers, the pin is now bent to conform to the curve of the resected mandible. The two stumps at each end of the pin are now ready to be threaded into the mandible stumps.

With an olive-shaped drill bit drill holes are made through the cancellous part of the mandible at its stump end to allow insertion of the pin stumps in the mandible stump. The opening in the mandibular stump on each side is made large enough to be filled with bone cement prior to insertion of the pin; following this, methyl methacrylate is packed into the space created by the drill on each side of the mandible stump. While the methyl methacrylate is setting it is poured into a plastic syringe and the latter used to stuff the bone cement into the mandible. Then the Steinmann pin is inserted at each end up to the nut at the stump of the mandible (4). The bone cement is now allowed to set in the mandibular canal over the Steinmann pin, and additional cement is used to incorporate the nut at each end of the Steinmann pin with the mandible stump. It is applied to the nut and the mandible stump by hand to create a conical shape between the stump and the Steinmann pin incorporating the nut in this way within the bone cement to prevent the pin sliding out of the mandible at each end (5). The stumps of the bone are now held until the bone cement solidifies, and stabilization of the mandible, by internal fixation, is then complete. The two sides of the mandible will now move in harmony with the Steinmann pin bridging the bony defect. Closure of the surgical defect is performed in the usual way: the cheek mucosa is sutured to the mucosa of the floor of the mouth over the Steinmann pin; and the soft tissue

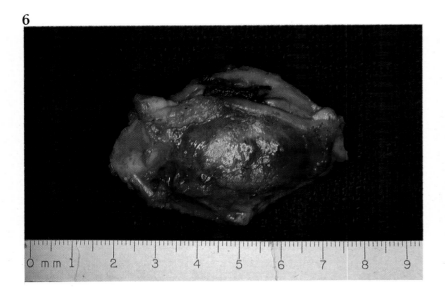

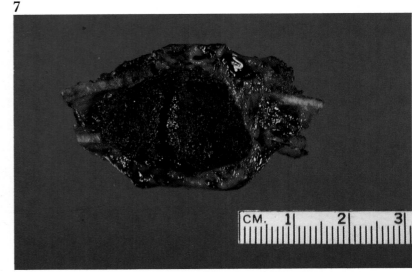

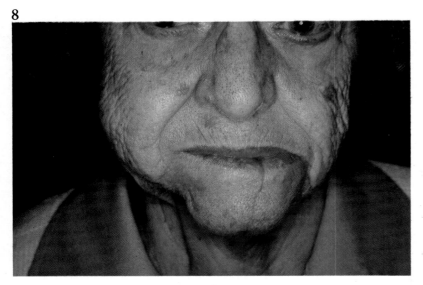

and the skin incision in the neck is closed as usual with a suction drain.

The surgical specimen (6) shows the excised metastatic tumor. The lesion is quite hemorrhagic and extends through the outer cortex of the mandible into the soft tissues. The cut surface of the surgical specimen shows a spongy, hemorrhagic tumor which has been completely resected (7).

The postoperative appearance of the patient approxi-

mately 2 months after surgery (8) shows satisfactory realignment of the arch of the mandible providing an excellent, temporary support for stabilization of the mandible. If the Steinmann pin causes no complications and is not exposed spontaneously, it may be left as it provides a good, functional result. However, the esthetic appearance is unsatisfactory due to lack of soft tissue support around the pin.

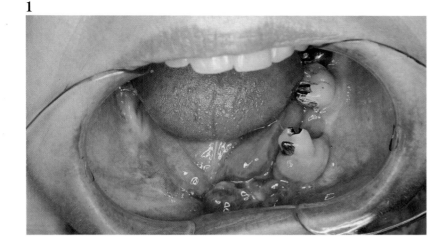

1

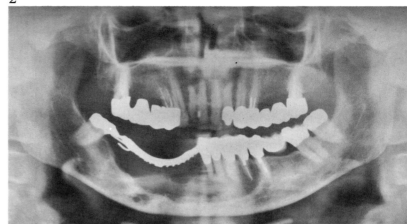

2

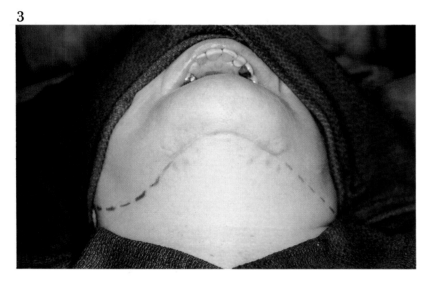

3

Mandibulectomy for ameloblastoma and reconstruction with teflon mesh prosthesis

Ameloblastoma is a malignant tumor of odontogenic origin most frequently involving the mandible. The patient presented here (1) had previously undergone two surgical procedures for attempted excision of ameloblastoma involving the body of the mandible on the right side. The second procedure was for extension of disease involving the soft tissues in the anterior floor of the mouth. Intraoral examination shows an ulcerated, expansile lesion of both the symphysis and body of mandible on the right side (1), with expansion of both the lingual and the outer plate of the mandible and ulceration and soft tissue disease presenting at the alveolar process in the midline.

Radiographic examination of the mandible with a panoramic view shows a large, lytic lesion involving the body of the mandible on the right side with extension of disease across the midline to involve the opposite side up to the premolar teeth (2). The outer cortex and lower part of the body of the mandible on the right side shows a multiloculated, cystic area with patchy bone destruction. The surgical procedure contemplated at this time required angle-to-angle resection of the mandible.

Preoperative evaluation by the dental team is absolutely essential for both intraoperative and postoperative dental management. The patient is given preoperative antibiotics and is brought to the operating room for surgical resection. Because of the presence of a previous scar in the submental region, the surgical procedure had to be undertaken using this scar and extending that incision on both sides as a visor flap (3). Since the previous scar was very close to the body of the mandible in the submental region, these lateral extensions also had to be taken close to the body of the mandible.

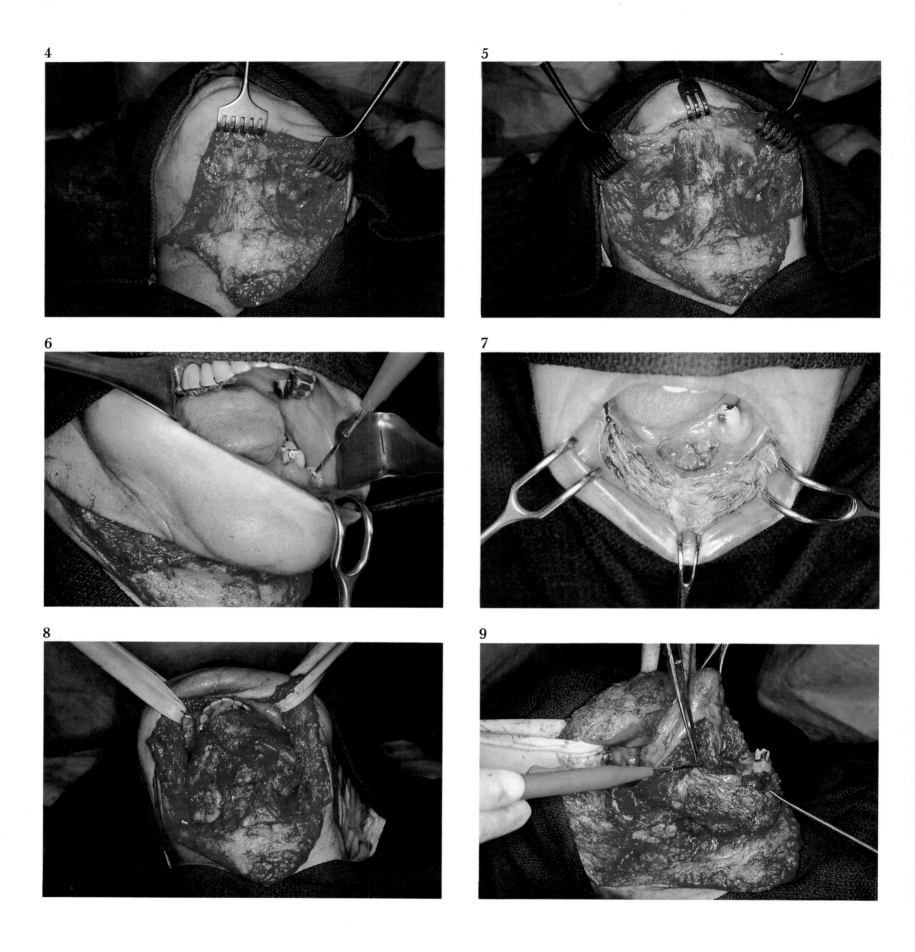

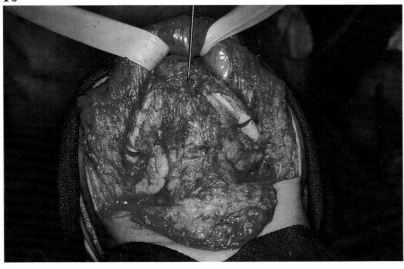

Taking the skin incision high meant that the skin flaps had to be elevated superficial to the platysma on both sides, since the mandibular branch of the facial nerve on both sides, lying deep to the platysma, would have to be dissected and reflected up together with the platysma (4). The skin flap is therefore elevated superficial to the platysma on both sides. An incision is now made in the platysma well below the site of the skin incision, and a meticulous search made to identify the mandibular branch of the facial nerve on both sides. These are then reflected, cephalad, along with the upper part of the platysma which remains attached to the facial skin (5). The mandibular branch of the facial nerve is retracted cephalad to remain in continuity with the platysma and the facial musculature on the visor flap, which is now elevated in the central compartment up to the body of the mandible. The skin flaps are elevated laterally on both sides up to the angle of the mandible to aid retraction of the visor flap. Inferiorly, the lower skin flap is elevated to expose the region of the thyroid cartilage, and a skin suture applied to the lower skin flap which is sutured to the drapes to provide exposure.

Attention is now focused on the intraoral incision (6). The lower lip is retracted with Richardson and loop retractors, and using needletip electrocautery an incision is made in the gingivolabial sulcus extending from the retromolar gingiva on one side to that on the opposite side. The mucosal incision is made in such a way that a considerable margin of the alveolar mucosa is left on the specimen. Dissection continues, using electrocautery, through the gingivolabial sulcus, leaving a generous portion of the soft tissues attached to the mandible (7). During this dissection, a finger is kept in the subcutaneous plane under the visor flap in the chin region to avoid inadvertent perforation of the skin. Once an entry is made into the neck anterior to the symphysis of the mandible, the rest of the mobilization of the visor flap is completed laterally detaching the entire visor flap from the mandible.

Two Penrose drains are now passed through the visor flap which is elevated and retracted cephalad to expose the entire mandible in the neck (8). If exposure of the mandible is inadequate, then further lateral mobilization of the visor flaps on both sides is undertaken.

With the visor flap retracted cephalad, the mandible and the tongue are retracted inferiorly into the neck (9). A mucosal incision is made through the floor of the mouth and the undersurface of the tongue around the intended surgical specimen using electrocautery. At this point the genioglossus musculature and the rest of the musculature of the floor of the mouth is divided as much as possible. Using electrocautery the site of proposed transection of the bone on both sides is demarcated.

Using a sagittal saw, the body of the mandible is divided on both sides through the previously outlined marks (10); this allows retraction of the surgical specimen downwards to aid division of the remaining musculature in the floor of the mouth, which consists of the remaining genioglossus, geniohyoid, myelohyoid and hyoglossus muscles.

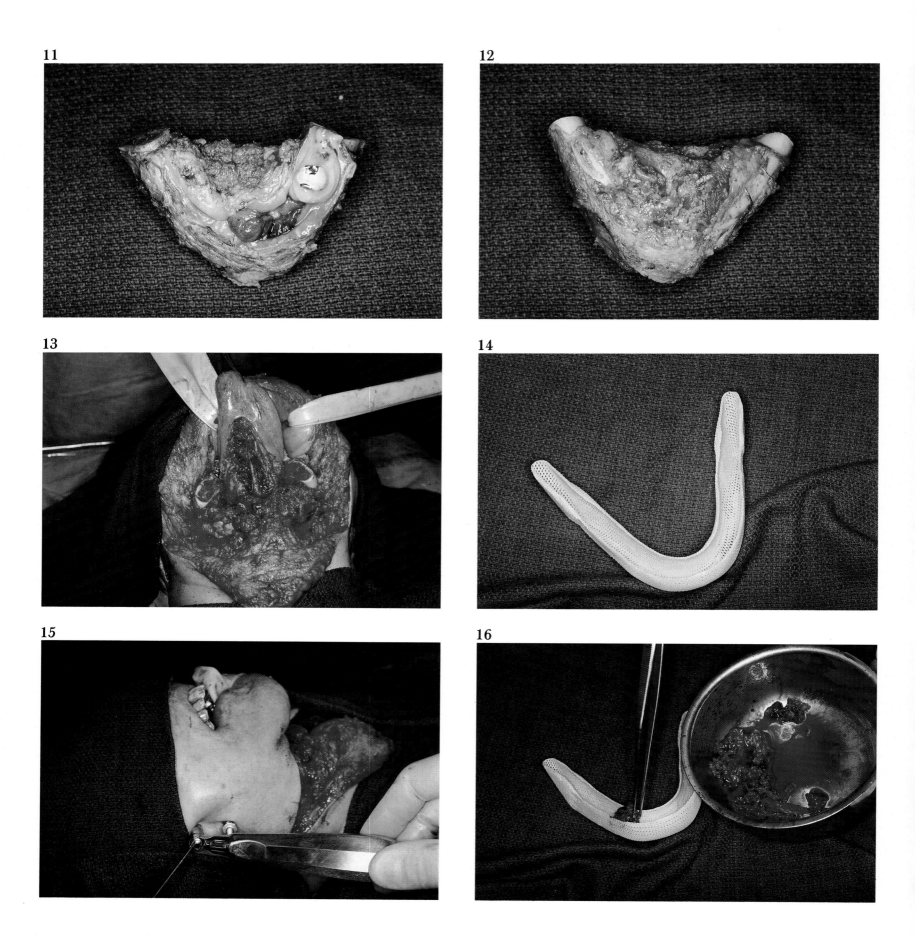

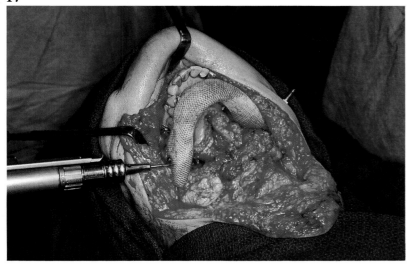

The surgical specimen as seen from the oral aspect **(11)** shows satisfactory excision of the arch of the mandible with a generous amount of soft tissue in the floor of the mouth where soft tissue disease was present.The undersurface of the specimen **(12)** shows a through-and-through resection of the muscular diaphragm of the floor of the mouth in the region of the symphysis and the genial tubercle.

The surgical defect in **(13)** shows the stumps of the mandible on both sides as well as the divided musculature of the floor of the mouth and tongue following removal of the surgical specimen. The stumps at this point are checked out for adequacy of resection by obtaining smears from the cancellous bone to rule out ameloblastoma, and when confirmed the reconstruction begins.

Reconstruction of the mandible in this patient was accomplished using a teflon-coated, polyvinyl chloride (PVC) mesh prosthesis with cancellous bone chip grafts obtained from the iliac crest **(14)**. The prosthesis comes prefabricated in three sizes, large, medium and small. The appropriate size is selected depending on the configuration of the patient's mandible. Using heavy scissors, the prosthesis is cut to the appropriate size necessary for replacement in the patient. In cross-section, the prosthesis is hollow and U-shaped, the hollow providing a tray to hold the cancellous bone chips. After the prosthesis is appropriately trimmed so that its proximal ends fit snugly over the remaining stumps of the ascending rami of the mandible on both sides, it is taken out and held on the operating table.

The dental surgical team now scrubs in and proceeds with insertion of retention screws and nuts in the ascending rami on both sides as shown in **(15)**; this aids fabrication and retention of external mandibular fixation with a helmet type of splint. The latter is made of methyl methacrylate, but at this point only the screws are inserted. The prosthesis will then be fabricated incorporating the screws on both sides after complete closure of the incision.

The screws are inserted through stab wounds in the skin and are driven through the subcutaneous tissue and parotid gland right into the ascending ramus of the mandible; a finger is placed here to ensure that the screw does not extend through the soft tissues and mucosa medial to the mandible into the oral cavity. The screw itself goes through the outer cortex and the cancellous part of the ascending ramus up to the inner cortex. A nut threaded on the outer end prevents it from sliding in further, and two screws are placed on each side to maintain adequate stabilization.

The technique of harvesting cancellous bone chips is standard, and they are now obtained from the iliac crest **(16)**. An incision is made along the lateral aspect of the iliac crest extending from the anterior superior iliac spine and extending posteriorly up to halfway through the iliac crest. The skin incision is deepened through the aponeurosis and the muscular attachments to expose the bony iliac crest. Using a sagittal saw, an incision is made into the iliac crest on its outer lip, and a similar parallel incision is made along the medial lip of the upper surface of the iliac crest. The two incisions are joined at the two edges, and a segment of the upper surface of the iliac crest is removed to gain access to the cancellous part of the iliac bone.

Using sharp, angled curettes, the cancellous bone from within the ilium is curetted out and harvested in a sterile container. A generous portion of the bone should be obtained since it must be sufficient to fill the entire prosthetic device for reconstruction of the mandible. Some bleeding is encountered during harvesting of the cancellous bone, but this is to be anticipated. After adequate quantities of cancellous bone chips are obtained, the bony defect in the iliac bone is stuffed with (Avitene) microfibrillar collagen. The segment of the iliac crest excised before is replaced, and the aponeurotic attachments to the ilium is now resutured with chromic catgut interrupted sutures. A suction drain is placed in the wound, and the wound for harvesting the bone graft on the iliac crest is closed in layers.

Attention is now focussed back to the mandible defect. The bone chips will be placed free within the tray of the prosthesis, but this is not done until after the prosthesis is adequately screwed to the ascending rami of the mandible.

Using a drill and very fine drill bit, two holes are made in the stumps of the mandible on both sides **(17)**. The prosthesis will be fixed to these stumps with screws driven through the previously made holes to stabilize the prosthesis. Alternatively, wires may be used to fix the prosthesis.

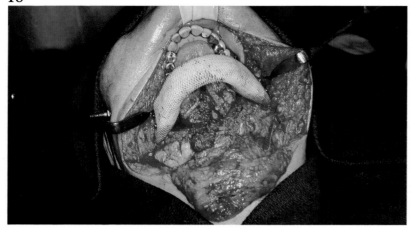

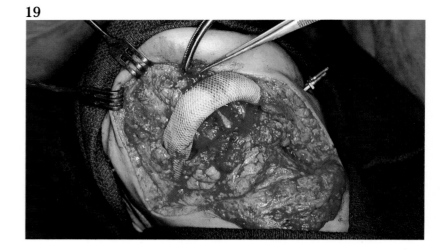

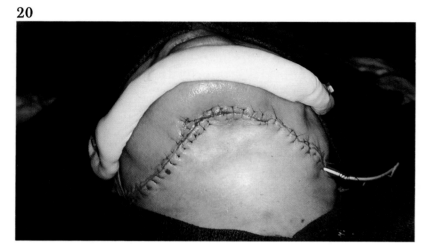

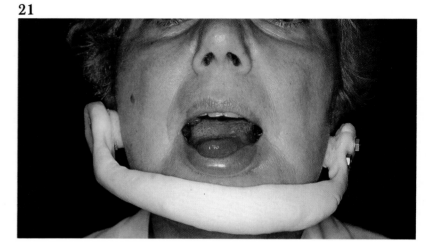

As shown in **(18)**, the prosthesis is now completely fixed and immobile, moving only with the ascending rami of the mandible on both sides. Care should be taken to avoid kinking of the prosthesis. Any sharp edges are trimmed off otherwise they may project through the mucosal suture line in the oral cavity. If the prosthesis is too high vertically, it should be reduced by trimming in a transverse plane to prevent ulceration and excessive stretch on the oral suture line.

The previously harvested bone chips are now placed in the tray which is filled snugly with the bone chips from one stump of the mandible to the opposite stump **(19).** Overstuffing is to be avoided, but too few bone chips are also undesirable. After the entire tray is filled with the bone chips, the wound is irrigated with Bacitracin solution, and suction drains are placed in it. The oral cavity is closed with interrupted 2-0 chromic catgut sutures, two layers being desirable. An initial soft tissue layer approximates the musculature of the tongue and the floor of the mouth to the musculature and soft tissues of the lip and cheek on the inner aspect of the visor flap. The second layer consists of mucosal closure approximating the mucosa of the cheek and lip to that of the floor of the mouth and tongue. The neck wound is irrigated again with Bacitracin solution, two suction

drains placed in and brought out through each end of the incision. The platysma and skin are then closed in layers. Following complete closure of the oral and skin wound, the external splint is fabricated with bone cement, which is used to create an external appliance as shown in **(20).** This device incorporates the two external screws from the ascending ramus of the mandible on each side. Sufficient space is left between the skin and the splint to accommodate soft tissue swelling postoperatively. A complimentary tracheostomy is performed for pulmonary toilet in the immediate postoperative period.

If primary wound healing is achieved in the mucosa of the oral cavity and the skin externally, the splint is left for a period of 8–10 weeks **(21).** Radiographs are taken at that time to visualize new bone formation and incorporation of the mandibular prosthesis. If there is sufficient stability the splint is removed and the patient allowed to move her jaw. This method of reconstruction of the mandible using a prosthetic device is suitable in situations where using vascularized bone is not feasible or advisable. However, the serious risks of this operation are exposure of the prosthesis and sepsis leading to its removal.

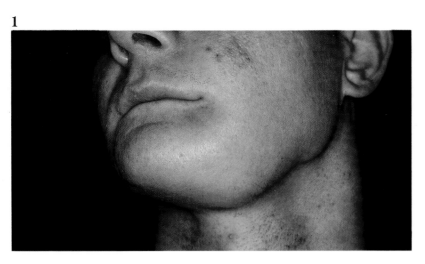

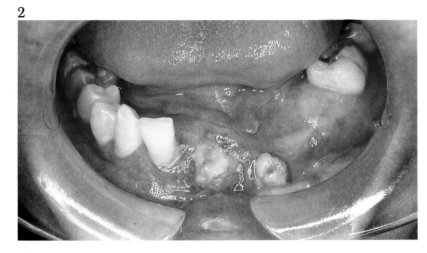

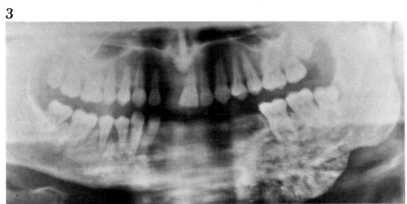

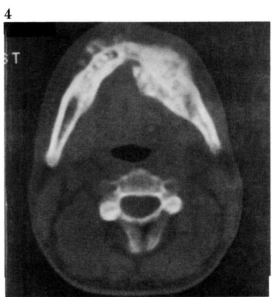

Radical resection of mandible for osteogenic sarcoma

Primary osteogenic sarcoma of the mandible is an infrequently encountered malignant tumor of the mandible. The patient presented here (1) had previously received chemotherapy and radiation therapy in a total dose of 6700 rads to the primary osteogenic sarcoma presenting in the body of the mandible on the left side. The tumor had shown initial shrinkage with chemotherapy, but no response to radiation therapy.

The intraoral view (2) shows a large expansile lesion involving the symphysis and the body of the mandible on the left side, with expansion of its outer and lingual plate and ulceration of the alveolar process in the midline, where a necrotic tumor can be seen. The overlying soft tissues as well as the skin of the chin adhered to the

tumor requiring sacrifice for a satisfactory *en bloc* resection.

The radiographic appearance of the tumor (3) shows the presence of an osteoblastic lesion involving the body of the mandible on the left side as seen on the panoramic view of the mandible. The tumor extends to involve the region of the symphysis and even the body of the mandible on the right side. However, the posterior part of the body of the mandible on right hand side and the angle of the mandible on the left hand side are radiographically normal.

The CT scan of the mandible shows an osteoblastic, expansile lesion (4). There is significant periosteal reaction with new bone formation, a diagnostic feature for osteogenic sarcoma.

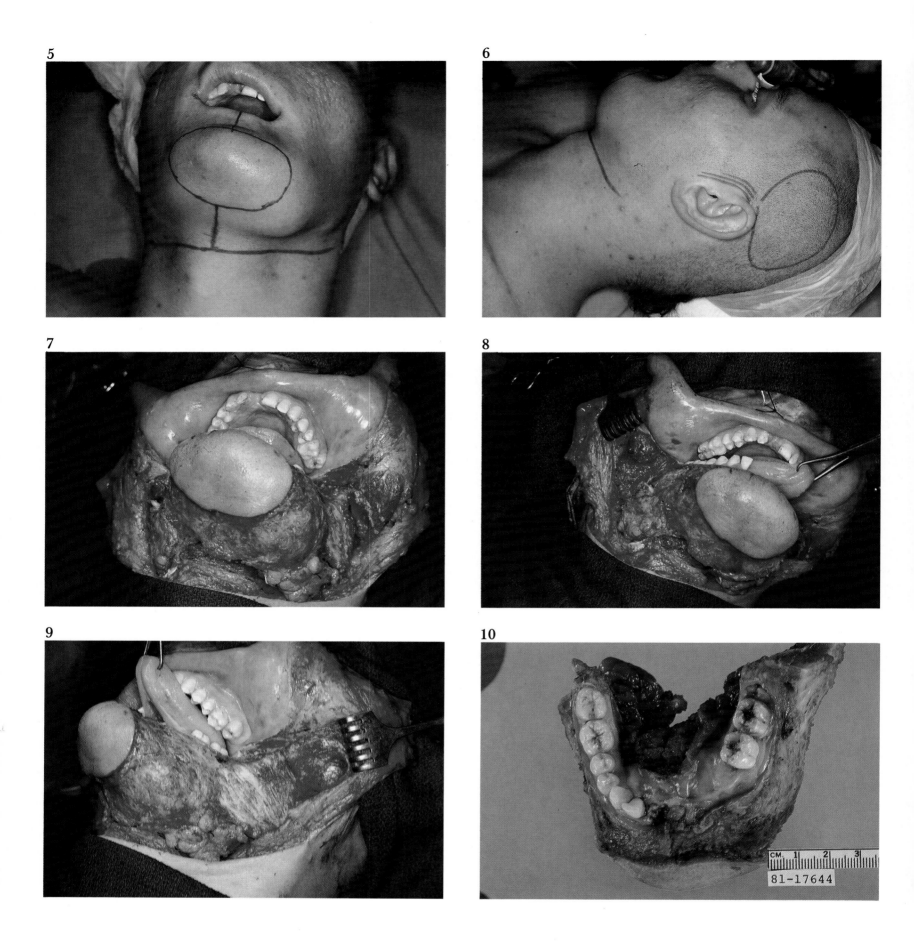

11

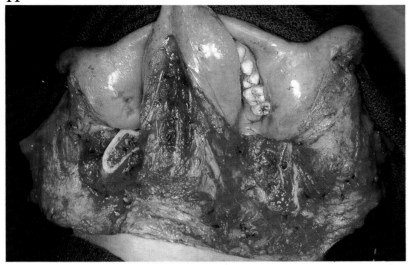

The plan of surgical excision required a through-and-through resection of the chin including segmental mandibulectomy extending from the angle of the mandible on the left side up to the posterior aspect of the body of the mandible on the right side. All the intervening soft tissues and a generous portion of the musculature of the floor of the mouth would be sacrificed with this resection. Because of the heavy amount of radiation given to the patient previously and the presence of infection in the oral cavity due to the ulcerated necrotic tumor, it is not advisable to proceed with immediate reconstruction of the mandible. Instead, the latter would be stabilized by internal fixation and the soft tissue and skin loss would be replaced using a distant flap for the chin. The mandible could then be reconstructed at a second stage.

The surgical incisions are outlined here (5). A lower lip-splitting midline incision is taken and extended, caudad, to make a circular incision encompassing the area of the skin of the chin to be sacrificed. The vertical incision then continues from the lower border of the circular incision up to the hyoid bone, where a transverse incision is taken along the upper neck skin crease extending from the mastoid process on one side to that on the opposite side.

The plan of reconstruction included coverage of the excised skin of the chin using a hair-bearing island flap of the scalp obtained from the temporal region (6). The vascular pedicle for this skin flap consisted of the superficial temporal artery and its accompanying vein. The mucosal defect in the oral cavity would be closed primarily by suturing the mucosa of the undersurface of the tongue to that of the posterior aspect of the lower lip.

The skin incisions have been taken and the cheek flap on both sides are elevated, carefully preserving the mandibular branch of the facial nerve on both sides to maintain competency of the lower lip (7). The cheek flap is elevated intraorally by making a mucosal incision in both gingivolabial and gingivobuccal sulci all the way up to the retromolar gingiva. A similar incision is taken on the opposite side, and both lower cheek flaps are elevated. The skin incision encompasses the circular disc of skin covering the chin which will be sacrificed with the mandible. The contents of the submandibular triangle on both sides are dissected for removal *en bloc* with the primary tumor. The tendons of the digastric muscles on both sides are divided to aid sacrifice of the anterior belly of these digastric muscles, achieving a through-and-through resection.

Attention is focussed on the right side of the mandible (8). The masseter muscle is detached by carefully elevating it over the outer cortex of the ascending ramus of the mandible using electrocautery, approximately 1 cm being exposed on the right side to aid surgical division of the mandible.

Attention is now focussed on the left side of the mandible where the masseter is detached almost up to the mandibular notch to expose the ascending ramus of the mandible beyond the angle (9). An incision is made in the mucosa of the floor of the mouth and undersurface of the tongue leaving generous soft tissue and mucosal margins around the gross tumor. At the proposed site of excision, the mandible is divided using a sagittal saw, on the left side cephalad and on the right side just distal to the angle of the mandible. Then the specimen is retracted anteriorly, and the musculature of the floor of the mouth and undersurface of the tongue is divided using electrocautery to deliver the surgical specimen, which shows (10) complete *en bloc* resection of the tumor. The division of the mandible extends from the ascending ramus of the mandible on the left side to its angle on the right side. All the anterior soft tissues including the skin of the chin is resected. Intraorally, a generous portion of the musculature of the anterior floor of the mouth is excised with the primary tumor, and all margins of resection around the latter are satisfactory.

The surgical defect is shown in (11). The stumps of the mandible, the musculature of the tongue, and the transected stumps of the musculature of the floor of the mouth over the hyoid bone are visible. Temporary stabilization of the mandible at this point will be achieved using the Steinmann pin bone cement technique described previously (p. 207).

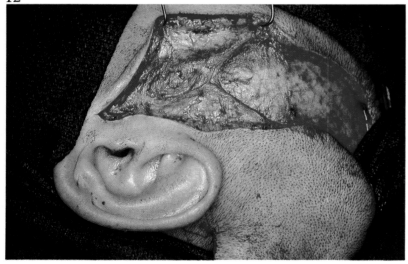

12

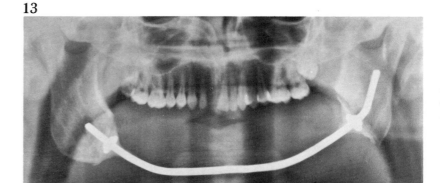

13

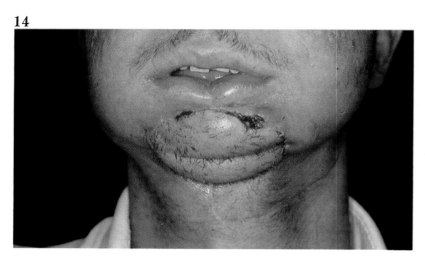

14

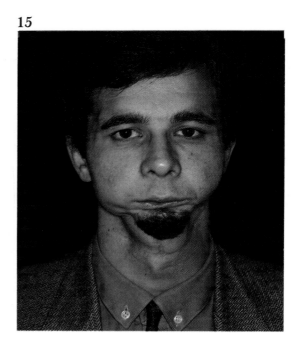

15

The previously outlined scalp flap from the temporal region is now elevated, and its vascular pedicle carefully dissected preserving the superficial temporal artery and its accompanying vein without any trauma to the vascular pedicle (12). Each of the unnecessary branches of these vessels are carefully divided without compromising the integrity of the main vessels. It is absolutely vital to mobilize the vascular pedicle up to the lobule of the ear before the flap is transferred in the region of the chin, as otherwise kinking of the vascular pedicle will seriously compromise the blood supply of the flap. Although the arterial perfusion of the flap is very generous, its venous drainage is not optimal, so patency must be maintained.

A tunnel is now created in a subcutaneous plane through the cheek. The island pedicle flap is passed through the tunnel into the defect of the excised chin. The vascular pedicle should be carefully inspected to avoid any rotation or kink in its placement. Once this is confirmed, the scalp flap is closed to the edges of the skin of the chin in two layers. The mucosa of the inner surface of the cheek and the lip is sutured to the mucosa

of the floor of the mouth and tongue with interrupted chromic catgut sutures. Suction drains are placed in the neck wound, and it is closed in layers. No external fixation is necessary since the mandible is well splinted by internal fixation.

The postoperative panoramic view of the mandible (13) shows the Steinmann pin with bone cement used for internal fixation of the two mandible stumps. Note that the stumps keep their normal configuration due to the Steinmann pin.

The postoperative appearance of the patient at approximately 3 weeks after surgery is shown in (14). Note that the scalp flap is fully viable. Edema and induration in the irradiated tissues of the skin of the cheek in the lower part can be seen clearly (14).

The postoperative appearance of the patient at 6 months after surgery is shown in (15). The growth of the tuft of hair on the scalp flap over the chin helps to achieve some facial contour. At this point, consideration may be given to secondary mandible reconstruction with vascularized bone graft.

10: The Neck

Surgery of the neck largely consists of operative procedures designed for removal of clinically apparent metastatic lymph nodes or those suspected to contain microscopic, metastatic disease. In addition, there are various masses arising in the lateral aspect of the neck which need surgical exploration and excision, including benign tumors such as a lipoma and congenital conditions such as branchial cleft cyst. Operative procedures for both neurogenic and neurovascular tumors are dealt with in the next volume.

Excision of subfascial lipoma of the neck

The patient presented here (1) had a soft, mobile swelling lying anterior and deep to the sternomastoid muscle in the upper part of the neck. A transversely oriented, oblique skin incision superimposed over a skin crease in the upper part of the neck is most desirable for exposure of this area. The angle of the mandible is shown outlined in black, while the proposed line of incision is shown along the upper skin crease in the neck. The incision should be at least two fingers below the angle of the mandible to avoid inadvertent injury to the mandibular branch of the facial nerve.

The skin incision has been taken and is deepened through the platysma to expose the underlying sternomastoid muscle and the presenting tumor (2). Both upper and lower skin flaps will have to be elevated deep to the platysma muscle to expose the tumor in its entirety, using electrocautery.

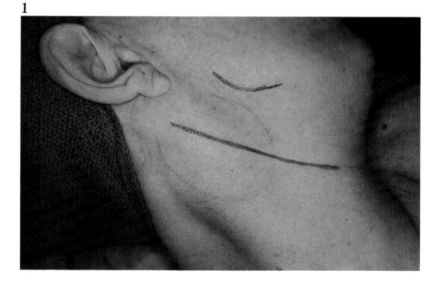

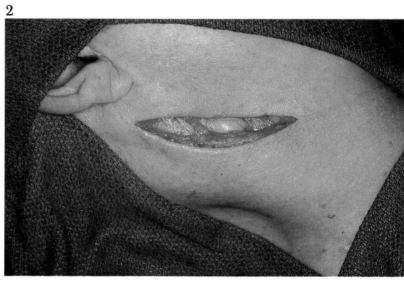

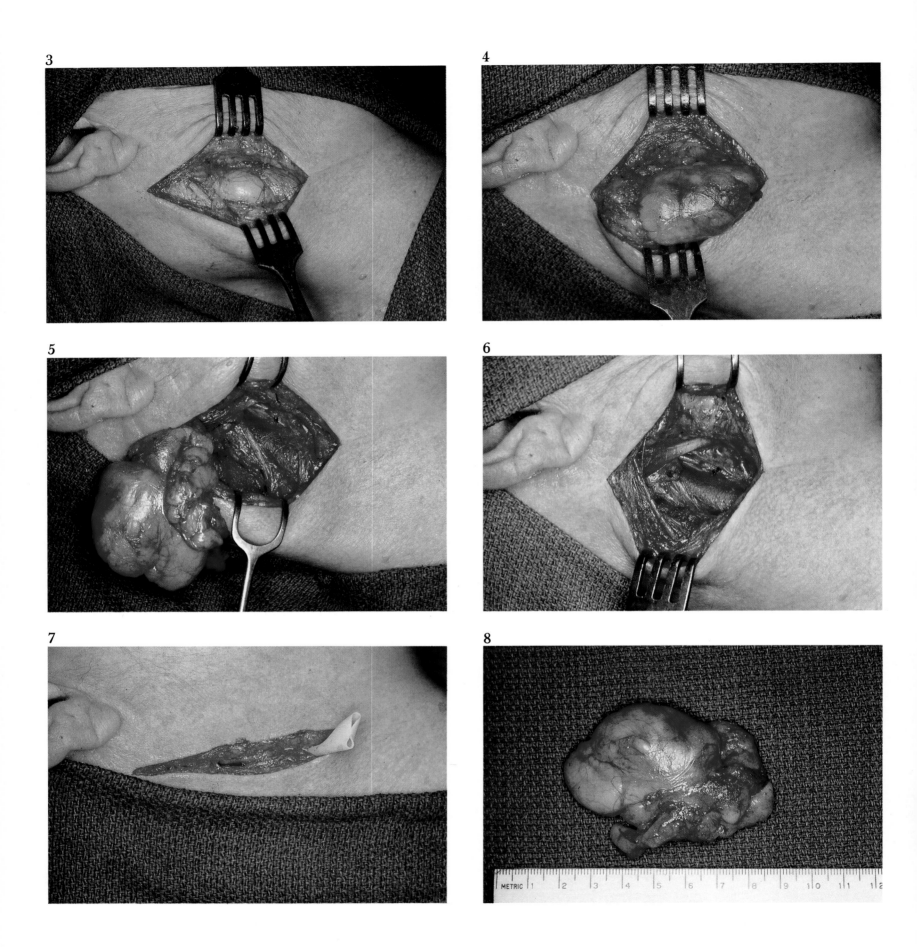

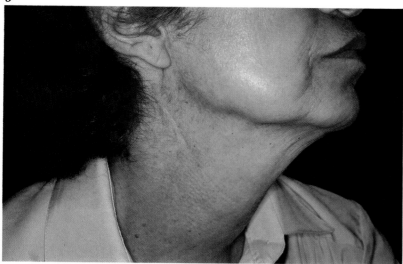

9

During elevation of the flap and mobilization of the tumor, the greater auricular nerve presents itself overlying the anterior aspect of the sternomastoid muscle **(3)**; this should be carefully preserved by retraction posteriorly, as sacrifice would result in numbness of the skin of the upper part of the neck and lower half of the external ear.

Dissection now continues remaining close to the tumor by carefully working around its pseudocapsule **(4)**. Fibrous bands of attachment adherent to the capsule and minor vessels that enter the lipoma are divided. Dissection is first undertaken anteriorly and the tumor is separated from the underlying soft tissues.

As the dissection proceeds the internal jugular vein is exposed **(5)**. The accessory nerve is also identified anterolateral to the internal jugular vein as it leaves the jugular foramen. Meticulous attention should be paid during sharp dissection in this area to carefully identify and preserve the nerve. Several minor vessels entering the tumor capsule are identified, clamped, divided and ligated.

The surgical field following removal of the lipoma **(6)** shows the sternomastoid muscle with intact greater au-

ricular nerve retracted laterally. The internal jugular vein with accessory nerve is also seen in the depth of the exposed field. The posterior belly and tendon of the digastric muscle are seen in the upper part of the surgical field. After complete hemostasis is achieved, the wound is irrigated with Bacitracin solution, a small Penrose drain inserted and brought out at the anterior edge of the skin incision **(7)**, which is then closed in two layers using 3-0 chromic catgut interrupted sutures for platysma and simple 5-0 nylon sutures for skin. The Penrose drain is left in for a period of 24–48 hours depending upon the amount of serosanguinous drainage.

The surgical specimen **(8)** shows the tumor removed *in toto* with an intact capsule and a portion of adjacent fibrofatty tissue and lymph nodes which remain attached to the lipoma.

The postoperative appearance of the patient at approximately 3 months after surgery shows satisfactory healing of the wound **(9)**. The scar overlies a skin crease in the upper part of the neck, but in time it will merge with the skin lines giving an acceptable esthetic result.

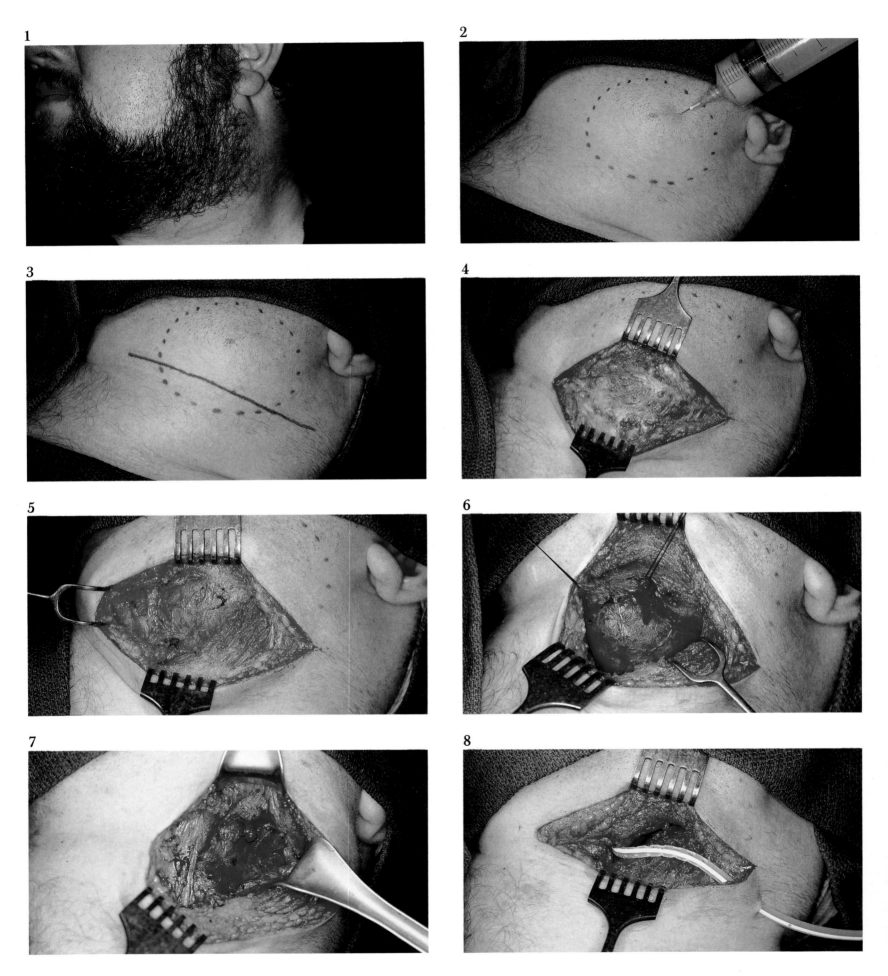

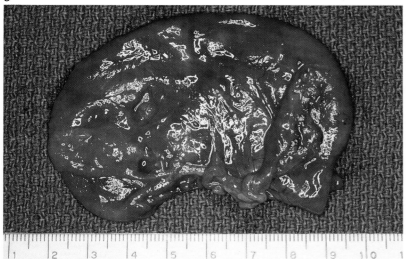

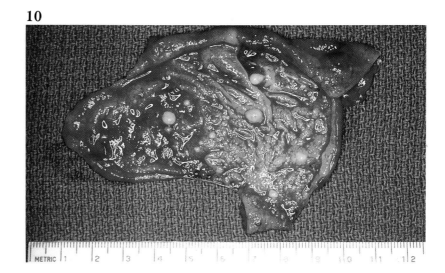

Excision of branchial cleft cyst

A branchial cleft cyst classically presents in the upper part of the neck below the angle of the mandible and anterior to the sternomastoid muscle. It is congenital and occurs as a result of sequestration of a branchial pouch which may present in adulthood as a cystic mass. The patient presented here (1) shows a large branchial cleft cyst presenting anterior to the sternomastoid muscle in the classical location. On palpation, this mass is soft and cystic, and it may show varied inflammatory reaction depending upon the presence or absence of recent infection within it.

Aspiration of the cystic mass may yield either clear straw-colored fluid or occasionally turbid, purulent material as seen in this patient (2). Under the microscope, the fluid shows cholesterol crystals. If the cyst is very tense, then removal of some of its contents by aspiration will aid its mobilization at surgical excision.

A transverse incision is taken along the skin crease in the upper part of the neck remaining at least two finger-breadths below the angle of the mandible (3), and must be long enough to provide sufficient exposure for adequate mobilization. The incision is deepened through the platysma and dissection begins in the subplatysmal plane carefully identifying the marginal branch of the facial nerve which is retracted cephalad with the upper skin flap (4). By alternate blunt and sharp dissection, and by mobilizing the mass from its posterior aspect, the anterior border of the sternomastoid muscle is identified, and separated from the cyst throughout the entire width of the incision (5). Both upper and lower skin flaps are now retracted to bring further exposure of the cystic mass.

A loop retractor is now placed anterior to the sternomastoid muscle (6) which is retracted posteriorly allowing further exposure to aid mobilization of the cystic mass. Careful attention should be paid to prevent inadvertent rupture of the cyst since it will contaminate the field and lead to an infected wound. By alternate blunt and sharp dissection, and by ligation of the capsular vessels, the mass is mobilized. Extension of the cyst in the form of a branchial cleft tract may occasionally be seen going up to the lateral pharyngeal wall, but mostly it is a single, unilocular cyst with no tract to the pharyngeal wall.

The surgical field following removal of the branchial cleft cyst is shown in (7). Note that the sternomastoid muscle is retracted posteriorly exposing the lateral pharyngeal wall seen in the depth of the surgical field. Complete hemostasis is obtained by ligating and/or coagulating all the bleeding points, and the wound is irrigated with Bacitracin solution.

A suction drain is introduced through a separate stab incision (8), and secured in position with a non-absorbable, cutaneous suture. The incision is closed in two layers using 3-0 chromic catgut interrupted inverting sutures for platysma and 5-0 nylon interrupted sutures for skin. Blood loss during this procedure should be minimal and in most patients the drain can be removed within 48 hours.

The surgical specimen of the collapsed cyst shows both the exterior wall and the internal surface with its secreting epithelium and several calcified cholesterol stones (9, 10).

Surgical treatment of cervical lymph nodes for carcinoma

The cervical lymph nodes are distributed in two sets of regional lymphatics, the superficial lymph nodes and the deep cervical lymph nodes. For practical purposes, the lymph node groups are divided into several anatomical groups as shown in (1), each of which drain certain specific sites in the head and neck area. These groups, therefore, serve as first-echelon lymph nodes which are involved by metastatic tumor when regional spread occurs from that particular site. For the pathologist to interpret accurately the location of the lymph nodes in a surgical specimen, certain anatomical landmarks are necessary; so for ease of description, and to establish a common language between the pathologist and the clinician, these lymph node groups are divided into several levels (2).

Level 1 includes those lymph nodes in the submandibular triangle, which include those in the submental region, those adjacent to the submandibular gland above the digastric muscle, and prevascular lymph nodes adjacent to the facial artery and vein.

Levels 2, 3 and 4 represent deep jugular lymph nodes along the internal jugular vein extending from the base of the skull to the supraclavicular region. These are divided into three levels: the upper third is level 2, the middle third up to the tendon of the omohyoid muscle is level 3, and those in the deep jugular chain caudad from the omohyoid tendon and up to the clavicle are level 4.

Level 5 are lymph nodes in the posterior triangle of the neck, and contain those along the accessory chain, the supraclavicular region lateral to the sternomastoid muscle, and those in the floor of the posterior triangle of the neck. Leveling of lymph nodes in this way is not universally practiced, but it gives a uniform description of them to establish a common language of understanding between the surgeon and the pathologist.

Leveling of lymph nodes is prognostic for primary carcinomas of the oral cavity, as the prognosis is significantly worse with increasing level of involvement of lymph nodes by metastatic cancer. This is generally in a sequential fashion, levels 1 and 2 being involved first, followed by levels 3, 4 and eventually level 5. It would be rare to find involvement of level 5 from an oral primary carcinoma in the absence of metastatic disease at levels 1 through 4.

The American Joint Committee (AJC) for cancer staging and end results reporting, stages the lymph nodes in the neck in a way that directly reflects tumor burden; the current staging system and descriptions of palpable lymph nodes are shown in (3). N_0 stands for absence of clinically palpable metastatic lymph nodes in the neck.

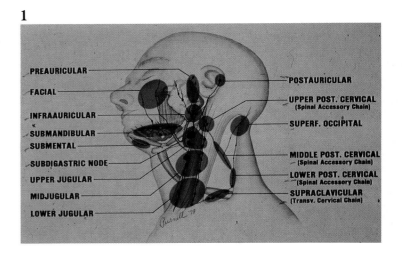

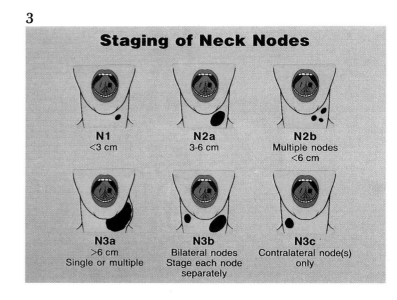

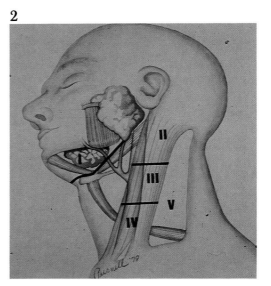

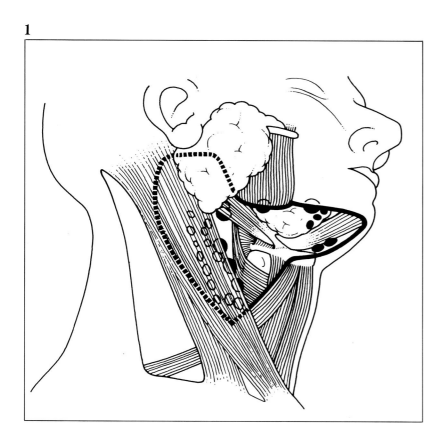

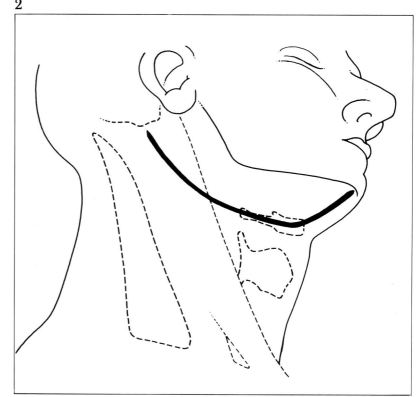

Supraomohyoid neck dissection

This operation entails removal of cervical lymph nodes from the submandibular triangle, the jugulodigastric and upper jugular lymph nodes, and midjugular lymph nodes remaining cephalad to the tendon of the omohyoid muscle.

The areas that would be cleared of the cervical lymph nodes are shown in (1), so those at levels 1, 2 and 3 are completely cleared. This operation is not therapeutic, but it is an excellent staging procedure for patients with primary carcinomas in the oral cavity with clinically negative neck where there is risk of microscopic metastases in the cervical lymph nodes. If microscopic metastases are confirmed by a supraomohyoid neck dissection, further treatment to the neck will be necessary.

The operation can be performed in conjunction with removal of the primary tumor from the oral cavity either

en bloc, or as a separate procedure, where the primary tumor in the oral cavity can be treated through a peroral approach while the supraomohyoid triangle can be dissected through a separate transverse incision in the upper part of the neck (2). The incision is taken in a skin crease at the level of the hyoid bone, and extends from the mastoid process up to the hyoid bone in the midline at which point it turns cephalad towards the chin. If the primary tumor is to be resected perorally, this incision should be satisfactory. Alternately, if the primary tumor of the oral cavity is to be removed *en bloc* with the contents of the supraomohyoid triangle of the neck, then a lower cheek flap will have to be elevated; this requires extension of the incision to divide the lower lip in the midline.

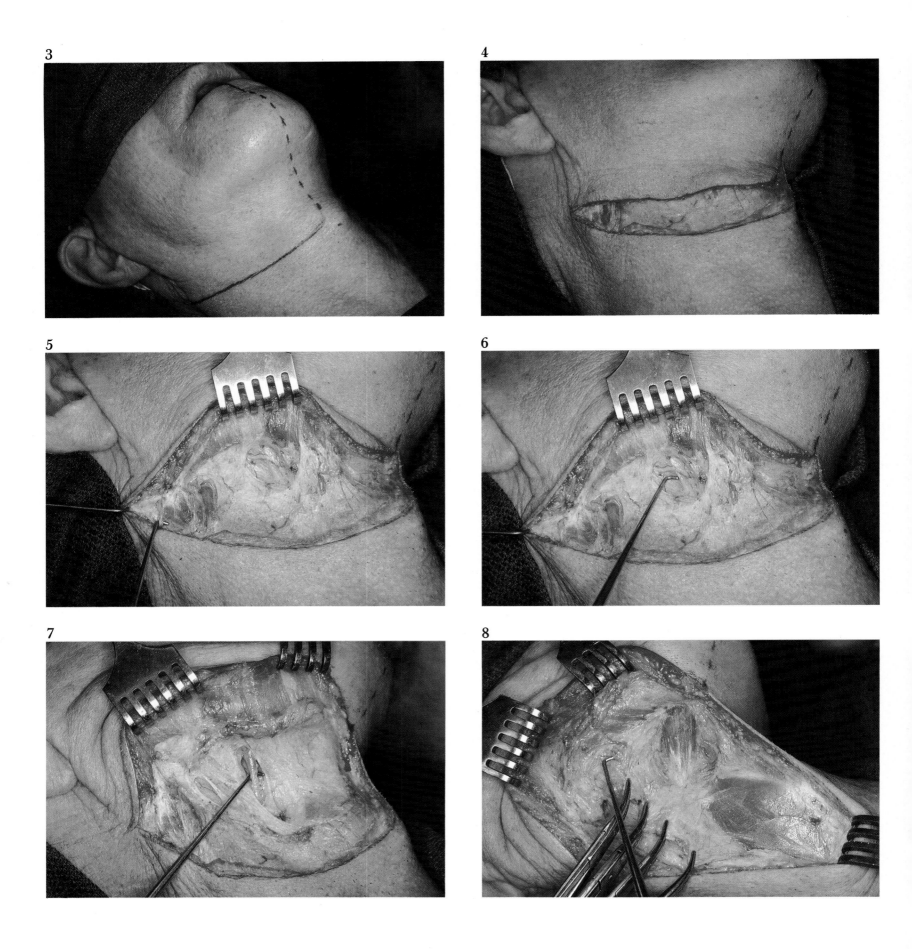

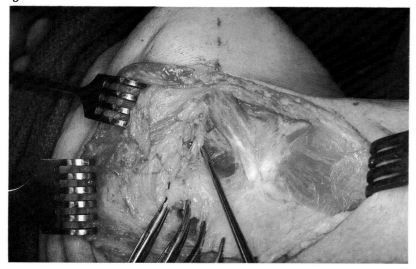

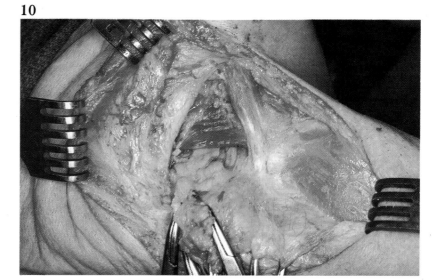

The skin incision is shown here (3) as previously described, with alternate extension in the midline shown by the dotted line. The patient's neck is extended and rotated to the opposite side to put the skin at the site of surgery under tension.

The skin incision is deepened through the platysma throughout its length (4). Since the incision is quite low in the neck, using electrocautery to divide the platysma has no risk of injury to the mandibular branch of the facial nerve. However, in the posterior aspect of the skin incision attention should be paid to avoid injury to the greater auricular nerve which can be safely preserved.

The upper skin flap is elevated first remaining close to the platysma and carefully identifying the marginal branch of the facial nerve. Posteriorly the greater auricular nerve overlying the sternomastoid muscle will appear and it should also be carefully identified and preserved (5). It is demonstrated here with a nerve hook.

Attention is now focussed on careful identification, dissection and preservation of the mandibular branch of the facial nerve which will directly overlie the submandibular salivary gland (6). This dissection should be performed sharply, either using a scalpel or scissors, since use of electrocautery in the vicinity of the mandibular branch can produce temporary paralysis of this nerve. In identifying and preserving the mandibular branch of the nerve, it may become necessary to sacrifice the cervical branch of the facial nerve. Once the nerve is identified and dissected along its course, it is retracted cephalad along with the upper skin flap by shifting the nerve with the flap and suturing soft tissues, caudad, with those of the upper cheek flap to form an envelope.

Alternatively, one may elect to identify the posterior

facial vein first as shown in (7). The vein is divided and its stump is suture-ligated at its upper end, with the platysma of the upper cheek flap carefully preserving the marginal branch of the facial nerve between the stump of the vein and the platysma muscle. Dissection now proceeds along the lower border of the body of the mandible, and the fascial attachments between the sternomastoid muscle and the angle of the mandible are divided.

As dissection proceeds anteriorly along the lower border of the body of the mandible, the prevascular facial lymph nodes will come into view as shown in (8). These are meticulously dissected and removed in continuity with the rest of the specimen, and during this the facial artery and its accompanying veins will be exposed, then divided between clamps and ligated. Dissection now continues anteriorly along the lower border of the body of the mandible all the way up to the attachment of the anterior belly of the digastric muscle. Soft tissues between the mandible and anterior belly of digastric are separated. At this point, brisk hemorrhage is likely to be encountered from several vessels which provide blood supply to the anterior belly of the digastric muscle and the myelohyoid muscle.

The nerve and vessels to the myelohyoid muscle, however, enter parallel to each other in a fascial envelope which is identified as shown in (9), clamped, divided and ligated. Once all the nerve filaments and vessels along the free border of the myelohyoid muscle are divided, the muscle will come into full view.

Gentle traction on the submandibular salivary gland with several hemostats (10) now allows mobilization and delivery of the submandibular gland from its bed. A

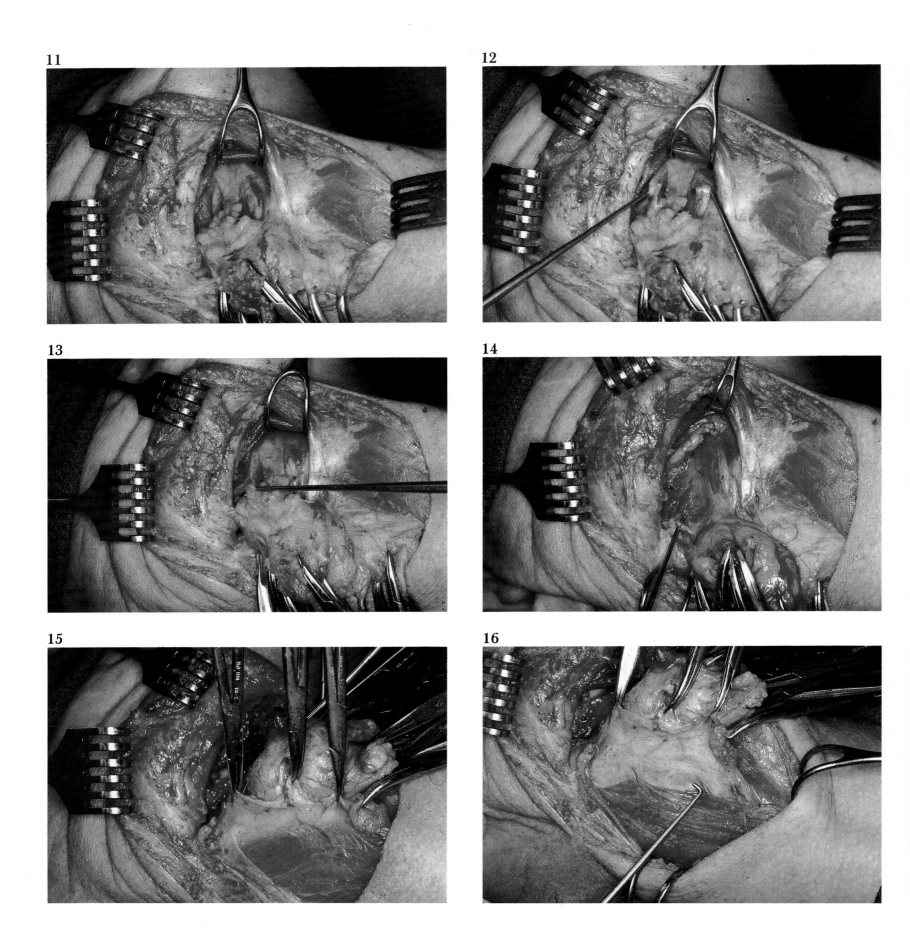

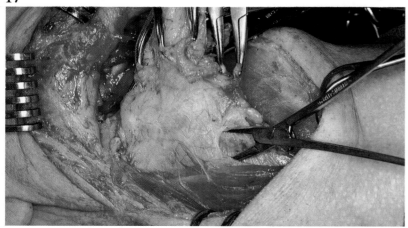

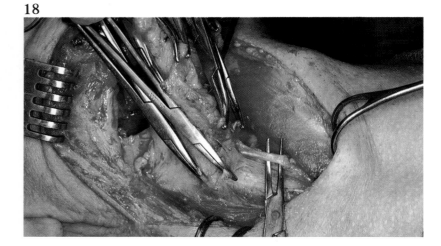

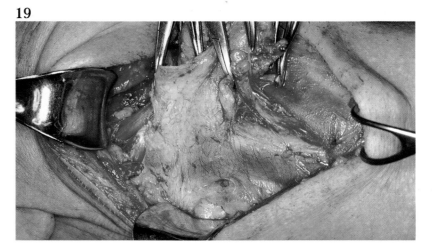

loop retractor is now placed along the free border of the myelohyoid muscle which is retracted medially towards the chin of the patient **(11)**. This gives exposure of the undersurface of the floor of the mouth and brings into view the secretomotor fibres to the submandibular salivary gland as they come off the lingual nerve as well as the Wharton's duct with accessory salivary tissue along the duct. At this juncture, alternate fine blunt and sharp dissection is necessary to clearly identify the Wharton's duct, and both the lingual, as well as the hypoglossal nerve in the floor of the mouth as it enters the tongue from beneath the tendon of the digastric muscle before entry into the tongue musculature.

Both the lingual and the hypoglossal nerve are shown here **(12)** with the Wharton's duct in the middle showing small amounts of salivary gland tissues along its length. Once the lingual nerve is clearly identified, the secretomotor fibres to the submandibular gland are divided. The latter are shown here **(13)** as they come off the lingual nerve. There is usually a small blood vessel accompanying this nerve so it is divided between clamps and ligated. Similarly, the Wharton's duct is divided between clamps and its distal stump ligated. The entire submandibular gland is now retracted posteroinferiorly, and loose areolar tissue between the salivary gland and the the digastric muscle is divided. As one approaches the posterior belly of the digastric muscle, the proximal part of the facial artery as it enters the submandibular salivary gland is exposed **(14),** then divided between clamps and ligated. The entire contents of the submandibular triangle are now dissected off and retracted inferiorly.

Attention is now focussed on the region of the tail of the parotid gland and the anterior border of the upper part of the sternomastoid muscle. The fascia along the anterior border of the sternomastoid muscle is grasped with several hemostats and retracted medially to provide tension along the anterior border **(15)**. Using electrocautery, the anterior border of the sternomastoid muscle is cleared off its facial attachments, by ligating or electrocoagulating several tiny vessels as they enter

the upper part of the sternomastoid muscle (branches from the occipital and superior thyroid arteries). Further retraction of the specimen medially will expose the carotid sheath as shown in **(16)**. The latter is incised and dissection now proceeds cephalad towards the base of the skull.

A hemostat is used to separate the fascia along the carotid sheath which is divided and retracted medially **(17)**. This dissection continues cephalad up to the posterior belly of the digastric muscle which is retracted upwards to expose the upper end of the jugular vein entering the jugular foramen. Several pharyngeal veins as well as branches of the superior thyroid vein may have to be divided in order to mobilize the specimen.

One of the pharyngeal veins shown in **(18)** will be divided to facilitate mobilization of the specimen. The sternomastoid muscle is now retracted posteriorly exposing the jugular vein in its entirety. The latter is still covered by the carotid sheath as well as a fascial envelope containing upper deep jugular and jugulodigastric lymph nodes **(19)**. The sternomastoid muscle is retracted posteriorly to expose lymph nodes in the accessory chain at the apex of the posterior triangle; these are meticulously dissected out and retracted anteriorly with the rest of the surgical specimen.

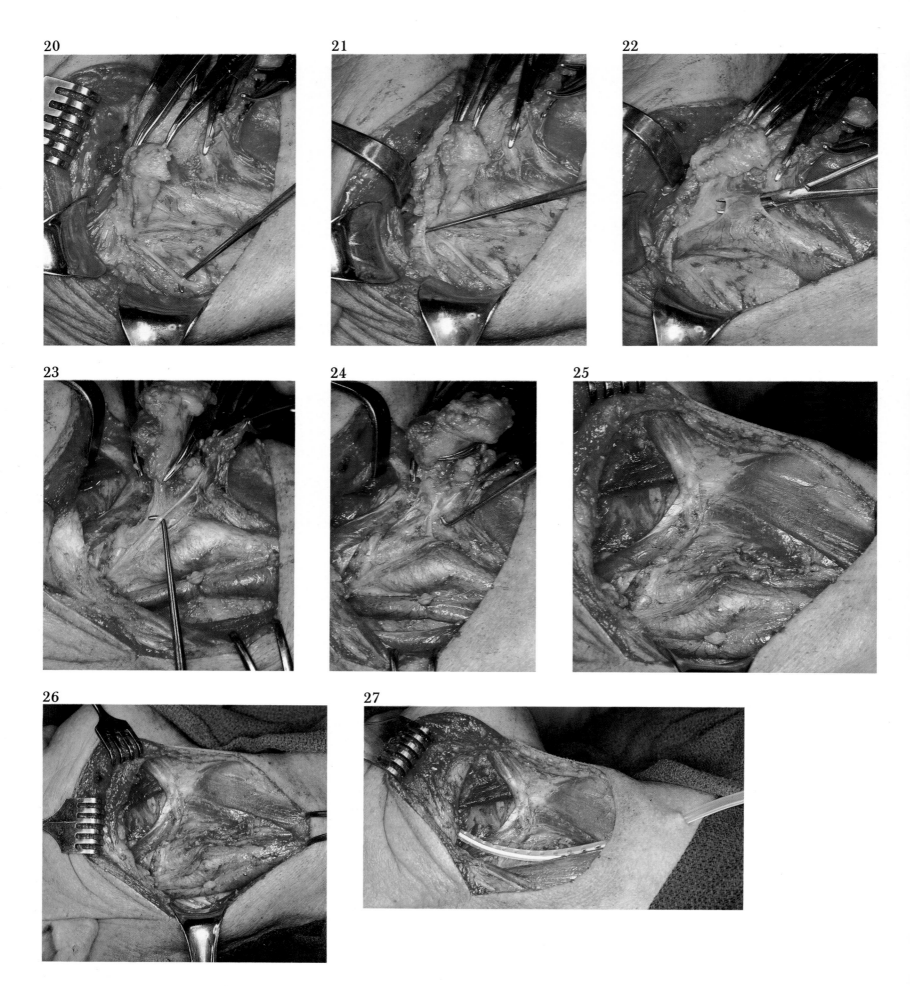

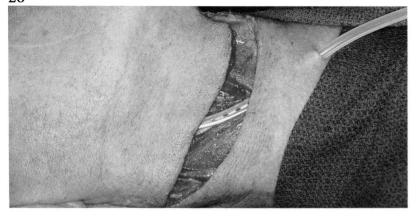

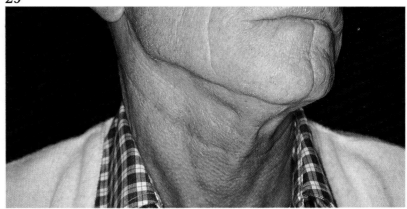

While dissecting the lymph nodes at the apex of the posterior triangle of the neck, extreme care should be exercised to identify and carefully preserve the accessory nerve as well as branches of the cervical plexus **(20).** Once the accessory nerve is identified, the rest of the lymph nodes in its vicinity are dissected out and reflected anteriorly along with the rest of the surgical specimen exposing the upper end of the jugular vein.

Most of the lymph nodes in the apex of the posterior triangle are now dissected out and pulled anteriorly showing further exposure of the internal jugular vein. The occipital artery is shown in (**21**).

The highest root of the cervical plexus is exposed as shown, with further dissection of the eleventh nerve and removal of lymph nodes in the jugulodigastric region nearly complete. The posterior boundary of the supraomohyoid neck dissection in this area is rather arbitrary, since no specific anatomical landmarks exist for the posterior triangle lymph nodes, so clinical judgment must be exercised to decide on the extent of their removal.

Dissection of the accessory chain lymph nodes posterior to the internal jugular vein at the apex of the posterior triangle is now complete **(22).** The entire jugular vein is exposed with the posterior belly of the digastric muscle retracted cephalad. The facial vein is now divided as it enters the internal jugular vein and is ligated. Dissection continues anteriorly carefully identifying and preserving the hypoglossal nerve as well as the ansa hypoglossi, the nerve supply to the strap muscles.

The ansa hypoglossi is shown here **(23)** as it comes off the hypoglossal nerve and runs anteroinferiorly. Dissection also continues along the medial aspect of the carotid sheath exposing the carotid bulb as shown here. The surgical specimen mobilized so far consists of the contents of the submandibular triangle, lymph nodes from the jugulodigastric and the posterior triangle of the neck, as well as the upper deep jugular lymph nodes. The specimen is reflected.

Dissection is now continued caudad towards the apex of the supraomohyoid triangle, the junction where the superior belly of the omohyoid muscle crosses the ster-

nomastoid muscle. A loop retractor is placed to expose the lower part of the carotid sheath from where midjugular lymph nodes are dissected out and reflected cephalad. In so doing, the external jugular vein will have to be divided and ligated. Dissection continues further medially exposing the origin of the superior thyroid artery **(24);** this will be preserved, but the superior thyroid vein will have to be sacrificed since this was previously divided from the internal jugular vein. The final attachments of the specimen in the region of the thyrohyoid membrane and the insertion of the strap muscles over the hyoid bone is divided with electrocautery. The specimen is now delivered.

The surgical field shows complete clearance of the supraomohyoid triangle **(25).** The anatomical landmarks are well demonstrated here with the anterior and posterior bellies of digastric and myelohyoid muscles. The lingual and hypoglossal nerves as well as the marginal branch of the facial nerve are seen in the submandibular triangle. The superior belly of the omohyoid, sternohyoid and the stylohyoid muscles as well as the bifurcation of the carotid artery are also in clear view. Note that the lymph nodes along the internal jugular vein are all dissected off with the specimen.

The posterior and inferior views of the surgical field **(26)** show the accessory nerve as well as branches of the cervical plexus, and the lower end of the supraomohyoid triangle where the sternomastoid and the omohyoid muscles cross each other. The wound is now irrigated with Bacitracin solution.

A single suction drain is inserted through a separate stab incision and is placed parallel to the anterior border of the sternomastoid muscle up to the submandibular triangle **(27).** The drain is secured in place with a silk suture to the skin at the site of entry **(28),** and the incision closed in two layers using 3-0 chromic catgut interrupted sutures for platysma and 5-0 nylon interrupted sutures for skin. Blood loss during this operative procedure should be minimal. There is essentially no esthetic or functional deformity following this operation **(29).**

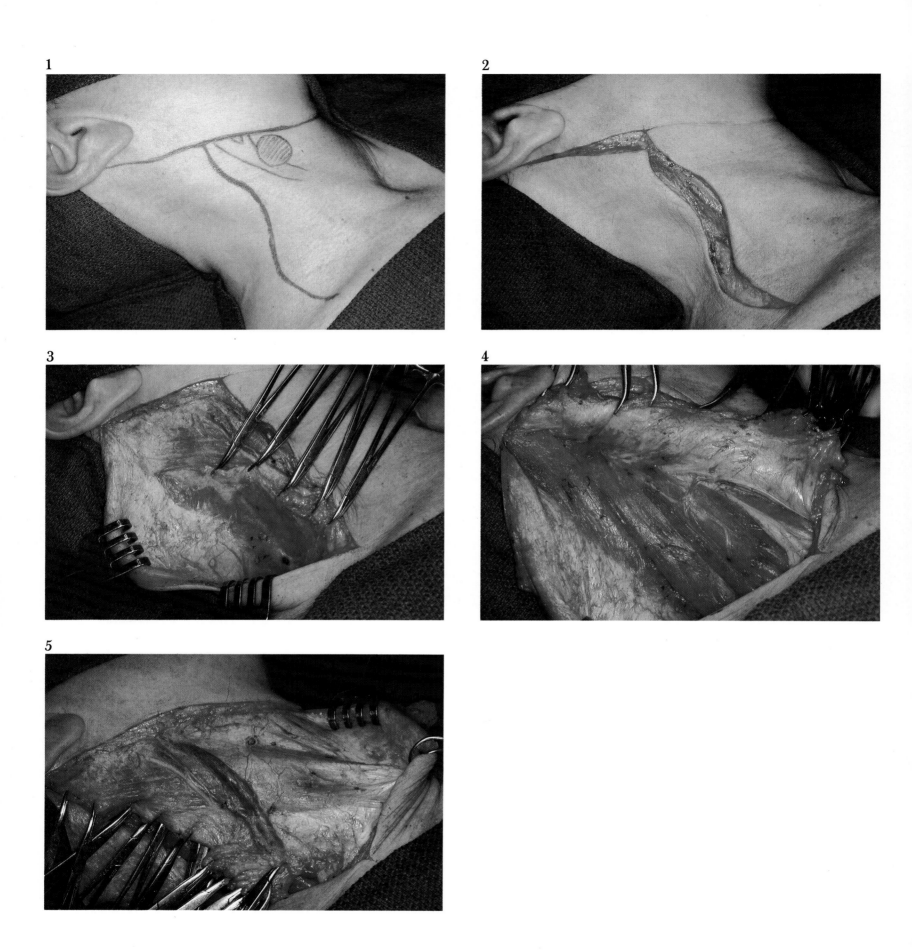

Classical radical neck dissection

The classical radical neck dissection still remains the operation of choice for clinically apparent, metastatic cervical lymph nodes. Although a variety of incisions are described for completing a radical neck dissection, a T-shaped incision is preferable (1). The transverse limb of the T begins at the mastoid process and follows an upper neck skin crease remaining at least two finger-breadths below the angle of the mandible. The upper neck incision is taken along the skin crease across the midline up to the anterior border of the opposite sternomastoid muscle. At about the midpoint of the transverse incision, but remaining well over the sternomastoid muscle, the vertical limb of the T incision is begun. This vertical limb is curvaceous and ends at the mid clavicular point. The incision provides adequate exposure for completion of a radical neck dissection; it is suitable both for bilateral radical neck dissections and for a pectoralis major myocutaneous flap since the vertical limb can be safely extended down on the anterior chest wall for elevation of the myocutaneous flap. Since the blood supply to the three skin flaps resulting from this incision is adequate, marginal necrosis at the trifurcation of the skin incision is rarely seen. The trifurcation of the incision is shown marked out on the skin here in relation to the carotid artery. The trifurcation point should be kept posterior to the carotid artery when feasible. This incision provides the necessary exposure by elevation of the posterior, anterior and superior skin flaps.

The dissection begins with elevation of the posterior skin flap (2). The posterior half of the transverse incision begins at the mastoid process, and the rest of the vertical incision is completed as shown here. The anterior and superior skin flaps are not elevated at this time. The skin incision is made with a scalpel, but the rest of the dissection is carried out with electrocautery. The skin incision is deepened through the platysma, but if grossly enlarged lymph nodes are present, and there is suspicion of extension of disease beyond the capsule of the lymph nodes, the platysma muscle is sacrificed. Electrocautery aids rapid elevation of the posterior skin flap. Several skin hooks are employed to retract the posterior skin flap, while countertraction is provided by the second assistant over the soft tissues in the neck. The plane of dissection is along the undersurface of the platysma muscle. The posterior skin flap is elevated until the anterior border of the trapezius muscle is identified, and exposed all the way from the mastoid process down to the clavicle.

Rake retractors are now employed to retract the posterior skin flap (3). Soft tissues anterior to the trapezius muscle are now grasped with several hemostats which are used to provide traction on the surgical specimen.

Dissection proceeds along the floor of the posterior triangle of the neck, exposing each succeeding muscle with anterior elevation of the specimen. The superior attachment of the sternomastoid muscle is detached from the mastoid process and retracted anteriorly. The plane of dissection continues just anterior to the anterior border of each succeeding muscle in the posterior triangle of the neck. The splenius capitis and levator scapulae muscle are then exposed, and several small veins will have to be ligated as this dissection proceeds anteriorly. In the lower part of the neck, the transverse cervical artery and its accompanying vein are identified, divided between clamps and ligated. Likewise, the posterior belly of the omohyoid muscle is divided in the floor of the posterior triangle of the neck and its anterior stump is retracted medially. Dissection continues medially exposing the posterior scalene muscle. The lower end of the external jugular vein is divided between clamps near the clavicle and its stump is ligated.

As the scalene muscles are exposed, roots of the cervical plexus will come into view (4). However, these are left intact until the phrenic nerve is identified lying on the anterior aspect of the scalenus anticus muscle. The cutaneous branches of the cervical plexus are then transected, leaving very short stumps to prevent injury to the phrenic nerve. The cervical roots carry with them small blood vessels and these require clamping and ligation prior to transection. In the lower part of the posterior triangle of the neck, the brachial plexus will come into view. Dissection over this is easy because there is a plane of loose areolar tissue between the cervical lymph nodes and the supraclavicular fat pad contained within the deep cervical fascia. Dissection of the posterior triangle of the neck is now complete.

The specimen mobilized so far is allowed to drop posteriorly (5). A dry gauze pad is placed on the musculature of the posterior triangle of the neck over which the surgical specimen is allowed to rest. Attention is now focussed on the anterior skin flap. The transverse skin incision is completed by extending it from the trifurcation point up to the medial end, deepening through the platysma. The anterior skin flap is retracted medially using skin hooks and rake retractors. Electrocautery elevates this skin flap through the loose plane of areolar tissue lying deep to the platysma muscle.

Several cutaneous vessels are encountered during elevation and these are electrocoagulated. The skin flap is elevated up to the midline of the neck in its upper part, and retracted inferiorly up to the medial end of the sternomastoid muscle at its attachment to the manubrium sterni. A large loop retractor is used to expose the sternal end of the sternomastoid muscle which facilitates complete elevation of the anterior skin flap. Using elec-

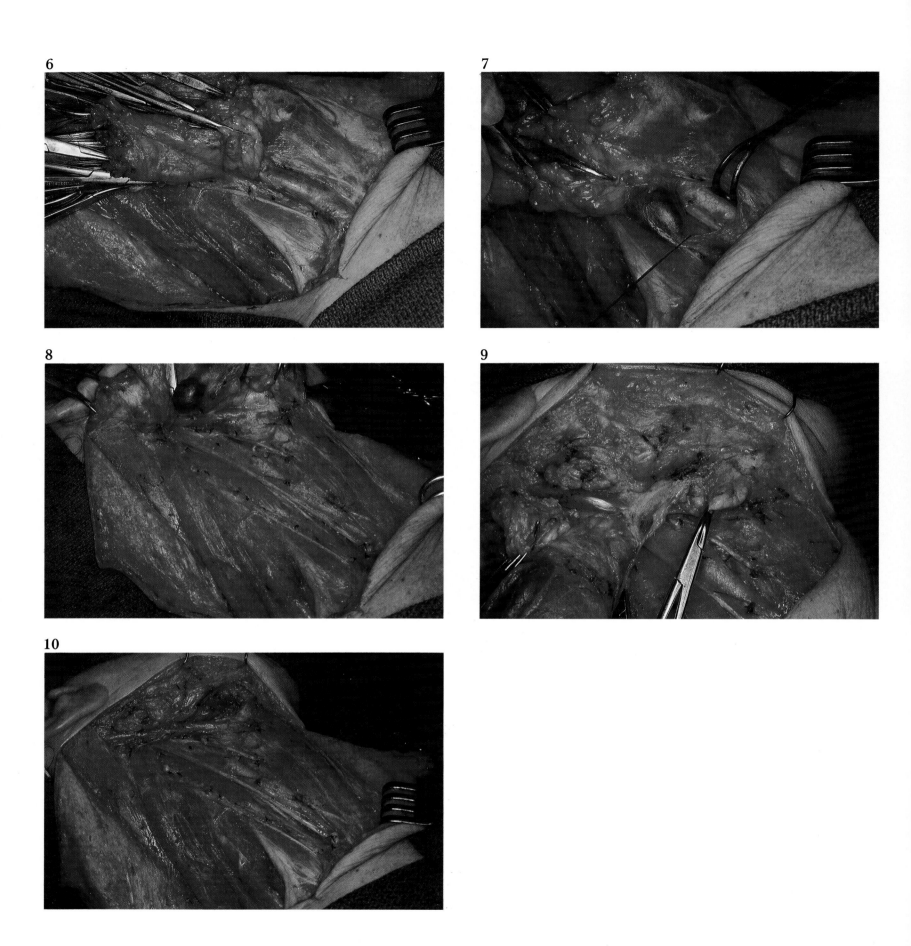

trocautery and a cutting current, the tendon of the sternomastoid muscle is divided from the sternal end, and the rest of the muscular attachment on the manubrium and the clavicle is divided using coagulating current with electrocautery.

Several small vessels enter the anterior skin flap as it is elevated near the clavicle; these are branches from the first perforating branch of the internal mammary artery, and are divided and ligated. Once the sternomastoid muscle is detached from both its sternal and clavicular ends, it is grasped with hemostats and retracted cephalad. There is a plane of loose areolar tissue containing fat between the carotid sheath and the posterior aspect of the sternomastoid muscle, so the latter can be divided with electrocautery. Using a sharp knife the fascia overlying the carotid sheath, medial to the carotid sheath, and lateral to the strap muscles is divided.

By alternate blunt and sharp dissection, the areolar tissue on the carotid sheath is divided circumferentially around the internal jugular vein **(6),** which will necessitate clamping and ligation of the proximal end of the transverse cervical artery and vein. Small lymphatic vessels present in the right side of the neck also have to be divided and ligated. On the left side of the neck, the thoracic duct requires special attention, and should be identified meticulously, dissected, carefully divided and ligated in order to prevent chyle leak and fistula. Lymph nodes contained in loose areolar tissue behind the internal jugular vein are dissected and pulled out to remain in continuity with the rest of the specimen. During this dissection, a careful eye should be kept on the phrenic nerve which should be out of the way.

The fascia along the medial aspect of the carotid sheath and the lateral border of the strap muscles is now incised, and a small loop retractor placed on the strap muscles to expose the common carotid artery and the vagus nerve **(7).** The internal jugular vein should not be ligated until after both the artery and nerve are identified and retracted medially, when it is doubly ligated, divided in between and its proximal stump suture-ligated.

The middle thyroid vein may often be seen at this point entering the medial aspect of the internal jugular vein, and is divided and ligated. Dissection now proceeds along the lateral border of the carotid sheath remaining posterior to the vein but anterolateral to the vagus nerve. This is a relatively avascular plane and one can safely divide the carotid sheath along this plane all the way up to the base of the skull. As dissection proceeds cephalad, minor vessels in the carotid sheath and on the vessel wall cause bleeding which is easily controlled with electrocoagulation **(8).**

Dissection of the lateral aspect of the carotid sheath in the upper part of the neck brings the hypoglossal nerve into view. At this juncture, the highest branches of the cervical plexus are now divided. The dissection is carried cephalad along the medial border of the superior belly of the omohyoid muscle up to the hyoid bone from which it is detached. Small blood vessels running along the ansa hypoglossi will have to be divided and ligated. The superior thyroid artery is preserved but the superior thyroid vein will have to be divided and ligated. A dry gauze pad is now placed on the surgical field and the entire specimen is allowed to rest over the gauze pad.

The superior skin flap is now developed as usual **(9).** For details of this part of the operation, follow the initial steps described in supraomohyoid neck dissection (p. 227 *et seq*). The mandibular branch of the facial nerve is carefully identified and preserved, and the facial vessels divided and ligated. The contents of the submandibular triangle are dissected off carefully preserving the lingual and hypoglossal nerves, retracted inferiorly and still kept attached to the rest of the specimen. Several pharyngeal veins along the digastric tendon and the posterior belly of the digastric muscle will also have to be divided and ligated. Finally, the tail of the parotid gland is transected along the superior border of the posterior belly of the digastric muscle. In dividing the tail of the parotid gland, the posterior facial vein and several arterial branches of the occipital artery are divided, and require ligation.

The posterior belly of the digastric muscle is now retracted cephalad with a deep, right-angled retractor, bringing into view the occipital artery which runs across the internal jugular vein anteriorly at right angles to it. If the occipital artery is high behind the digastric muscle, it may be left alone, but if it is quite low it will have to be divided and ligated. The adipose tissue and lymph nodes lateral to the internal jugular vein under the sternomastoid muscle are dissected off, and the rest of the muscle and tendon detached from the mastoid process. The accessory nerve is identified, divided and its proximal stump is ligated as there is a small vessel running with the nerve. Finally, the upper end of the jugular vein is skeletonized, and the internal jugular vein is doubly ligated and divided. The surgical specimen is now delivered.

The surgical field following radical neck dissection **(10)** shows clearance of all five levels of lymph nodes as previously described. The wound is now irrigated with Bacitracin solution. Meticulous hemostasis must be achieved by ligating and/or coagulating all bleeding points prior to closure of the wound. Two suction drains

11

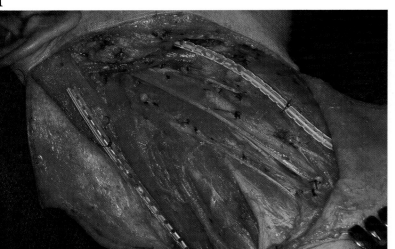

13

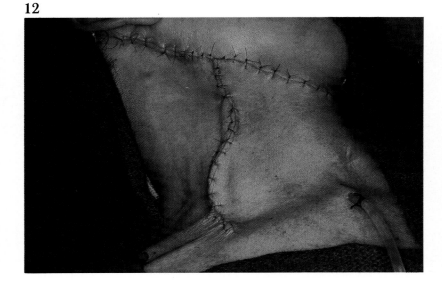

12

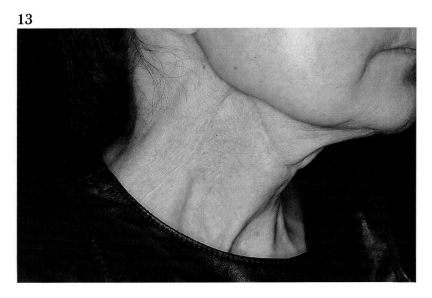

are now inserted through separate stab incisions **(11)**. One drain overlies the anterior border of the trapezius muscle in the posterior triangle, and is retained there through a loop of chromic catgut suture between the skin flap and the trapezius muscle; another is maintained over the strap muscles, anteriorly, and is retained by a loop of catgut suture. The rest of the skin wound is closed in two layers using 3-0 chromic catgut interrupted sutures for platysma and 5-0 nylon sutures for skin **(12)**. It is vital for the suction drains to be attached to suction equipment while the wound is being closed.

As soon as the last skin sutures are applied, the wound should be made airtight allowing the skin flaps to remain completely down and adherent to the deeper tissues by suction through the drains. If suction in this manner is not maintained, minor venous oozing will allow the flaps to remain elevated causing collection of hematoma and clotting of blood in drainage tubes which will, in turn, open up new venous hemorrhage leading to a large hematoma. The suction drains are necessary for approximately 4–5 days at which point minimal serous drainage will allow their removal.

The postoperative appearance of the patient approximately 6 months after surgery is shown in **(13)**. Note that the skin incision has healed well. Patients undergoing classical radical neck dissection require an intensive program of postoperative physiotherapy to regain shoulder function and avoid a painful and stiff shoulder joint.

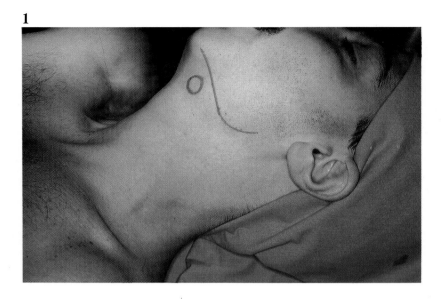

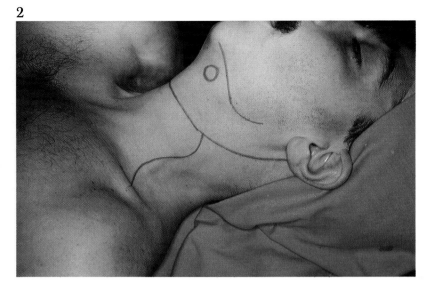

Modified radical neck dissection sparing the accessory nerve

This type of neck dissection is recommended when elective neck dissection is contemplated for massive primary carcinomas of the oral cavity, oropharynx or hypopharynx, and when there is no clinical involvement of the cervical lymph nodes. This operation can also be employed for patients with a limited extent of clinically apparent metastatic disease in the anterior triangle of the neck as depicted in the patient shown here (1). This patient had a primary carcinoma of the tongue treated previously and he now presents with a 1 cm, clinically apparent metastatic lymph node in the submandibular triangle. The location of the lymph node is shown in relation to the outline of the lower border of the mandible. In patients with such a limited extent of metastatic disease, sparing the 11th nerve is considered feasible since metastatic disease in the posterior triangle of the neck is unlikely.

The skin incision, as previously outlined for radical neck dissection, is marked out (2). The transverse incision is at least two fingerbreadths below the angle of the mandible with a curvaceous, vertical limb remaining posterior to the carotid artery.

The posterior skin flap is elevated first remaining just on the undersurface of the platysma (3). Meticulous attention should be paid as the lateral aspect of the skin

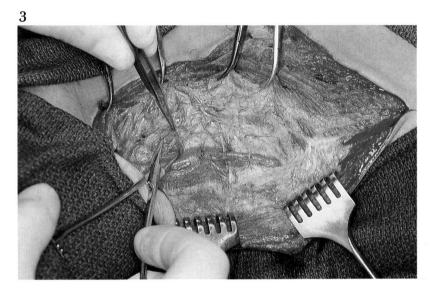

flap is reached near the anterior border of the trapezius muscle as the accessory nerve enters the muscle in this region. The flap is elevated well over the anterior border of the trapezius muscle to expose at least 1 cm of its anterolateral surface. On occasion, elevation of the superior part of the skin flap may have to be withheld if the accessory nerve is found entering the trapezius muscle high in the neck rather than its usual lower location. At this point the accessory nerve is identified as it enters the trapezius muscle, using a hemostat and spreading technique to prevent any direct injury to the nerve.

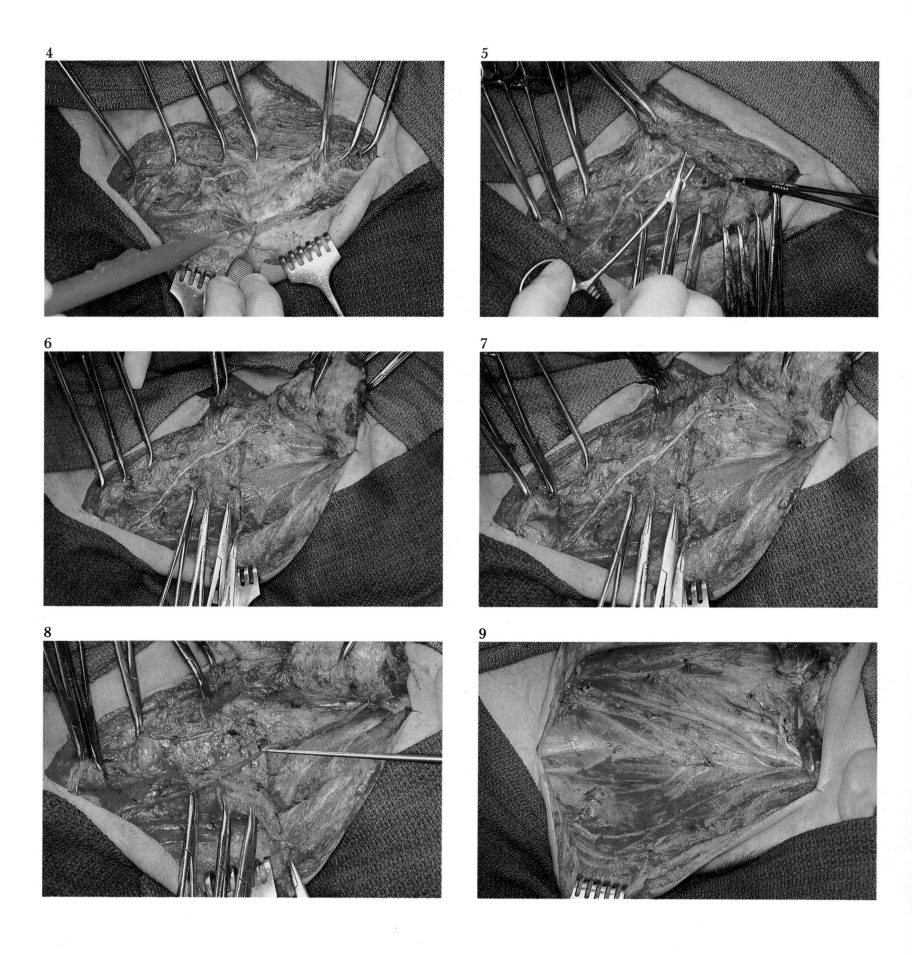

10

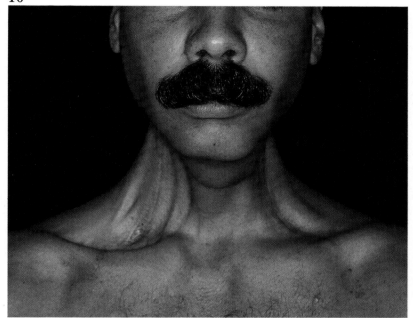

11

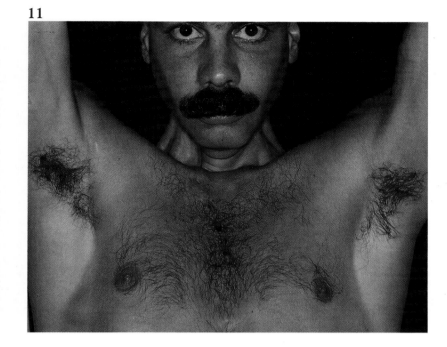

Once identified, the nerve is traced cephalad by careful and meticulous sharp dissection. It will become apparent that the specimen of the contents of the posterior triangle of the neck is being split into two halves which are opened up as dissection proceeds **(4)**. Dissection of the accessory nerve through the posterior triangle of the neck is continued until the nerve exits from behind the sternomastoid muscle. At this point the muscle may have to be divided in order to trace the nerve further cephalad **(5)**. The posterior half of the sternomastoid muscle is divided, carefully keeping the nerve in view at all times during its division.

The upper portion of the divided sternomastoid muscle is retracted cephalad, while the lower posterior part is retracted caudad **(6)**. Dissection of the accessory nerve behind and through the sternomastoid muscle now proceeds cephalad as the sternomastoid branch of the nerve comes into view, and is divided aiding its further dissection until it leaves the jugular foramen.

Dissection of the nerve continues further cephalad near the upper end of the jugular vein in a plane deep to the posterior belly of the digastric muscle **(7)**. The entire nerve is now exposed from its exit at the skull base to its entry in the trapezius muscle. This, however, necessitates division of both the contents of the posterior triangle and the posterior half of the sternomastoid muscle in the upper part of the neck. The nerve is completely free at this point.

Using a nerve hook, the nerve is lifted up and the dissected contents of the posterior triangle of the neck are pushed from behind the nerve and pulled out anteriorly **(8)**. The specimen from the dissected posterior triangle is shown here being pushed from behind the nerve into the anterior aspect of the surgical field to remain in continuity with the rest of the specimen. The nerve is allowed to rest on the exposed, clean musculature of the floor of the posterior triangle of the neck.

The rest of the neck dissection continues as described in classical radical neck dissection **(9)**. All other steps of the operative procedure are exactly the same, removing all other structures as described before. The surgical field at the conclusion of the operation is similar to a classical radical dissection except for the accessory nerve which is preserved in its entirety as seen in the lower part of the surgical field. Suction drains are placed in the wound after irrigation and the incisions are closed in the usual way.

The postoperative appearance of the patient is shown in **(10)**, 6 months after bilateral modified radical neck dissections sparing the eleventh nerves. Note the absence of dropped shoulder. The contour of the trapezius muscle is preserved, demonstrating that the nerve supply to the muscle is maintained intact so the shoulder function is not compromised. The patient is able to raise his shoulders all the way up, demonstrating the function of the trapezius muscle, which has been preserved **(11)**.

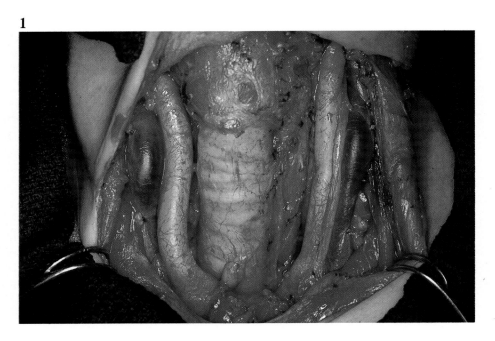

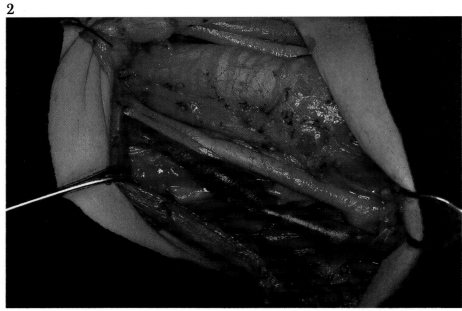

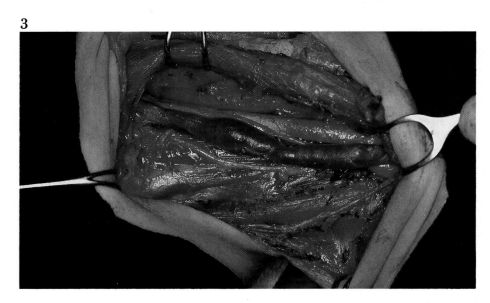

Modified neck dissection preserving the sternomastoid muscle, internal jugular vein and accessory nerve (functional neck dissection)

This operation is usually indicated in patients who present with clinically apparent, metastatic lymph nodes from well-differentiated carcinomas of the thyroid gland. It is not a satisfactory operation for metastatic squamous cell carcinoma or metastatic adenocarcinoma of salivary gland origin.

The surgical exposure shown here (1) shows clearance of the central compartment of the neck following a radical, total thyroidectomy. Complete dissection of the tracheoesophageal groove lymph nodes is accomplished, but the right lower parathyroid gland is preserved as seen in the lower part of (1). Both carotid sheaths are opened and the deep jugular nodes in the central compartment of the neck on the right side are also cleared. The sternomastoid muscle on the left side is retracted laterally showing clearance of the cervical lymph nodes in the central compartment. The surgical field in this exposure is seen directly from above with the larynx cephalad and the suprasternal notch caudad.

The side view of the surgical field (2) is seen from patient's left side, with the chin in the right upper corner. Complete clearance of the tracheoesophageal groove lymph nodes is demonstrated here, but the recurrent nerve is carefully preserved. Lymph nodes medial to and along the jugular vein are all cleared and excised *en bloc* with primary lesion. The sternomastoid muscle is retracted laterally exposing the contents of the carotid sheath and demonstrating total clearance of lymph nodes from the anterior triangle of the neck.

The surgical field with the sternomastoid muscle now retracted anteriorly demonstrating the carotid sheath with its contents clearly dissected (3). All the lymph nodes lateral to the carotid sheath and from the posterior triangle of the neck are completely removed. Note that the vagus, phrenic and accessory nerves in the lower part of the surgical field overlying the trapezius muscle are carefully preserved.

Since this operation has to be performed with the sternomastoid muscle intact, it is often difficult to keep the surgical specimen in continuity as a monobloc resection. Generally, the contents of the anterior triangle of the neck and the primary tumor are resected *en bloc*, while those of the posterior triangle may be removed as a second specimen. Wound closure with suction drains is similar to previous surgical procedures on the neck.

The postoperative appearance of the patient is shown in (4), approximately 6 months after bilateral modified neck dissections with total thyroidectomy for papillary carcinoma of the thyroid with bilateral neck node metastasis. Note that the surgical procedure in this patient was performed through two parallel incisions, one in the upper part of the neck at the level of the hyoid bone extending from one mastoid process to the other, and a second incision along the collar line in the lower part of the neck extending from the trapezius muscle on one side to that on the opposite side.

4

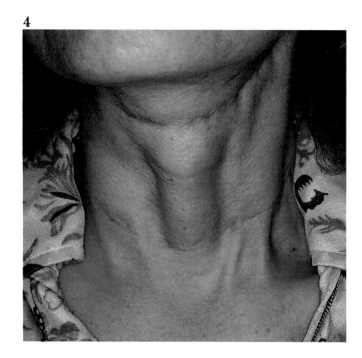

Comparative evaluation of clearance of cervical lymph nodes by various types of neck dissections

The following four diagrams show clearance of lymph nodes in various parts of the neck by the previously described four types of neck dissections.

Supraomohyoid neck dissection

As discussed previously, the supraomohyoid neck dissection clears lymph nodes presenting in the submental, submandibular and carotid triangles (1). These include the jugulodigastric and upper and midjugular lymph nodes. Thus, lymph nodes at levels 1, 2, and 3 are cleared when this neck dissection is performed.

Functional neck dissection (modified neck dissection preserving the sternomastoid muscle, internal jugular vein and accessory nerve)

This type of neck dissection provides clearance of both the anterior and posterior triangles of the neck although the surgical removal of the specimen may not be in a monobloc fashion (2). This is probably not a satisfactory operation for clinically apparent cervical lymph node metastasis from squamous cell carcinoma of the head and neck region; it is best advocated for metastatic carcinoma to cervical lymph nodes from well-differentiated thyroid cancer. The lymph nodes from both anterior and posterior triangles of the neck are excised by elevating and retracting the sternomastoid muscle back and forth.

Modified neck dissection sparing the accessory nerve

This operation is essentially comparable to a classical radical neck dissection in terms of clearance of lymph nodes, except for preservation of the accessory nerve (3), and best advocated in patients with a limited extent of metastatic disease in the anterior triangle of the neck.

Classical radical neck dissection

This is the operation of choice at the moment for clinically apparent cervical lymph node metastasis (4).

1

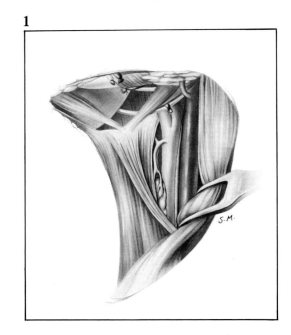

2

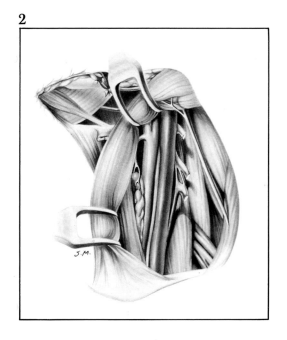

3

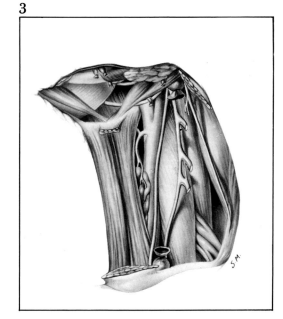

4

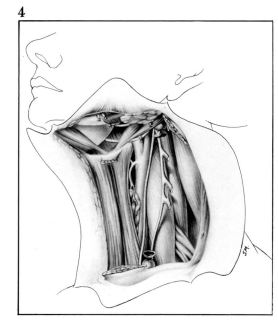

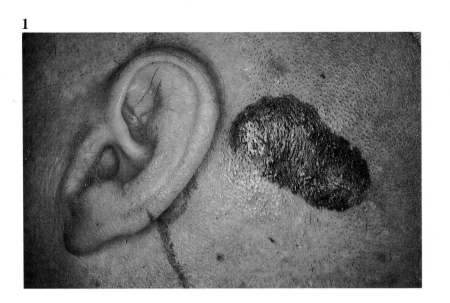

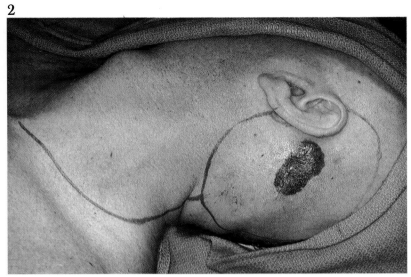

Excision of melanoma of scalp with posterior neck dissection

Lymphatic drainage from the scalp posteriorly is such that both the occipital and postauricular lymph nodes are likely to be involved by metastatic tumor. Therefore, excision of tumors posteriorly in the scalp requires a neck dissection with clearance of the occipital and postauricular group of lymph nodes in conjunction with lymph nodes in the posterior triangle of the neck.

The patient presented here (1) has a 2.5 × 4.5 cm malignant melanoma of the postauricular scalp, which had extended to Clark's level IV in the depth of infiltration.

The plan of surgical excision entailed a wide excision of the melanoma in conjunction with left neck dissection (2). A circular disk of skin is excised around the primary tumor, and from its lower part, a hockeystick type of incision is brought along the trapezius and the clavicle up to the suprasternal notch. Neck dissection proceeds from the supraclavicular region cephalad towards the primary site in the usual way. The technical details of classical radical neck dissection are given on page 233. When the surgical specimen reaches the upper part of the neck, the trapezius muscle is detached and reflected posteriorly to give access to the occipital triangle for removal of occipital lymph nodes. Monobloc dissection of the latter often may not be possible with the rest of the neck dissection specimen because of the presence of trapezius muscle which has to be reflected.

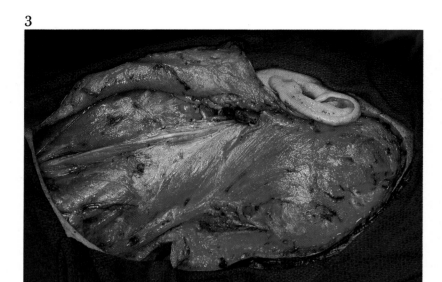

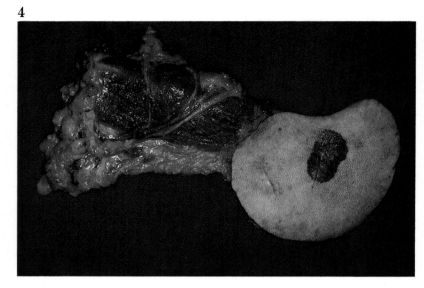

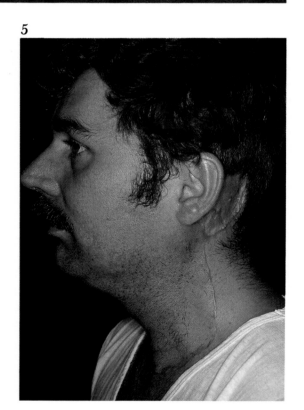

The surgical field is shown in (3) following removal of the primary melanoma in conjunction with classical radical neck and posterior neck dissections excising the occipital and postauricular group of lymph nodes. The detached trapezius muscle is resutured at its normal anatomical position.

The surgical specimen in (4) shows the primary tumor with a large area of skin around the primary tumor and lymph nodes removed by both radical and posterior neck dissections.

The postoperative appearance of the patient several months after surgery (5) shows a well-healed skin graft at the primary site as well as the incision.

Posterior neck dissection is an operation indicated for patients who present with tumors of the scalp with a high potential of lymph node metastasis to postauricular and occipital regions. The operative procedure is tedious because of the anatomical location of the occipital lymph nodes that require reflection of the trapezius muscle. Clearance of occipital lymph nodes in continuity with the rest of the neck dissection is often not possible because of the need to reflect the trapezius muscle to excise the occipital lymph nodes.

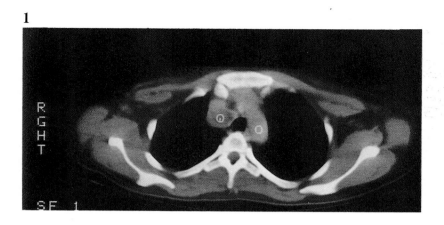

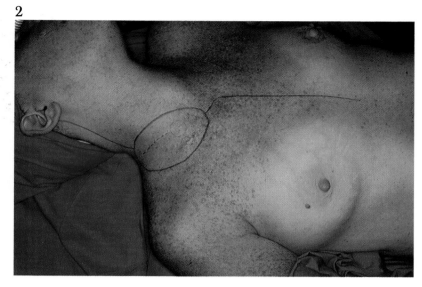

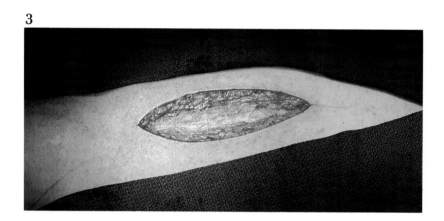

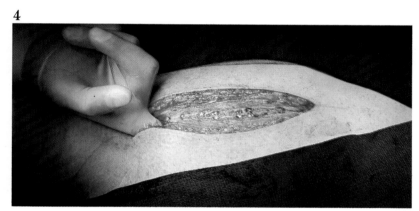

Neck dissection in continuity with mediastinal lymph node dissection

The clinical presence of lymph node metastases in the lower part of the neck with contiguous involvement of superior mediastinal lymph nodes often demands both neck and mediastinal lymph node dissection. Such operative procedures may be necessary in patients presenting either with thyroid carcinoma or occasionally with melanoma. The patient presented here had a primary melanoma of the skin of the lower part of the neck with clinically apparent cervical lymph node metastasis in the supraclavicular region, and extension of metastatic disease to the superior mediastinal lymph nodes. The patient had previously undergone excision of the primary lesion, and a biopsy of a lymph node had recently been performed through a separate incision.

The CT scan through the superior mediastinum at the level of the arch of aorta (1) shows a large centrally necrotic metastatic mass in the right side of the superior mediastinum. The rest of the mediastinum was clear of any other abnormality, and metastatic disease elsewhere was also ruled out.

The plan of surgical procedure (2) included a right neck dissection with sacrifice of a large area of skin at the site of the primary tumor in continuity with superior mediastinal node dissection. The skin incision is outlined here beginning from the mastoid process, going along the trapezius muscle to meet an area of wide skin excision in the supraclavicular region. The skin incision then continues medially to the suprasternal notch where a straight vertical limb is extended down over the manubrium up to the xyphoid process.

Median sternotomy for mediastinal node dissection is undertaken first (3). The skin incision is taken from the suprasternal notch down to the xyphoid process and deepened through the subcutaneous tissue up to the anterior surface of the sternum. Hemostasis is obtained with electrocoagulation or tying the blood vessels.

Using digital blunt dissection in the suprasternal notch, a space is created in the superior mediastinum behind the manubrium sterni (4), by detaching the strap muscles from the posterior aspect of the manubrium.

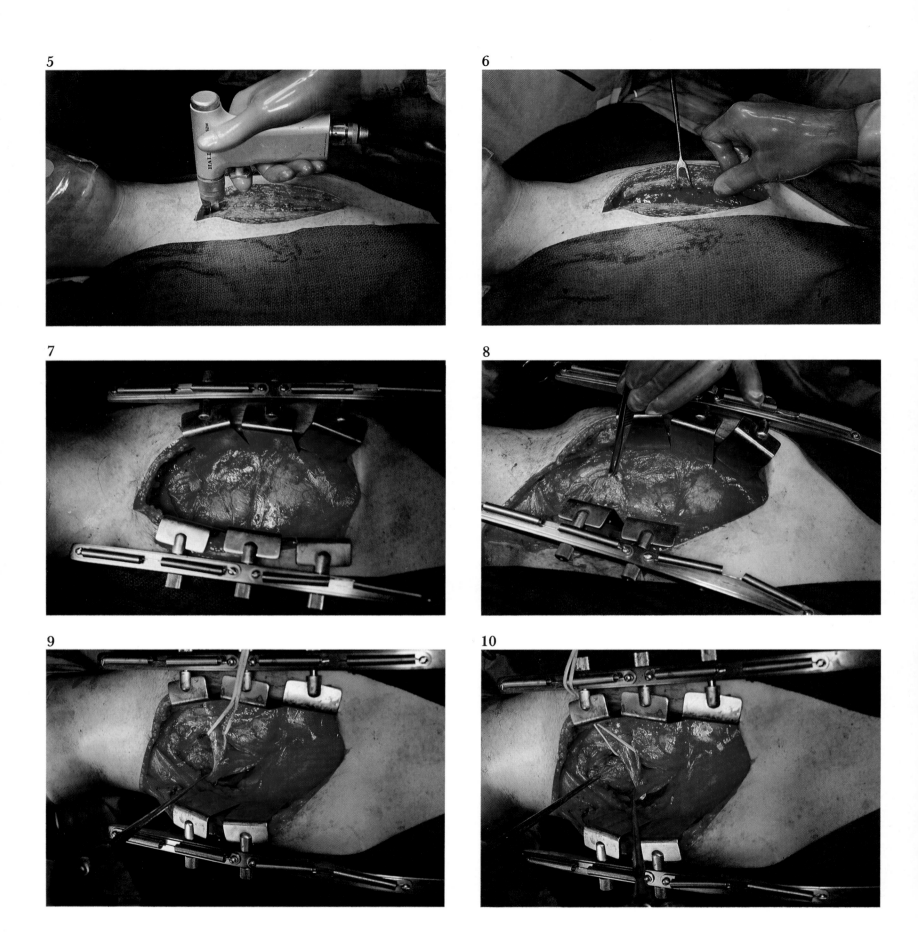

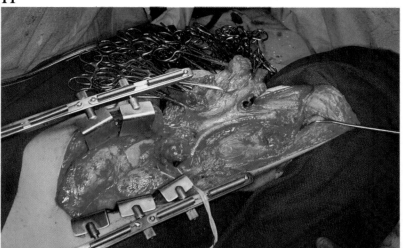

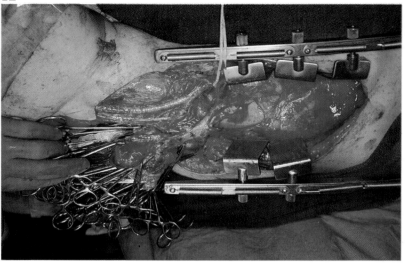

Digital dissection posterior to the manubrium creates a space for insertion of the sternal saw, which is used to divide the sternum (5). A median sternotomy is performed extending from the suprasternal notch down to the xyphoid process. During division of the sternum, it is lifted up with the distal lip of the sternal saw to prevent injury to the mediastinal structures beneath.

Brisk hemorrhage occurs from the divided ends of the sternum, but this is easily controlled by bone wax applied to the raw cut edges of the manubrium (6).

Then a self-retaining sternal retractor is used to expose the mediastinum (7). Careful and meticulous dissection through the mediastinal fat and lymph nodes is undertaken, denuding both left and right innominate veins and the superior vena cava. The complete mass of fibrofatty tissue and lymph nodes are dissected and swept towards the right side.

Dissection of the mediastinal lymph nodes begins with identification of the left innominate vein (8). Lymph nodes from the region of the superior vena cava are mobilized and dissected towards the right side (9). This dissection is tedious and should be carefully undertaken to prevent inadvertent injury to the innominate veins. Both these and the superior vena cava are cleared of the lymph nodes as demonstrated here. Note that all the tissues are dissected and reflected superiorly towards the right side.

At this point, dissection continues to mobilize the large mass of lymph node metastases present between the innominate artery and right innominate vein (10). A cuff of the parietal pleura of the right side is removed since the mass is adherent to the pleura, and once this is accomplished superior mobilization of the metastatic nodes is possible along the innominate artery.

The view of the surgical field from the opposite side (left side of the patient) in (11) shows the mass of metastatic lymph nodes overlying the innominate artery in the superior mediastinum. At this point, excision of the primary site is completed in continuity with right radical neck dissection. However, the specimen remains attached at the root of the neck to the mediastinal nodes, near the origin of the common carotid artery from the innominate artery.

Further dissection along the innominate artery at its bifurcation (12) shows the takeoff of the common carotid artery and the subclavian artery. Note the defect in the parietal pleura on the right side showing the lung in the right pleural cavity. The big mass of metastatic nodes lying inferior to the innominate artery and posterior to right innominate vein is now dissected out and reflected cephalad towards the neck dissection specimen.

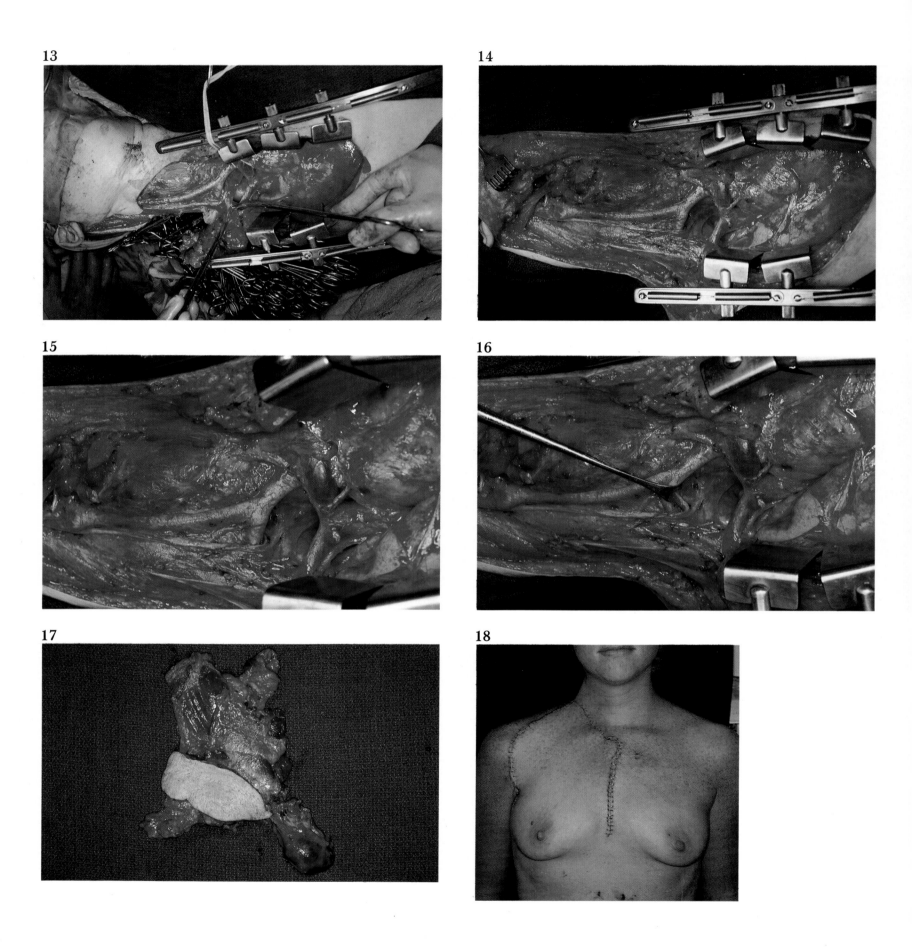

As dissection proceeds towards the root of the neck, the vagus nerve comes into view with its recurrent laryngeal branch as it winds around the subclavian artery to return into the neck (13). Remaining attachments of the surgical specimen in this area are divided carefully avoiding any injury to the vagus or recurrent nerves.

The surgical field following radical neck dissection is shown in (14) in continuity with superior mediastinal lymph node dissection. Note the intact great vessels of the mediastinum which include the left and right innominate veins and superior vena cava, and the right innominate artery with its common carotid and subclavian branches.

A closeup view of the area of tumor removal is shown in (15). The mass of metastatic lymph nodes was located inferior to both the innominate and subclavian arteries, and superior and posterior to the right innominate vein and superior vena cava.

Retraction of the subclavian artery (16) clearly shows the recurrent laryngeal branch of the right vagus nerve turning cephalad behind the artery. The surgical specimen (17) shows a large area of skin at the site of the primary melanoma in continuity with right radical neck and superior mediastinal lymph node dissection.

The surgical defect is irrigated with Bacitracin solution, and a right thorocostomy tube drainage with underwater seal established. The pleural defect is repaired with primary closure, the median sternotomy is closed with heavy, silver peristernal wires, and the skin incision in the chest is closed in layers. The surgical defect in the neck requires coverage with a rotation advancement flap obtained from the anterior chest wall. The flap incision begins at the lateral aspect of the skin defect and is taken down along the deltopectoral groove and the lateral aspect of the breast. The skin flap is elevated superficial to the pectoralis major muscle, and is advanced cephalad and rotated medially to cover the surgical defect. The postoperative apperance of the patient at approximately 1 week after surgery (18) shows primary healing of the incisions.

Radical neck and mediastinal lymph node dissection is thus a safe operation that can be accomplished without difficulty.

Further Reading

Index

All references are to page numbers

The companion volume, to be published soon, will deal with the following:

1. The Oral Cavity
2. Oropharynx
3. Hypopharynx and Cervical Esophagus
4. Larynx and Trachea
5. Thyroid and Parathyroids
6. Salivary Glands
7. Endoscopic Procedures
8. Neurovascular and Soft Tissue Tumors
9. Reconstructive Surgery
10. Microvascular Free Tissue Transfer